The
Doctor *of*
Nursing Practice
Essentials

A New Model for Advanced
Practice Nursing

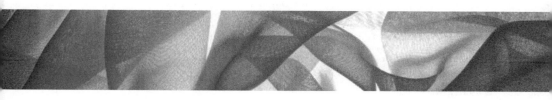

Edited by

Mary E. Zaccagnini, DNP, RN, ACNS-BC, AOCN

Clinical Assistant Professor
University of Minnesota, School of Nursing
Minneapolis, Minnesota

Kathryn Waud White, DNP, RN, CRNA

Chief Nurse Anesthetist
Minneapolis Veterans Affairs Medical Center
Minneapolis, Minnesota

JONES AND BARTLETT PUBLISHERS
Sudbury, Massachusetts
BOSTON   TORONTO   LONDON   SINGAPORE

World Headquarters

Jones and Bartlett Publishers
40 Tall Pine Drive
Sudbury, MA 01776
978-443-5000
info@jbpub.com
www.jbpub.com

Jones and Bartlett Publishers
Canada
6339 Ormindale Way
Mississauga, Ontario L5V 1J2
Canada

Jones and Bartlett Publishers
International
Barb House, Barb Mews
London W6 7PA
United Kingdom

Jones and Bartlett's books and products are available through most bookstores and online booksellers. To contact Jones and Bartlett Publishers directly, call 800-832-0034, fax 978-443-8000, or visit our website, www.jbpub.com.

Substantial discounts on bulk quantities of Jones and Bartlett's publications are available to corporations, professional associations, and other qualified organizations. For details and specific discount information, contact the special sales department at Jones and Bartlett via the above contact information or send an email to specialsales@jbpub.com.

The authors, editor, and publisher have made every effort to provide accurate information. However, they are not responsible for errors, omissions, or for any outcomes related to the use of the contents of this book and take no responsibility for the use of the products and procedures described. Treatments and side effects described in this book may not be applicable to all people; likewise, some people may require a dose or experience a side effect that is not described herein. Drugs and medical devices are discussed that may have limited availability controlled by the Food and Drug Administration (FDA) for use only in a research study or clinical trial. Research, clinical practice, and government regulations often change the accepted standard in this field. When consideration is being given to use of any drug in the clinical setting, the health care provider or reader is responsible for determining FDA status of the drug, reading the package insert, and reviewing prescribing information for the most up-to-date recommendations on dose, precautions, and contraindications, and determining the appropriate usage for the product. This is especially important in the case of drugs that are new or seldom used.

Production Credits
Publisher: Kevin Sullivan
Acquisitions Editor: Amy Sibley
Associate Editor: Patricia Donnelly
Editorial Assistant: Rachel Shuster
Associate Production Editor: Katie Spiegel
Marketing Manager: Rebecca Wasley
V.P., Manufacturing and Inventory Control: Therese Connell
Composition: Paw Print Media
Cover Design: Kristin E. Parker
Cover Image: © Sofiaworld/Dreamstime.com
Printing and Binding: Malloy, Inc.
Cover Printing: Malloy, Inc.

Library of Congress Cataloging-in-Publication Data
The doctor of nursing practice essentials : a new model for advanced practice nursing / [edited by] Mary E. Zaccagnini, Kathryn Waud White.
     p. ; cm.
  Includes bibliographical references and index.
  ISBN 978-0-7637-7346-5
  1. Nursing—Study and teaching (Graduate)--United States. 2. Doctor of philosophy degree—United States. I. Zaccagnini, Mary E. II. White, Kathryn Waud.
  [DNLM: 1. Education, Nursing, Graduate. 2. Nurse Clinicians—education. 3. Nurse Practitioners—education. WY 18.5 D6367 2011]
  RT75.D56 2011
  610.73071'1—dc22
                              2009054073
6048

Printed in the United States of America
14 13 12 11   10 9 8 7 6 5 4 3

This book is dedicated to all of our current and future DNP colleagues, especially those who so graciously gave of their time and volunteered to author this book.

—Kathy & Mary

This book is also dedicated to my sister Karen, who passed away suddenly while I was writing this book.

—Mary

CONTENTS

PART II DOCTOR OF NURSING PRACTICE ROLES 347

PART III THE DOCTOR OF NURSING PRACTICE SCHOLARLY PROJECT 449

Health care is in a whirlwind of change, and advanced practice nurses are right in the center of that change. The societal forces driving the transformation of health care have been dissected, researched, and exhaustively discussed, debated, and documented. Now, with the development of the Doctor of Nursing Practice program of study and the American Association of Colleges of Nursing's *Essentials of Doctoral Education for Advanced Nursing Practice*, we have the opportunity to place these ideas into action—to bring them into nursing practice in a way never before done. This book provides a roadmap for creating change in health care and the tools to make those changes.

It is important to mention that this book was authored solely by nurses who practice at an advanced level and who have achieved the Doctor of Nursing Practice degree. Some fulfill traditional advanced practice roles, and some have expanded roles as administrators, educators, and entrepreneurs. Each of these nurses took hours out of his or her busy practice to author these materials. In that aspect, this book is unique. Additionally, this book is unique in that it lays out a step-by-step template or framework for the development of the scholarly project.

Purpose of the Book

This book is intended to serve as a core textbook for DNP students and faculty to use to achieve mastery of the American Association of Colleges of Nursing essentials as well as a shelf reference for practicing DNPs. The DNP essentials are all covered herein; each essential is covered in adequate detail to frame the foundation of the DNP educational program. This book provides the infrastructure for students, faculty, and practicing DNPs to achieve and sustain the highest level of practice.

This book gives students the foundation necessary to enter into the highest level of advanced practice nursing and develop that practice to the highest level possible for the benefit of their patients and the health of the country and the world. For faculty, this book provides a framework that can partner with their creativity to make a program their own unique program, different from others but all coming to the same endpoint: graduates who practice at the clinical doctorate level. For practicing DNPs, this book serves as a reference to reinforce their skills as they take on leadership roles in health care. The skills outlined in this book will help DNPs engage in advocacy, lead large and small organizations, integrate the skills of collaboration, use informatics to demonstrate the value of nursing interventions, document quality clinical competencies, and improve the health of the nation.

CONTRIBUTORS

Laurel Ash, DNP, RN, CNP
Assistant Professor
College of St. Scholastica
Duluth, Minnesota

Marcia K. Britain, DNP, RN, FNP-BC
NP/PA Education and Quality
  Coordinator
Department of Surgery
Mayo Clinic
Rochester, Minnesota

Deonne J. Brown Benedict, DNP, ARNP, FNP-BC
Founder, Charis Family Clinic
Assistant Professor
Seattle University College of
  Nursing
Seattle, Washington

Susan F. Burkart-Jayez, DNP, RN, ANP-BC
Occupational Health Program
  Manager
Samuel S. Stratton Veterans
  Medical Center
Albany, New York

Katherine H. Casey, DNP, RN, CNP, CCRN
Operations Manager NP/PA Services
Department of Surgery
Mayo Clinic
Rochester, Minnesota

Germaine M. Edinger, DNP, RN, CNS
Psychiatric CNS
North Memorial Health Care
Robbinsdale, Minnesota

Sandra R. Edwardson, PhD, RN, FAAN
Professor and Director of DNP
  Program
School of Nursing
University of Minnesota
Minneapolis, Minnesota

Carole R. Eldridge, DNP, RN, NEA-BC
Dean, Campus Director, and
  Associate Professor
St. John's/SBU College of Nursing
  and Health Sciences
Southwest Baptist University
Springfield, Missouri

Joy Elwell, DNP, RN, FNP-BC
Assistant Professor, Nursing, and
  Director
College Health Service
Concordia College
Bronxville, New York

Don R. Hirschman, DNP, MHA, RN, CRNA
Director of Anesthesia, Associate
  Eye Surgery Center
Anesthetist, Wichita Veterans
  Administration Hospital
Wichita, Kansas

Catherine J. Miller DNP, RN, C-NP (Pediatric)
Assistant Professor
College of St. Scholastica School of
  Nursing
SMDC-Duluth Children's Clinic
Duluth, Minnesota

Angela Mund, DNP, RN, CRNA
Clinical Director, Nurse Anesthesia
  Area of Study
School of Nursing
University of Minnesota
Minneapolis, Minnesota

Garrett J. Peterson, DNP, RN, CRNA
Minneapolis Veterans Affairs
  Medical Center
School of Nursing
University of Minnesota
Minneapolis, Minnesota

Sandra Petersen, DNP, RN, GNP-BC
Program Director
Master's in Nursing Leadership
UTMB School of Nursing
Galveston, Texas

Michelle Riley, DNP, RN
Director, NNAAP and MACE
  Examinations
National Council of State Boards of
  Nursing
Chicago, Illinois

Deborah Ringdahl, DNP, RN, CNM
Clinical Assistant Professor
School of Nursing
University of Minnesota
Minneapolis, Minnesota

Diane Marie Schadewald, DNP, RN, CNP, WHNP, FNP
Clinical Assistant Professor
School of Nursing
University of Minnesota
Minneapolis, Minnesota

Kathleen Sgro, DNP, MBA, RN
President, Alterna-Care Home
  Health Agency
Springfield, Illinois

Gwendolyn Short, DNP, C-FNP, MPH
Clinical Assistant Professor
School of Nursing
University of Minnesota
Minneapolis, Minnesota

Catherine Tymkow, DNP, APN, WHNP-BC, CNE
Associate Professor
College of Health and Human Services
Governors State University
University Park, Illinois

Kathryn Waud White, DNP, RN, CRNA
Chief Nurse Anesthetist
Minneapolis Veterans Affairs Medical Center
Minneapolis, Minnesota

Mary E. Zaccagnini, DNP, RN, ACNS-BC, AOCN
Clinical Assistant Professor
University of Minnesota, School of Nursing
Minneapolis, Minnesota

REVIEWERS

Brian Bullard, MBA, MPH, MA
Joy Elwell, DNP, FNP-BC
Nancy Granberry, DNP, RN
Connie Delaney, PhD, RN, FAAN, FACMI
Kathy Fagerlund, PhD, RN, CRNA
Carol Flaten, DNP, RN
Jane K. Gardner, DNP, RN
Linda Halcon, PhD, RN, MPH
Josh Hamilton, DNP, RN-C, FNP-C, PMHNP-C, CNE
Don R. Hirschman, DNP, RN, CRNA
Karen V. Lamb, DNP, GCNS, BC
Ruth Lindquist, PhD, RN, APRN, BC, FAAN
Georgia Nygaard, DNP, RN, CNP
Jeanne Pheiffer, DNP, RN, MPH, CIC
Mary Rowan, PhD, CNM, RN
Diane Twedell, DNP, RN
Connie Zak, DNP, RN, MBA, APRN, BC

Imagining the DNP Role

Sandra R. Edwardson

Doctoral preparation in nursing has had a long development. From programs designed to prepare nursing faculty to the Doctor of Nursing Practice (DNP), the profession has experienced several forms of doctoral education. Before describing the development of the DNP concept, this section summarizes its roots in doctoral education.

Beginning in the mid-1950s with the first pre- and postdoctoral research grants and the research fellowship program of the Division of Nursing Resources (precursor of the Division of Nursing within the U.S. Public Health Service), nursing leaders have gradually won recognition at both the federal and university levels. Although the first emphasis was on preparing faculty and developing research programs, the call for clinical or professional programs was ever present.

Stevenson and Woods (1986) identified four generations of nurses with doctorates:

- 1900–1940: EdD or other functional degree offered through colleges of education to prepare nursing faculty
- 1940–1960: PhD in basic or social science with no nursing content
- 1960–1970: PhD in basic science with minor in nursing through nurse scientist programs offered in conjunction with basic science programs
- 1970–present: PhD in nursing or DNS
- 2000 and beyond: Programs projected to contain "greater specificity within nursing" and "formalized postdoctoral programs" (p. 8)

To this chronology, we can now add the practice doctorate. Since the formal approval of the DNP by the American Association of Colleges of Nursing (AACN) in October 2004, the AACN has reported that, by April 2009, 92 programs had been launched, with even more in the planning stages. Although many of the programs are offered by schools that also offer research doctorates, 43 of the programs are the only doctoral program in the school (AACN, 2009). Clearly the degree has made it possible for many schools unable or unwilling to offer research degrees to move into doctoral education. Because the accreditation process had just begun, it is not clear how many of these new programs will warrant accreditation.

From the beginning, the primary reason for wanting doctoral preparation in nursing was to develop the knowledge necessary for practice and to gain credibility within the academy. Some of the early programs were DNS (Doctor of Nursing Science) programs. In their earliest incarnations, the DNS programs were established as substitutes for the PhD (Meleis, 1988). This was because some states allowed the PhD to be offered only through the main campus of the system or because the school was a baccalaureate-granting institution (Downs, 1989). In other cases, university officials believed that there was insufficient research and scholarship in nursing to justify a PhD degree. Therefore, some of the early schools seeking permission to establish PhD programs lacked a mechanism for doing so and chose the DNS as an option.

Early thinkers recommended PhD preparation for generation of new knowledge and DNS programs to prepare individuals to apply that knowledge (Cleland, 1976; Peplau, 1966). This was in keeping with the statements of the Association of Graduate Schools and the Council of Graduate Schools, who distinguished PhD from professional degrees: "The professional Doctor's degree should be the highest university award given in a particular field in recognition of completion of academic *preparation for professional practice*, whereas the Doctor of Philosophy should be given in recognition of *preparation for research* whether the particular field of learning is pure or applied" (Council of Graduate Schools in the United States, 1966, p. 3).

Over time the purpose of DNS programs tended to move toward research preparation. Noting the number of articles describing the differences and similarity in types of nursing doctoral programs, Starck, Duffy, and Vogler (1993) proposed that the DNS prepares individuals "in a specialized area of practice for the purpose of testing and validating application of" knowledge that extends and generates nursing practice protocols (p. 214). They advocated for content including healthcare practices; biologic, psychosocial, economic, legal, and ethical knowledge; and research methods for investigating clinical problems.

An analysis of the curricula of PhD and DNS programs showed that there was more clinical emphasis in the latter, but the differences between the programs as they were implemented were very subtle (Edwardson, 2004). Florence Downs (1989), the long-term editor of *Nursing Research*, conducted an informal review of topics by PhD and DNS authors in the journal. It revealed essentially the same number of manuscripts on clinical topics by each. Her bottom line was that she was less concerned about the structure and content of the programs than with the quality and excellence of them.

Practice Doctorates

There are subtle although uncertain distinctions between professional degrees such as the DNS and practice degrees such as the DNP. Recently, the Council of Graduate Schools appointed a task force to examine the growth of professional programs, but it too has been grappling with defining exactly what they are (Rawitch, 2008). European and Australian universities have also attempted to make meaningful distinctions between professional and research degrees. In those countries, professional doctorates have been attempts to make the doctorate more focused on the application of knowledge to the solution of societal problems (Maxwell, Shanahan, & Green, 2001).

In the United States, professional doctorates have existed for many years in fields such as in education (e.g., the EdD). Although subtle, the major distinction between a professional and a practice degree seems to be in the goals. In the view of Starck, Duffy, and Vogler (1993), the DNS has as its purpose the testing and validation of knowledge to extend and generate nursing practice protocols. In other words, the purpose is to extend the knowledge generated by research doctorates by testing it in practice. The practice doctorate, on the other hand, is the highest-level preparation for the actual practice of the discipline. Holders of practice doctorates are in the business of applying knowledge as they provide direct service to clients. In so doing, they may also do systematic inquiry similar to that of holders of professional or research degrees, but the primary purpose of the degree is to prepare practitioners.

The first nursing doctoral degree dedicated solely to practice was the Doctor of Nursing (ND) established at Case Western Reserve University in 1979 (Case Western Reserve University, n.d.). It began as an entry-level nursing degree but evolved into a program offering preparation for advanced practice. Few other schools embraced the ND degree, and by the late 1990s, there was only one institution (the University of Colorado) that offered an entry-level program.

There are many examples of practice-focused degrees in other disciplines, including entry-level degrees such as the Doctor of Medicine (MD) and Juris Doctor (JD) and advanced practice degrees such as the Doctor of Psychology (PsyD). In the early part of the 21st century, existing practice-focused degrees in nursing were mainly advanced practice doctoral degrees. They included the ND at Case Western Reserve University, Rush University, and the University of South Carolina; a Doctor of Nursing Science (DNSc) at the University of Tennessee, Memphis; the Doctor of Nursing Practice (DNP) at the University of Kentucky, and the Doctor of Nursing Practice (DrNP) at Columbia University.

The DrNP (now DNP) offered by Columbia provides greater depth and breadth of knowledge and practice than existing master's programs in clinical science, informatics, and research methods. It is also designed to prepare students to admit, co-manage, and discharge patients from hospitals. They are expected to be able to provide care from the outpatient to the inpatient setting and vice versa (Mundinger, 2005). Few if any schools have adopted the model of admitting patients to acute care settings.

The AACN's Role in Creating the DNP

This brief review of our history brings us to 1999. In that year, the board of the American Association of Colleges of Nursing appointed a task force to revise quality indicators for doctoral education and to address the differences among three types of nursing doctorates: PhD, DNSc/DNS/DSN, and ND degrees. The task force was able to prepare a revised version of the *Indicators of Quality in Research-Focused Doctoral Programs in Nursing* (2001), but found that for all of its attempts to make distinctions between research degrees (PhD) and professional degrees (DNS, DNSc, DSN), the faculty of programs that offered the DNS/DSN degrees saw the need for a common set of quality indicators for both. The task force members concluded that there may be differences in the roles for which the graduates are prepared and in the curricular content of the programs, but that the basic requirements for quality programs were viewed as the same for research and professional degrees.

Based on its analysis, the quality indicators task force constructed Figure 1 to describe what was happening in the field. Although the task

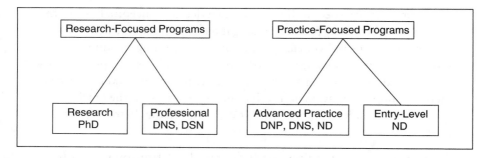

■ Figure 1 Proposed classification of nursing doctorates.
Source: Edwardson, 2004.

force was able to address the research half of the model, there was insufficient time and clarity to deal with the practice-focused half of the model. There seemed to be only one true entry-level doctorate left at the time (the ND), although the discussion suggested that there were a number of AACN member deans who thought that the idea ought to be resurrected. Other programs, such as those at the University of Kentucky, Columbia, and University of Tennessee–Memphis, had emerged to give nurses advanced practice preparation at the doctoral level, but they too differed in goals and structure.

Because of the lack of clarity concerning the right half of the model, the quality indicators task force recommended appointment of a second group to study it, and the Task Force on the Practice Doctorate in Nursing was established to focus on that issue alone (AACN, 2004). There were several resources available for the group's work, but the task force also found it necessary to gather some information on its own.

Marion and colleagues (2003) pointed out discernible differences between practice-focused and research-focused programs. Practice-focused programs place less emphasis on theory, meta-theory, and research methods than do research-focused programs. Capstone projects are designed to solve practice problems or inform practice, with an emphasis on scholarly practice and outcome evaluation. Clinical practica or residencies are required (Marion, Viens, O'Sullivan, Crabtree, Fontana, & Price, 2003).

After considering published definitions and consulting with leaders in health care and nursing education, the task force defined *practice* as follows:

The term practice, specifically nursing practice, as conceptualized in this document refers to any form of nursing intervention that influences health care outcomes for individuals or populations, including the direct care of individual patients, management of care for individuals and populations, administration of nursing and health care organizations, and the development and implementation of health policy. Preparation at the practice doctorate level includes advanced preparation in nursing, based on nursing. (AACN, 2004)

There was controversy about including in the definition roles other than nurse practitioner, clinical nurse specialist, nurse–midwife, or nurse anesthetist. But the task force concluded that caring for populations and seeing to the arrangements under which nursing is practiced were equally important as direct clinical care for advancing the health of the public. Omitted from the definition was preparation for nursing education. This omission is consistent with PhD and practice education in other disciplines, in which preparation concentrates on the specific specialty or subspecialty, and preparation for faculty roles is something that is added as a separate discipline. In short, the task force concluded that nursing faculty need substantive expertise in the subject matter of the discipline and not just pedagogical theory and practice.

Another topic of considerable discussion was the title of the degree. Whereas many in the task force might have preferred the simple Doctor of Nursing or DN label, a search of titles revealed that DN was reserved for the Doctor of Naprapathy (National College of Naprapathic Physicians, n.d.). Similarly, the ND degree title was in use by Doctors of Naturopathy (American Association of Naturopathic Medicine, n.d.) in some states and not available to us. It was finally concluded that there should be only one title and that it should be Doctor of Nursing Practice. It was thought to be the most descriptive title despite the assumption of some that it referred only to nurse practitioners. The task force recommended that the ND be phased out.

A transitional plan was also proposed. Knowing that most of the graduates of the programs would want or need specialty certification, it was clear that the education sector could establish the educational preparation for the role but had no control over the certification process. Therefore, the recommendation was that the many bodies that certify nurses set the year 2015 as the time when initial certification would require the DNP degree.

A final discussion focused on quality control. Whereas the quality of PhD programs is the responsibility of graduate schools, professional and practice degrees are typically awarded by professional schools without the built-in quality control mechanisms provided by graduate schools. For this reason, the task force recommended that an accreditation process similar to that for master's and baccalaureate programs be established to ensure quality in DNP programs. The Commission on Collegiate Nursing Education (CCNE) took up the challenge immediately, developed the criteria, and began reviewing DNP programs in the fall of 2008.

Factors Propelling the Practice Doctorate

From the outset, the DNP had significant opposition. Several nationally recognized leaders in nursing objected based on the fears that the degree would detract from the hard-fought growth and recognition of research in nursing and of nursing in the academy. Meleis and Dracup (2005) argued that the MS and PhD degrees are widely understood and accepted and that a new doctoral degree would amount to second-class citizenship. They believed that the nursing doctorate should be dedicated to advancing and translating knowledge and that separating the practice and research foci could thwart knowledge development and interfere with establishing evidence for quality and safety in health care. Having been among those who fought most vigorously for the acceptance of nursing as a bona fide academic discipline, they feared the DNP would lead to remarginalization within the academy.

Many factors led to the perceived need for the DNP. First was the growing complexity of the healthcare environment, coupled with the rapid expansion of knowledge required for practice. Groups such as the Institute of Medicine, the Robert Wood Johnson Foundation, and others urged health profession educators to meet this growing complexity with educational programs that acknowledge the high levels of scientific knowledge and practice expertise required to ensure high-quality patient outcomes. The Institute of Medicine, for example, emphasized the need for all health professions programs to prepare students able to deliver patient-centered care as members of interdisciplinary teams that emphasize evidence-based practice, quality improvement, and informatics (Institute of Medicine, 2003a).

Another Institute of Medicine report observed how management decisions in healthcare organizations had expanded the responsibilities of chief nursing executives, increased the scope of responsibilities for all nursing managers, and led to the loss of midlevel nurse managers (Institute of Medicine,

2003b). The result has been that nurses at all levels need increased knowledge and administrative skills to provide the needed leadership. The Institute of Medicine recommended preparation of nursing leaders for all levels of management and encouraged nursing managers to participate in executive decisions (Institute of Medicine, 2003b).

Another factor propelling the DNP was the movement to doctoral entry levels in related health professions such as pharmacy and physical therapy. These professions had recognized the need for advanced preparation in order to realize fully their potential contribution to health care. Lest it appear that this was a keeping-up-with-the-Joneses rationale, there were others who saw the need for doctoral preparation of practitioners. For example, a landmark study by the National Research Council of the National Academies noted the following: "The need for doctorally prepared practitioners and clinical faculty would be met if nursing could develop a new non-research clinical doctorate, similar to the M.D. and Pharm.D. in medicine and pharmacy, respectively" (National Research Council, 2005, p. 74). But the DNP, which is designed for nurses who are already licensed practitioners, is unlike the doctoral degrees in other health disciplines that are required for entry into the professions.

Leaders of national nursing, medical, and healthcare organizations with whom the Task Force on the Clinical Doctorate met confirmed the need for nurses able to deal with the increasing complexity and sophistication of health care. In response to concerns that the DNP might amount to degree creep, they were sympathetic with the need for additional preparation and expressed confidence that such preparation would add value (AACN, 2004).

As noted earlier, there were eight clinically focused programs in existence when the Task Force on the Clinical Doctorate began its work. The task force's survey of these programs showed considerable variation among the programs in design but also revealed some commonalities. The commonalities included content related to advanced clinical practice (including both patient and practice management); organizations, systems, and leadership skills; research methods; and basic scientific underpinnings for practice (AACN, 2004).

Yet another issue propelling the development of the DNP was the way master's programs had responded to the inexorable growth in scientific knowledge and technological sophistication. To fulfill their obligation to provide adequate preparation and to meet the requirements of specialty certification bodies, nursing schools had gradually expanded their master's curricula. In many schools, programs required upward of 50% more credits than typical for master's programs, increasing the cost and time for completing the program. At one school, for example, the minimum credits required from high school graduation to program completion for a family nurse practitioner degree and a PharmD degree were equal. This suggested that it was time to recognize the preparation with an appropriate degree.

Of course, curriculum length should not be the only criterion for a new degree. Despite the expanded credit requirements of master's programs, practicing nurse practitioners continued to ask for additional preparation in health policy, management, informatics, evaluation of evidence, and advanced diagnosis and care management (Lenz, Mundinger, Hopkins, Clark, & Lin, 2002). Therefore, the Task Force on the Clinical Doctorate and its successor, the Task Force on the Essentials of the DNP, both recommended curricula that would not only meet the requirements of existing master's programs but would also respond to the Institute of Medicine's call for greater facility with evidence-based practice, quality improvement, and informatics (Institute of Medicine, 2003a). This is in keeping with the position of the National Organization of Nurse Practitioner Faculties, which called for additional preparation in business practices, information management, health literacy, end-of-life care, genetics, mental health concepts, caring for older adults, and managed care (Bellack, Graber, O'Neil, Musham, & Lancaster, 1999).

Some have objected to the DNP based on the assumption that it was preparation to replace physicians. This was especially troublesome to the American Medical Association (AMA), which saw the emergence of the degree as an attempt to educate nursing students with skills equivalent to primary care physicians. Its House of Delegates passed Resolution 214 in June 2008, which said "that our AMA adopt a policy that those nurses who are Doctors of Nursing Practice must only be able to practice under the supervision of a physician and as part of a medical team with the final authority and responsibility for the patient under the supervision of a licensed physician" (AMA, 2008a). Resolution 232 from the same meeting declared that "the title 'Doctor,' in a medical setting, [should] apply only to physicians licensed to practice medicine in all its branches, dentists and podiatrists" and that the organization should serve to protect, through legislation, the titles "Doctor," "Resident," and "Residency" (AMA, 2008b).

Some nurses, too, feared that the growing role of advanced practice nurses in primary care could lead to abandoning the unique role and contribution of nurses. Yet there is growing evidence that advanced practice nurses can and do provide services that allow for the full expression of the nurse's role while also filling gaps for needed services in the system (Brooten, Kumar, Brown, et al., 1986; Brooten, Youngblut, Deatrick, et al., 2003; Lenz, Mundinger, Kane, et al., 2004; Naylor & McCauley, 1999). Nurses are proving to have important roles in filling the need for primary and chronic care for all population groups, but especially the growing number of elderly and those living longer with chronic illnesses.

Finally, the shortage of doctorally prepared nursing faculty has been a growing concern within the discipline as schools find themselves turning away qualified applicants partly because of a shortage of faculty. Although the number of PhD programs grew substantially throughout the 1990s, most schools graduated fewer than four or five new PhDs per year (Edwardson, 2004). Schools, including those with PhD programs, had employed master's-prepared practitioners to fill the need for faculty prepared to supervise beginning and advanced nursing students. Although the DNP was specifically designed as advanced preparation for the *practice* of the discipline, many saw DNPs as one way to fill the void for faculty with advanced practice expertise. They could supplement PhD-prepared faculty whose time is increasingly consumed with the scholarship so necessary for the growth and contribution of the discipline. As O'Sullivan and colleagues (2005) argued, the myth that a practice doctorate would have an adverse impact on the PhD degree was countered by the reality that it will help "to preserve the integrity of the PhD as a true research degree" (p. 7).

The Future

The nursing profession has followed a long and varied path for preparing its practitioners. The DNP graduates hold promise for investigating and solving some of the vexing problems facing our healthcare system and delivering the highest level of nursing practice. As knowledge workers, nurses can no longer rely on tradition and task orientation as their substantive base. Rather, they need facility with obtaining and maintaining the most current and evidence-based knowledge to inform their practice. The DNP has been designed to give its practitioners the tools for navigating complex systems and mining the latest available knowledge. Early indications are that DNP-prepared nurses are up to the task.

References

American Association of Colleges of Nursing. (2001). *Indicators of quality in research-focused doctoral programs in nursing.* Washington, DC: Author.

American Association of Colleges of Nursing. (2004). *AACN position statement on practice doctorates in nursing.* Washington, DC: Author.

American Association of Colleges of Nursing. (2009). *The doctor of nursing practice.* Retrieved from http://www.aacn.nche.edu/Media/FactSheets/dnp.htm

American Association of Naturopathic Physicians. (n.d.) *What is naturopathic medicine?* Retrieved from http://www.naturopathic.org

American Medical Association. (2008a, June). *House of Delegates Resolution 214 (A-08): Doctor of Nursing Practice.* Retrieved from http://AMA_Resolution_214_Doctor_of_Nursing _Practice.pdf

American Medical Association. (2008b, June). *House of Delegates Resolution 232 (A-08): Protection of the titles "Doctor," "Resident" and "Residency."* Retrieved from http://www.ama-assn .org/ama1/pub/upload/mm/471/232.doc

Bellack, J. P., Graber, D. R., O'Neil, E. H., Musham, C., & Lancaster, C. (1999). Curriculum trends in nurse practitioner programs: Current and ideal. *Journal of Professional Nursing, 15*(1), 15–27.

Brooten, D., Kumar, S., Brown, L. P., Butts, P., Finkler, S. A., Bakewell-Sachs, S., et al. (1986). A randomized clinical trial of early discharge and home follow-up of very low birth weight infants. *New England Journal of Medicine, 315*(15), 934–939.

Brooten, D., Youngblut, J. M., Deatrick, J., Naylor, M., & York, R. (2003). Patient problems, advanced practice nurse interventions, time and contacts among five patient groups. *Journal of Nursing Scholarship, 35*(1), 73–79.

Case Western Reserve University. (n.d.). *DNP: The future of advanced nursing practice.* Retrieved from http://fpb.case.edu/DNP

Cleland, V. (1976). Develop a doctoral program. *Nursing Outlook, 2*(6), 631–635.

Council of Graduate Schools in the United States. (1966). *The doctor's degree in professional fields. A statement by the Association of Graduate Schools and the Council of Graduate Schools in the United States.* Washington, DC: Author.

Downs, F. S. (1989). Differences between the professional doctorate and the academic/research doctorate. *Journal of Professional Nursing, 5*(5), 261–265.

Edwardson, S. R. (2004). Matching standards and needs in doctoral education in nursing. *Journal of Professional Nursing, 20*(1), 40–46.

Institute of Medicine. (2003a). *Health professions education: A bridge to quality.* Washington, DC: National Academies Press.

Institute of Medicine. (2003b). *Keeping patients safe: Transforming the work environment of nurses.* Washington, DC: National Academies Press.

Lenz, E. R., Mundinger, M. O., Kane, R. L., Hopkins, S. C., & Lin, S. X. (2004). Primary care outcomes in patients treated by nurse practitioners or physicians: Two-year follow-up. *Medical Care Research and Review, 61*(3), 332–351.

Lenz, E. R., Mundinger, M. O., Hopkins, S., Clark, J., & Lin, S. (2002, September). Patterns of nurse practitioner practice: Results from a national survey. Presented at the State of the Science Conference, Washington, DC (Unpublished data).

Marion, L., Viens, D., O'Sullivan, A., Crabtree, C., Fontana, S., & Price, M. (2003). The practice doctorate in nursing: Future or fringe? *Medscape.* Retrieved from http://www.medscape.com/viewarticle/453247

Maxwell, T. W., Shanahan, P., & Green, B. (2001). Introduction: New opportunities in doctoral education and professional practice. In B. Green, T. W. Maxwell, & P. Shanahan (Eds.), *Doctoral education and professional practice: The next generation?* (pp. 1–13). Armidale, New South Wales, Australia: Kardoorair.

Meleis, A. I. (1988). Doctoral education in nursing: Its present and its future. *Journal of Professional Nursing, 4*(6), 436–446.

Meleis, A., & Dracup, K. (2005, September 30). The case against the DNP: History, timing, substance, and marginalization. *Online Journal of Issues in Nursing, 10*(3). Manuscript 2. Retrieved from www.nursingworld.org/MainMenuCategories/ANAMarketplace/ANA Periodicals/OJIN

Mundinger, M. O. (2005). Who's who in nursing: Bringing clarity to the doctor of nursing practice. *Nursing Outlook, 53*(4), 173–176.

National College of Naprapathic Medicine. (n.d.) *What is naprapathic medicine?* Retrieved from http://www.naprapathicmedicine.edu/what.htm

National Research Council of the National Academies. (2005). *Advancing the nation's health needs: NIH research training programs.* Washington, DC: National Academies Press.

Naylor, M. D., & McCauley, K. M. (1999). The effects of a discharge planning and home follow-up intervention on elders hospitalized with common medical and surgical cardiac conditions. *Journal of Cardiovascular Nursing, 14*(1), 44–54.

O'Sullivan, A., Carter, M., Marion, L., Pohl, J., & Werner, K. (2005, September 30). Moving forward together: The practice doctorate in nursing. *Online Journal of Issues in Nursing, 10*(3). Manuscript 4. Retrieved May from www.nursingworld.org/MainMenuCategories /ANAMarketplace/ANAPeriodicals/OJIN/TableofContents/Volume102005/No3Sept05 /tpc28_416028.aspx

Peplau, H. E. (1966). Nursing's two routes to doctoral degrees. *Nursing Forum, 5*(2), 57–67.

Rawitch, A. B. (2008). *Dean dialogue: How can graduate deans and CGS provide leadership for professional doctorates?* Retrieved from http://www.cgsnet.org/portals/0/pdf/mtg_sm08Rawitch.pdf

Starck, P. L., Duffy, M. E., & Vogler, R. (1993). Developing a nursing doctorate for the 21st century. *Journal of Professional Nursing, 9*(4), 212–219.

Stevenson, J. S., & Woods, N. F. (1986). Nursing science and contemporary science: Emerging paradigms. In G. E. Sorensen (Ed.), *Setting the agenda for the year 2000: Knowledge development in nursing* (pp. 6–20). Kansas City, MO: American Academy of Nursing.

PART I

ESSENTIALS FOR PRACTICE

CHAPTER 1

Nursing Science and Theory: Scientific Underpinnings for Practice

Carole R. Eldridge

Many advanced practice nurses tend to be pragmatic in their view of nursing, focusing on whether or not something "works" in their practice and with their clients. They look for actions and their consequences, believing that every effect has a discernible, hopefully treatable, cause. Clinical practitioners are often inclined to discard nursing theory as too abstract for practical purposes and too broad to have meaningful application to daily nursing practice. This view, which seems to eschew the value of philosophical thought, is actually a philosophical stance of its own. Whether we appreciate it or not, every nurse operates from a philosophical and theoretical base. The mature doctor of nursing practice (DNP) acknowledges this and seeks to understand the values, beliefs, and ideas that inform his or her daily practice. Practicing at the doctoral level is a highly complex, rich, multileveled experience that demands deeper insights if we are to effectively help our clients and represent our profession.

As we explore the meaning of our practice as doctorally prepared advanced practice nurses, there are several questions to consider. What distinguishes the DNP from other types of advanced practice nurses when it comes to nursing science and theory? How does the DNP-prepared advanced practice nurse use scientific concepts and theory at the bedside? How might the DNP graduate manipulate theoretical and scientific concepts differently from other healthcare providers? What philosophies and values guide the decisions and actions of the DNP in the clinical setting? DNP-prepared advanced practice nurses bring specific expertise to their work, based on a very particular grounding in the scholarship of application. This chapter examines nursing science and theory, focusing on the concepts undergirding the doctor of nursing practice.

Nursing Science

What Is Nursing Science?

A definition of nursing science is best arrived at by first examining the definition of nursing itself. Nursing has been defined in multiple ways, depending on the particular philosophical or professional paradigm of those doing the defining. The view of nursing as a function is captured in Fawcett's (2000) definition of nursing as actions taken by nurses and the outcomes achieved by those actions. Parse (1997) offered a different focus when she wrote that nursing is a discipline organized around nursing knowledge, and that the practice of nursing is a performing art. Rogers (1994) wrote that it is not the practice of nursing that defines nursing, but rather it is the use of nursing knowledge to improve the human condition. King (1990) spoke of nursing as a process of interactions within and between systems. Reed (1997) proposed that, just as archeology is the study of ancient things and biology the study of living things, nursing is the study of promoting well-being.

Actions and outcomes, a discipline, special knowledge, an art, a process, a study of processes, and interacting systems represent just some of the varied definitions of nursing. Four metaparadigm concepts of nursing have gathered general, although not exclusive, acceptance in the nursing body of knowledge: person, environment, nursing, and health. *The Essentials of Doctoral Education for Advanced Nursing Practice* by the American Association of Colleges of Nursing (AACN) reflects nursing's conceptual heritage with this statement describing the focus of the discipline of nursing:

- The principles and laws that govern the life-process, well-being, and optimal function of human beings, sick or well;
- The patterning of human behavior in interaction with the environment in normal life events and critical life situations;
- The nursing actions or processes by which positive changes in health status are affected; and
- The wholeness or health of human beings recognizing that they are in continuous interaction with their environments. (Donaldson & Crowley, 1978; Fawcett, 2005; Gortner, 1980, as cited in AACN, 2006, p. 9)

These foundational concepts address nursing in its many facets, as a discipline with special knowledge of human beings, human behavior, health, and human interaction with the environment, as well as the actions and processes that affect health.

Defining the *science* in nursing science presents a few challenges of its own. Science is variously defined as the study of something, or the knowledge gained by that study, or the methodological activity required to gain the knowledge. Burns and Grove (2001) defined science as a body of knowledge, the research findings and theories that have been developed, tested, and accepted by a specific discipline, agreeing with numerous others who have said that science is a product (knowledge), as well as a process of methodical study. Barrett (2002) postulated that science is our ongoing effort to discover truth. As such, it is always evolving and being revised.

The attempt to define nursing science is further complicated by the debate over whether nursing is a pure or fundamental science, also called basic science, or an applied science. Pure science focuses on building knowledge without the concern shown by applied science for the practical applications of theories and concepts. In recent years, a number of influential nurse authors have promoted the idea that nursing is a basic science with its own body of knowledge focused on the human-environment (or universe)-health process (Parse, 1999).

The way scientific knowledge is obtained in a given field varies. Observation and measurement of the phenomena being studied, followed by description and explanation of the findings, is the most familiar form of scientific research. Experiments or interventions may be performed on the phenomena, and the impact recorded. Replication of scientific studies, with similar results each time, is required before the information gained can be included in the body of accepted knowledge. Research is the process we use to create science. Theories are often developed from research findings, and more research may be conducted to test the theories. Scientific theories form the framework that holds research together and builds scientific knowledge (Barrett, 2002; Burns & Grove, 2001).

In nursing, certain research methodologies and theoretical frameworks have been, and continue to be, developed that are unique to the discipline. Many nurse researchers believe that the progress of nursing as a discipline, science, and practice depends on developing distinctive, nursing-specific theories and research methods. Other factors and methods besides replicable laboratory studies can contribute to scientific knowledge; indeed, such things as abstract thought, intuition, judgment, and experience are essential to scientific advancement (Phillips, 1996).

In *The Essentials of Doctoral Education for Advanced Nursing Practice* (2006), the AACN adopted a definition of nursing science as an entity in itself, with a growing body of scientific knowledge, while acknowledging the value of incorporating knowledge from other sciences. Nursing science is unique, with a particular concern for the factors that affect human wellness, but it draws from any and all of the broader realms of theoretical and scientific thought that can contribute to the nursing body of knowledge. The document states:

> Preparation to address current and future practice issues requires a strong scientific foundation for practice. The scientific foundation of nursing practice has expanded and includes a focus on both the natural and social sciences. . . . In addition, philosophical, ethical, and historical issues inherent in the development of science create a context for the application of the natural and social sciences. Nursing science also has created a significant body of knowledge to guide nursing practice and has expanded the scientific underpinnings of the discipline. (p. 9)

Phillips (1996) emphasized that nursing science is not made up solely of facts. Instead, nursing science is a pattern, a particular way of obtaining, understanding, and using scientific knowledge. This pattern brings unity to the body of nursing knowledge. Silva (1999) questioned the necessity of requiring linear reasoning and logic in nursing science, believing that nursing science should encompass other ways of knowing besides mechanistic data-in, knowledge-out empirical processes. Some have argued for the dynamic coexistence of multiple paradigms or ways of knowing. Monti and Tingen (1999) proposed that multiple paradigms in nursing science are indicative of a flourishing science in which creativity, debate, diversity, and open inquiry serve to strengthen the exchange of multiple points of view and the growth of knowledge.

The definition of nursing science offered by Stevenson and Woods (1986) provides a point of view that is useful in emphasizing practical knowledge about the health problems DNP graduates encounter in practice: "Nursing science is the domain of knowledge concerned with the adaptation of individuals and groups to actual or potential health problems, the environments that influence health in humans and the therapeutic interventions that promote health and affect the consequences of illness" (p. 6).

How Nursing Science Differs from Medical Science

Much of the controversy about nursing science centers on the distinctiveness of nursing's body of knowledge, particularly its differentiation from medical science. The study and practice of medicine focuses on the diagnosis and *cross purposes?*

treatment of disease. Nursing focuses on the human response to illness and its treatment. Yet, medicine and nursing overlap at many points, and seemingly even more so in advanced practice nursing. Do medicine and nursing truly differ in anything besides mere scope of practice?

As a general rule, people enter the healthcare system because they have a problem. A sick person wants to know what is causing his or her symptoms, and wants the healthcare provider to make the symptoms go away. Medical providers seek to solve the diagnostic riddle and apply a treatment to cure the disease or, at the least, calm the symptoms. This approach is mechanistic, and could imply that humans are machines that can be fixed by identifying the problem and intervening at the point of the breakdown. In this context, nurses usually operate as assistants to physicians, or as providers operating under the approval and guidance of a physician (Parse, 1999). This paradigm confines nurses to the boxes drawn and controlled by medical thought and perspectives. If we follow the medical model, nursing science is an applied science that is concerned primarily with using the things learned in other disciplines.

If, however, we view nursing science as a basic science, we open new ways of thinking and acting as advanced practice nurses. Holistic theories and approaches address broad concepts of health, wholeness, caring, and healing of entire systems instead of being limited to the medical concept of curing a disease. Taking this broader, patient-centered, holistic view presents significant challenges in a healthcare system based on the medical model. The current healthcare system, however, is infamously dysfunctional, and the time has arrived for a reexamination of the ways we conceptualize and implement nursing.

When we start from the premise that nursing science is a unique body of knowledge containing theories and evidence intuited, observed, and tested by nurses involved in the processes of human health, we can follow where the evidence leads (Parse, 1999). This is the difference that advanced practice nurses can make, the contribution the DNP graduate should provide to nursing science. The advanced practice nurse begins with the human being, not with the disease, and with the individual human's unique values and goals. The person and the nurse embark on an experiential journey together, with the nurse's knowledge informing and guiding the person along a path that belongs only to the person within his or her special environment.

Every advanced practice nurse should be a nurse scientist, gathering evidence at the patient's side, making observations, having experiences, responding to the patient's experiences, and thinking about reasons, theories, or concepts that might organize the evidence. DNP graduates should examine their own thinking and that of others, testing the concepts and gathering new evidence as an essential part of the nursing process. Throughout the nursing–human interaction, the advanced practice nurse views the individual holistically, as a complex person with unique values and goals, never treating the patient as an object that can be passively acted upon by a benevolent, all-knowing medical and nursing force.

Nursing is commonly accepted as a human science that focuses on human experiences, and nursing's holistic framework is widely acknowledged, but this framework is not always thought to include medicine and the biomedical model. Nursing should incorporate, but not be limited to, biomedical science as part of its holistic approach to healing and health. Rather than merely performing delegated medical tasks, professional nurses incorporate medical treatments and cures within their broader approach to health and wellness, treating the whole person with nursing interventions that do not spring solely from a limited biomedical approach (Bunkers, 2002; Engebretson, 1997).

Fawcett (1999) painted a vision of nursing scholarship and advanced nursing practice that placed nurses squarely and constantly at the patient's side. In her vision, research and practice occur at the bedside by the nurse using nursing concepts, methodologies, and theories. Each interaction between the nurse and the patient is a research case that tests the nursing model guiding the encounter. Clinical data are examined to support, refute, or revise nursing theories. Every nurse and every patient contributes continuously to the ongoing development of nursing knowledge and nursing science. This vision can and should inform advanced nursing practice as we move into the future. It is nursing science that can and should distinguish the DNP from other midlevel healthcare providers and from physicians, and it is nursing knowledge and care that can and should foster health and wholeness in our patients.

Scientific Foundations of Nursing Practice

Philosophical Foundation

The philosophical underpinning of any scientific body of knowledge provides the bones upon which the body is built. Our philosophy is the overarching way we explain the world, the enduring beliefs we hold (Parker, 2006). The values we adhere to, whatever they are, frame the approach we take to science, theory, and research. Nurse scientists vary in their philosophical positions, but themes common to the profession include the concepts of holism, quality of life, and the relativity of truth based on each individual's perceptions (Burns & Grove, 2001). Advanced practice nurses have a responsibility to define and refine the philosophies and values informing our theories, our research, and our application of research.

Two major philosophic orientations have guided nursing's knowledge development: positivism or empiricism, which is the foundation for research in the hard or natural sciences, and antipositivism, which embraces the soft or interpretive human sciences (Kim, 1997). Contemporary empiricism, also known as postpositivism, recognizes that knowledge is developed within specific social and historical contexts. Postpositivism acknowledges the value of observable reality as well as the complex nature of human phenomena (Fawcett, 1997b; Schumacher & Gortner, 1992).

The discipline of nursing benefits from the philosophical body of knowledge available to all scientists, but we build our own philosophical positions based on individual and collective perceptions and experiences. These positions heavily influence the research we conduct and the way we frame that research (Burns & Grove, 2001). For example, one belief commonly held by advanced practice nurses is that the practical application of knowledge is the only worthwhile goal of scientific inquiry. With this in mind, doctorally prepared advanced nurse practitioners generally frame their research within middle-range theoretical concepts that are focused enough to be useful in clinical settings. Nursing metaparadigms provide insights that can guide practice approaches, but the middle-range nursing theories provide a bridge from grand theory to nursing practice, firmly within the realm of clinicians with practice-based value systems (Parker, 2006).

Ethical Knowledge

Ethical issues in health care are complex and varied, and ethical decisions can have significant impact on our patients' lives. Although most nurses face ethical dilemmas from time to time in individual practice, doctorally prepared advanced practice nurses should be prepared to actively address ethical decisions on an ongoing basis and from a broad professional and organizational perspective (Hamric & Reigle, 2005). DNP graduates understand the dominant ethical theories and are cognizant of their practical applications.

The American Nurses Association's Code for Nurses is based on the principle-based model of ethical decision making, which appeals to principles such as respect for persons and autonomy. Ethical reasoning using the principled approach begins with general rules and moves to specific instances. A contrasting ethical theory is the casuistic model, wherein ethical dilemmas are examined in context and compared to similar cases. The ethics of care, or care-based theory, is another ethical decision-making model relevant to nursing. Care-based theory focuses on responsibilities, not rights, and encourages ethical responses based on relationships and needs. Although all of the different ethical theories have inherent limitations, possessing an understanding of ethical reasoning will help the DNP guide patients and organizations through the process of moral decision making. At the core of most contemporary nursing theories that guide advanced practice there is wide agreement that the old medical ethics of paternalism are replaced in nursing by respect for the individual's autonomy (Hamric & Reigle, 2005).

The ethical conduct of both research and clinical practice are of great concern to many scientific disciplines and endeavors, including nursing. Although research on human subjects is essential to building knowledge about human response to health and illness, human research must not harm the subjects. Additionally, researchers need to report results with scrupulous honesty and full disclosure if their findings are to add useful information to the discipline's body of knowledge. Ethics regulations have been developed to protect human rights, guard intellectual property, and promote integrity in reporting (Burns & Grove, 2001).

Federal regulations require that research involving human subjects be subjected to an institutional review process. The review of such research is conducted by a research review board (RRB) or institutional review board (IRB), a committee that is responsible for ensuring that human rights and safety are protected and that research is carried out ethically and in compliance with federal guidelines. Although the composition and processes of specific institutional review boards vary, federal law requires that members have adequate expertise to review research. Members must not have conflicts of interest pertaining to the research they review (Burns & Grove, 2001).

An IRB can decide that research submitted to the committee is either exempt from review, appropriate for expedited review, or required to undergo a complete review. The decision about the level of review is based on the risk to human subjects inherent in the proposed research. A proposed nursing study that posed nothing more than a small cost of time or inconvenience to subjects, such as a survey about working conditions, would probably be considered exempt from review. That decision cannot be made by the researcher, however. The researcher must submit information about the proposed study to the IRB. Usually the chair of the IRB will decide whether the research proposal is exempt or should be presented to the full committee for review. No nurse researcher should conduct even the smallest human study in any institution without first obtaining approval from the institutional review board (Burns & Grove, 2001).

Doctorally prepared nurse practitioners are obligated to learn and follow the ethical codes applying to scientific research. Many apparently benign clinical practices have turned out eventually to have adverse consequences, and a clinical researcher can never assume that an intervention will not have a negative impact where human subjects are concerned.

The World Medical Association developed the "Declaration of Helsinki: Ethical Principles for Medical Research Involving Human Subjects." Originally based on the Nuremberg Code, a response to the Nazi medical experiments, the Declaration of Helsinki was adopted in Finland in 1964 and later amended numerous times, most recently in 2008. Although targeted primarily to physicians, the declaration encourages adoption by anyone conducting medical research on human subjects. The *Code of Ethics for Nurses with Interpretive Statements* (American Nurses Association, 2001) stipulates that nurses have an ethical obligation to protect human rights. When conducting nursing research, nurses must protect subjects' rights to privacy, self-determination, confidentiality, fair treatment, and protection from harm (Burns & Grove, 2001). DNP graduates should familiarize themselves with these principles before undertaking clinical research. Please see Chapter 8 for further discussion of ethics in advanced practice nursing.

Historical Knowledge

Knowledge of how the discipline of nursing achieved its current state is essential for understanding its philosophical, theoretical, ethical, and scientific foundations. History gives context to data, and facts interpreted outside of their context usually result in misinformation and erroneous conclusions.

Biophysical and Psychosocial Knowledge

As a human science, nursing benefits from knowledge accumulated in many other disciplines, including such important areas as biology, physiology, psychology, and sociology. Nurses are generally well educated regarding biophysical and psychosocial sciences in their nursing preparation, but the rapid changes and discoveries occurring in these fields necessitate constant updating of the advanced nurse practitioner's knowledge. Graduation with a DNP degree should be only one stage of an ongoing, lifelong quest for knowledge and growth. Providing safe, high-quality care is an imperative that requires current information, up-to-date clinical and technical skills, and familiarity with the latest research in the biological and human sciences. Professional development should never end, supported by lifelong learning that brings fresh insights from science and newly discovered evidence to the practice environment.

Analytical Knowledge

Analytical reasoning provides an important underpinning for scientific knowledge in any discipline. When we analyze an issue, we make judgments about it based on the evidence in our possession, using thought processes to make connections and derive meaning.

Organizational Knowledge

Organizational science brings an essential dimension to advanced nursing practice. Organizations, whether simple or complex, can only be fully understood as whole systems in motion, with intricate relationships among multiple parts. Small particles of organizations cannot be properly understood in isolation from one another. Organizational scientists look for patterns of behavior and interactions. Systems thinking is a framework for seeing wholes. Human beings, and organizations containing humans, are open systems that change in response to even very small occurrences (Senge, 1994; Wheatley, 2006).

Organizational structure is much more important to nursing practice than many nurses realize. Some DNPs choose organizational leadership as their area of clinical practice because they have learned that patient care at the bedside is intricately interwoven with the systems of management and administration that support, and sometimes hinder, health care. It is the business of doctorally prepared clinical nurse leaders to work within complex systems to secure and implement the resources and education needed to provide safe, high-quality patient care. We know, for example, that the majority of medication errors are not caused by any single person or event.

Instead, these errors are caused by problems inherent within the system of medication administration used by the organization. DNPs who want to protect their patients need to understand the organizational system, help to uncover the causes of inefficiencies and errors, and collaborate with others to improve and strengthen the system in order to support both providers and patients.

Knowledge of organizational structure and science is critical for understanding and affecting nursing effectiveness and outcomes. The advanced nurse practitioner who has a grasp on how complex systems affect nursing satisfaction and patient safety will be able to operate within the system to effect change. Organizational theories that DNP graduates should be familiar with include scientific management, bureaucratic management, administrative theory, the neoclassical approach, participative management, systems theory, the sociotechnical approach, and contingency or situational theory. Shared governance of nursing practice by the professional nurses who work in an organization is based on some of these theories and approaches.

Nursing Theory

Nursing Theory–Guided Practice

Nursing theory–guided practice is the recognition and use of models, concepts, and theories from nursing and other disciplines in our work with clients. Theories provide the base from which we seek to understand patients and their health problems, and from which we plan interventions to help them. Nursing theory improves our care by giving it structure and unity, by providing more efficient continuity of care, by achieving congruence between process and product, by defining the boundaries and goals of nursing actions, and by giving us a framework in which to examine the effectiveness of our interventions. When advanced practice nurses use theory to guide care, they achieve higher quality in their care while simultaneously elevating nursing's professional standards, accountability, and autonomy. Considering the often fragmented, inefficient, and disorganized care typical of the current healthcare system, we need nursing theory–guided practice to provide a coherent antidote (Kenney, 2006; Meleis, 1997; Smith, 1994).

Scientific research and practice require a framework. Whether the framework is explicitly described or merely implied does not change the fact that the framework exists. There are many theories and conceptual models to consider in advanced nursing practice, and the DNP's responsibility is to become knowledgeable about a broad range of theoretical frameworks in order to intelligently use them in clinical practice. Kenney (2006) believed that nurses should choose the appropriate model or theory of care for a particular client's situation as part of the initial assessment.

Burns and Grove (2001) offered a framework linking nursing research to the rest of nursing that proposed a continuum between the concrete world of nursing practice and the abstract realms of philosophy and theory. Because nurses have traditionally been expected to perform tasks, nursing thought has tended to be concrete and action-oriented. Skillful concrete thought is essential for planning and carrying out necessary interventions. Abstract thought, although it may seem to have less application to nursing's everyday work, is in reality required if we are to recognize the patterns and implications that underlie events, symptoms, and behaviors exhibited by our patients. In clinical practice, the advanced practice nurse must probe beneath the symptoms to find causes and relationships. Theory and research depend on abstract thought, and nursing theory and research are essential for developing the scientific knowledge that nurses need to provide evidence-based health care.

What makes a theory a nursing theory? Nurses use knowledge from many disciplines to frame nursing research, and the knowledge gained, while shared with others, is important to nursing and is used by nursing in distinctive ways. A theory that organizes nursing knowledge and offers a systematic way to explain or describe nursing practice is a nursing theory. Nursing theories clarify what we do and help establish the parameters of our profession (McEwen & Wills, 2006). The DNP graduate knows how to "integrate nursing science with knowledge from ethics, the biophysical, psychosocial, analytical, and organizational sciences as the basis for the highest level of nursing practice" (AACN, 2006).

Developing Middle-Range Theories and Concepts to Guide Practice

Theories are variously classified according to philosophy, perspective, and scope or scale. In nursing, grand theories have the widest scope and are the most abstract, aiming to explain or describe broad issues. Middle-range theories are specific descriptions, explanations, or predictions about a phenomenon of interest, more explicitly focused and concrete than grand theories. A middle-range theory has a limited number of concepts, and these concepts can be defined in operational terms for generating testable hypotheses. Because middle-range theories can be tested, they are the theories most amenable to clinical nursing research, putting them within the exploratory domain of the advanced practice nurse scientist (McEwen & Wills, 2006; Parker, 2006).

Nursing Theories

The many nursing theories that have been developed cannot be described here in detail, but we will examine some of the work of nurse theorists as it applies to advanced nursing practice. Before doing so, it is useful to consider how the DNP should select and implement theories in nursing practice.

Fawcett (1997a) wrote that nurses must first make a conscious decision to use theories in practice. The DNP should understand that nursing theory is what differentiates us from physicians and the medical model of practice. In the traditional medical model, humans are reduced to decontextualized pieces of data. In contrast, nursing practice occurs in the interactions between nurse and person. This process is human based and can only be properly guided by values and principles, theories, and philosophical orientation, not by discrete bits of data (Mitchell, Schmidt, Bunkers, & Bournes, 2006). Many nurse researchers and theorists believe that professional nursing is uniquely distinguished from other healthcare professions only by its use of nursing models and theories to guide practice (Kenney, 2006).

For example, when patients come to the DNP with problems caused by lifestyle choices, we unavoidably interact with the patients based on our values. If we follow the traditional medical model, we instruct the patient to change the behavior that is causing the illness and, if medications or treatments are available, advise the patient to use them. We define the goals of therapy and the state of health we want for the patient, and we expect the individual to follow our advice. If, on the other hand, we apply a nursing model, our interaction with the patient is entirely different. The nursing values of autonomy and nonjudgmental acceptance of the patient's choices will direct us to follow different processes of assessment and intervention. Depending on the theory we apply to the situation, we join our patients' struggles to define and create a state of health that is unique to them (Mitchell, 1999).

Using nursing theories means we must change the way we think and act in our work with clients. One of the decisions we must make as DNPs is whether we should use only one nursing model throughout our clinical practice. Using only one nursing theory to guide our care of every patient could limit our assessment and narrow our vision, so that we see only the things we need to see to fit the client into our chosen model. To create individualized care for each patient, we can benefit from knowing and using a variety of theories, selecting the conceptual models that are most suitable for particular situations. In doing so, however, we need to maintain congruence with the philosophical underpinnings, principles, and propositions that form the different theories (Kenney, 2006).

Kenney provided five steps that nurses should follow once the decision has been made to use theory-based nursing practice:

1. Consider your personal values and beliefs about nursing, clients, health, and environment.
2. Examine the underlying assumptions, values, and beliefs of various nursing models, and how the major concepts are defined.
3. Identify several models that are congruent with your own values and beliefs about nursing, clients, and health.
4. Identify the similarities and differences in client focus, nursing actions, and client outcomes of these models.
5. Practice applying the models and theories to clients with different health concerns to determine which ones best "fit" specific situations and guide nursing actions that will achieve desired client outcomes. (2006, pp. 306–307)

It is worth noting that the majority of nurse theorists developed their theories in an effort to improve the care nurses provide to clients. Nurse theorists were and are experienced practitioners whose theories grew out of their clinical experiences and their attempts to do a better job in the delivery of care. By reflecting on their practice and observations, nurse theorists recognize patterns and gain insights into concepts that lead to theoretical formation (Sitzman & Eichelberger, 2003). This is the same process the DNP student should follow in practice and research, forming middle-range theories that are testable at the bedside.

When studying and selecting a theoretical basis for nursing practice, the DNP should study the theory of interest in its entirety. The brief summaries provided here should serve only to pique the DNP student's interest in studying an appealing theory more thoroughly. The purpose of these summaries, which are presented in chronological order, is to consider how various theories can inform the DNP's practice. The majority of the theories will be familiar to the nurse involved in graduate studies, but should be viewed by the DNP student with a fresh focus on applying nursing theory in practice and developing middle-range theories from within a grand theoretical perspective.

FLORENCE NIGHTINGALE'S PHILOSOPHY

Although Florence Nightingale is not generally considered a theorist in the formal sense, her vision of nursing and her philosophy of care resonate with many modern nurses and often inform the work of advanced practice nurses. Nightingale, who wrote *Notes on Nursing* in 1859, put the patient at the center of her model, and taught that the goal of nursing is to meet the patient's needs and manipulate the patient's environment so that the patient can attain a healthy state. The work of nursing was not, in Nightingale's view, something delegated to nurses by physicians; rather, nursing was a management role, separate and distinct from medicine, with the job of managing the environment, observing the patient and the patient's interactions with the environment, and assisting the patient toward health. Nightingale perceived patients holistically, and considered the impact of environmental conditions on the person's physical, intellectual, psychological, and spiritual components. Nurses were defined as those who had responsibility for another person's health, and in this role nurses make health possible by arranging for clean, warm, properly lit, quiet surroundings and a correct diet (Dunphy, 2006; Lobo, 1995).

PEPLAU'S INTERPERSONAL MODEL

Like Nightingale, Hildegard Peplau believed that nursing concepts should come from making observations in nursing situations. Her book, *Interpersonal Relations in Nursing*, first published in 1952 and again in 1988, presented Peplau's ideas about nursing's roles, the interpersonal process, and how to study nursing as an interpersonal process. Peplau taught a system of theoretical development that combined inductive reasoning, based on observation, with deductive reasoning, based on known concepts. Peplau used qualitative methods to examine something of interest, and then used quantitative methods to test an intervention targeted at the problem (Belcher & Fish, 1995; Peden, 2006).

Peplau's interpersonal model pictures nursing as an interpersonal process between the nurse and patient, who are working toward mutually agreed-upon goals. The sequential steps taken to reach the goals are (1) orientation, in which the patient's problems are defined, (2) identification, in which the nurse and patient clarify expectations and figure out how to work together, (3) exploitation, in which the patient uses the services offered by the nurse that the patient finds useful, and (4) resolution, in which the patient's needs have been met and the patient moves toward independence. Even when conflict arises or things do not proceed smoothly, these therapeutic interactions can and should cause growth in both the nurse and the patient (Belcher & Fish, 1995).

VIRGINIA HENDERSON'S DEFINITION OF NURSING

Henderson, who developed and published her theory of nursing in the years from 1955 to 1966, sought to differentiate nursing from other healthcare work by defining it as the performance of health-enhancing activities that patients cannot do without help. She described 14 components of nursing care: breathe normally; eat and drink adequately; eliminate body wastes; move and maintain posture; sleep and rest; select suitable clothing; maintain body temperature; keep body clean and well-groomed; avoid dangers in the environment; communicate; worship according to one's faith; work to achieve a sense of accomplishment; recreation; and learn, discover, or satisfy curiosity. By assisting the patient with these basic components of care, the nurse works to help the patient become independent again (Furukawa & Howe, 1995; Gesse, Dombro, Gordon, & Rittman, 2006).

HALL'S CARE, CORE, AND CURE MODEL

Lydia Hall conceptualized the patient as a person, a body, and a disease, which she placed into overlapping, dynamic, and interactive circles of core (the person), care (the body), and cure (the disease). Her theory was honed over a period covering the latter half of the 1950s and the early 1960s. Nursing is concerned with all of these circles, with different parts of the model becoming the predominant nursing focus at different times. Practically speaking, Hall believed that nursing is most crucial after the patient's acute crisis has stabilized, when nurses should nurture and educate and assist the patient to make changes that will prevent a repeat of the original crisis (George, 1995; Touhy & Birnbach, 2006).

A central tenet of the care, core, and cure model is that intimate personal care such as bathing belongs exclusively to nursing, and that nursing is needed when an individual cannot take care of these bodily requirements unassisted. The professional nurse is able to perform personal care in such a way that it provides comfort but also engenders learning, growth, and healing. The nurse in this caring role is a nurturer, using these intimate inter-actions to take the client beyond cleanliness and comfort to health (George, 1995; Touhy & Birnbach, 2006).

OREM'S SELF-CARE DEFICIT THEORY OF NURSING

First published in an early form in 1959, three interrelated theories com-pose Dorothea Orem's self-care deficit theory of nursing: theory of self-care, self-care deficit theory, and theory of nursing systems. To understand her general theory, it is essential to grasp the six central concepts and one periph-eral concept within the overarching theory:

1. Self-care is initiating and performing activities on one's own behalf to maintain life, health, and well-being.
2. Self-care agency is the individual's ability to practice self-care.
3. Therapeutic self-care demand is the set of self-care activities needed to meet self-care needs.
4. Self-care deficit is the gap between self-care agency and self-care demand, between the self-care activities the individual can do and the self-care activities that are needed.
5. Nursing agency is the nurse's ability to meet the therapeutic self-care demands of others.
6. The nursing system is the package of nursing responsibilities, roles, relationships, and actions that is organized to meet the client's ther-apeutic self-care demand. (Foster & Bennett, 1995; Orem, 2006)

The self-care deficit nursing theory has been used extensively in nursing practice. As a general theory, it is relevant for guiding practice in any care set-ting or specialty area. Backscheider (1974) used Orem's theory to organize nursing care in a diabetic nurse management clinic, structuring the nursing system based on the nature of the clients' self-care deficits. Nursing agency overcomes the self-care deficits caused by, in this case, diabetes. Crews (1972) applied Orem's theory to nurse-managed cardiac clinics. The theory has been used to guide inpatient, outpatient, and community settings; across a variety of age groups and disease states; in the care of families and communities; to inform administration and management of nursing care; and as a basis for nursing research and education.

Orem believed that nursing is a practical science with both theoretical and practical knowledge. She taught that nursing is different from other disciplines and services because of its focus on human beings. The broad applicability of her theory to a variety of situations, and its focus on designing nursing care to meet clients' needs, makes the self-care deficit theory a useful theoretical base for the DNP's practice and research (Isenberg, 2006).

JOHNSON'S BEHAVIORAL SYSTEMS MODEL

Dorothy Johnson was influenced by Florence Nightingale in her early publications, including her 1959 proposal that nursing should draw on the basic and applied sciences in developing the science of nursing. In "The Significance of Nursing Care," Johnson (1961) reflected Nightingale again by writing that nursing care should support the patient's maintenance of equilibrium in the face of stressful, destabilizing stimuli. Based on systems thinking and developmental theories, Dorothy Johnson's 1968 behavioral systems model conceptualizes humans as open systems containing interdependent subsystems. The person is a behavioral system existing within an environment (both internal and external) of multiple components, and the human/system interacts with the environment in various ways. Johnson draws analogies between five core general systems principles and concepts of human development: wholeness and order form the basis for human identity and continuity; stabilization or balance is the basis of development; reorganization correlates with change and growth; hierarchic interaction is analogous to discontinuity; and dialectical contradiction provides the basis for motivation (Holaday, cited in Parker, 2006).

The behavioral system (person) in Johnson's model is composed of subsystems that perform specialized functions to meet a specific goal. The activities that a person employs to meet the system's goals differ based on the individual's values, motives, gender, age, self-concept, and other variables. The system's overall goal is to maintain equilibrium in the face of internal and external environmental pressures. Each subsystem works to achieve its own equilibrium, contributing to the balance or homeostasis of the whole person. Balance is attained and maintained by accommodation to the environment, and the individual with a large bank of possible accommodating behaviors will be more adaptable to changing forces (Holaday, 2006).

Nursing action is intended to help the person arrive at a state of equilibrium when possible. Johnson stated that whereas medicine sees the patient as a biological system, nursing sees a behavioral system instead. And, although nursing's responsibility is to assist the patient toward behavioral system balance, Johnson made it clear that individuals must make their own choices about the level of functioning and balance that they want to achieve. It is the nurse's responsibility to help the client understand the function and balance that is possible and how to achieve it, and then to guide progress toward the goals of the patient's choosing (Holaday, 2006).

When practicing with this model as a guide, the nurse assesses the client to determine the source of the problem and then uses nursing interventions to create change. In the behavioral systems model, the nurse might provide essential functions or help the patient obtain essential functions, negotiating a plan with the patient. Or, the nurse might act as a regulatory force, enacting controls to restore stability. A third possible intervention is to attempt to change the person's guiding set of concepts and choices in order to bring about actions that can repair the damage (Holaday, 2006).

Johnson's model has found useful application in studies of cancer patients, psychiatric patients, education, and administration, among others. The behavioral systems model establishes behavioral system balance as a clear goal for nursing, gives a way to identify the cause of the imbalance, and guides the nurse as an external force that helps the system achieve equilibrium.

ABDELLAH'S PROBLEM-SOLVING APPROACH

Faye Abdellah's theoretical stance, described in 1960, was nursing centered and focused on solving nursing problems. She developed 21 nursing problems as a way to help nurses systematically identify problems presented by clients. The problems, although written from the perspective of the nurse, bear similarities to Henderson's basic nursing care components, which were written from the patient's view. For example, instead of Henderson's "keep body clean and well-groomed," Abdellah identified the nursing problem as "to maintain good hygiene and physical comfort." In practice, the nursing problems are useful for directing the nurse's actions and for providing a structure for developing principles of care (Falco, 1995).

ROY'S ADAPTATION MODEL

Sister Callista Roy's adaptation model was first presented in 1964 as part of Roy's graduate work under the mentorship of Dorothy Johnson (Galbreath, 1995). In its final form the theory contains four essential elements: the person receiving nursing care, the environment, health, and nursing (Roy & Andrews, 1991). The person, or a group, is a holistic adaptive system. People and groups use coping processes to adapt to, interact with, transform, and be transformed by their environment. Human behavior results from adaptation in various modes. Health is integration and wholeness, and adaptation is used to support the process and state of health (Roy & Zhan, 2006).

Roy's model is broadly applicable to all types of nursing practice and nursing research. In particular, the adaptation model lends itself well to guide research and practice regarding the changes that occur in human development and aging. Life stages that require significant adjustment, such as adolescence and the older adult years, are good areas for research into appropriate interventions to support the processes of adaptation. The theory emphasizes finding ways to enhance the coping processes of the individual or group experiencing change. The DNP who bases practice on this model will seek to understand the patient's adaptation processes and work with patients to help them cope with their environment and adapt toward a state of health (Roy & Zhan, 2006).

LEVINE'S CONSERVATION MODEL

Writing in 1969, Myra Levine taught that nursing's role is to support the human process of adaptation to achieve the goal of conservation, which includes conservation of energy, structural integrity, personal integrity, and social integrity. Conservation protects the integrity and wholeness of living systems in the face of change. Levine illustrated the principle of conservation by referring to a thermostat. A thermostat does not respond until there is a change in the environment, at which time it activates the heating or cooling system until the temperature in the environment is restored to the set point. The thermostat conserves energy until it is needed to restore balance, just as a successful living system in a state of homeostasis is conserving energy until action is needed to bring the system back into balance (George, 1995).

The principles of conservation form the foundation of the model: people are always acting within a complex environment that affects behavior; people protect themselves by learning everything they can about the environment; nurses are active participants in a patient's environment; and nursing care works to restore and strengthen the patient's adaptive responses to survive within the environment, including responses that help the patient deal with disease and difficulties (Schaefer, 2006).

Levine believed that knowing and using a variety of nursing theories was essential, because there could never be a theory of nursing that was appropriate in every situation. Her conservation model has been used widely in practice, across the life span and in clinical settings ranging from community care to critical care. The model assumes that health is the goal, and that nurses should develop interventions that focus on conservation of the system's energy and integrity to achieve wholeness. The interventions will vary widely within this theory, depending on the problem, the person, and the environment (Schaefer, 2006).

ROGERS'S SCIENCE OF UNITARY HUMAN BEINGS

Evolving during the decades between 1961 and 1994, the science of unitary human beings is based on five assumptions about humans, described in Martha Rogers's 1970 publication *The Theoretical Basis of Nursing*: (1) a human is a unified whole, more than and different from the sum of its parts, (2) humans and their environment are continuously exchanging energy and matter in an open system, (3) human beings evolve in one direction and cannot go backward to a previous state, (4) life's patterns identify humans and reflect their wholeness, and (5) humans are capable of abstract thought. Theorist Rogers identified four building blocks based on the five basic assumptions: energy fields (human beings and their environment are energy fields of concern to nursing); openness and dynamic movement among energy fields; pattern, or distinguishing characteristics of an energy field; and pandimensionality, meaning without boundaries of space and time (Falco & Lobo, 1995; Malinski, 2006).

Rogers's three principles of homeodynamics are grounded on the five assumptions and four building blocks. Integrality is the first principle of homeodynamics, which is defined as the continuous interaction between humans and the environment. The second principle is resonancy, which addresses the continuous changes occurring between human and environmental fields and the identification of the fields by wave patterns. Helicy, the third principle, proposes that the changes occurring between human and environmental fields are moving in the direction of increasing diversity and complexity in unpredictable and nonrepeating ways (Falco & Lobo, 1995; Malinski, 2006).

Rogers believed that many theories could be developed from the science of unitary human beings. She devised the theory of accelerating evolution, postulating that human–environment field interactions become faster and more diverse over time. There can be no such thing as a static state of normalcy in a world of accelerating evolution. A second theory, of the emergence of paranormal phenomena, suggested that experiences we usually consider paranormal are actually glimpses of innovation in field patterns. Her third theory, manifestations of field patterning in unitary human beings, is focused on the process of evolution as a nonlinear movement forward to increasing diversity (Malinski, 2006).

In clinical practice, the science of unitary human beings leads to highly individualized nursing and healthcare services. Rogers was opposed to nursing diagnosis and care mapping schemata that try to standardize care. Instead, she taught that increasing diversity meant increasingly individualized care. She emphasized each person's right to choose his or her own path to health, and believed that noninvasive methods of treatment should form the basis for nursing practice. In Rogers's view, the goal of practice is to promote well-being, and nurses do this as part of a mutual process with clients (Malinski, 2006).

Rogers considered the nursing process too static, reductionistic, and sequential to apply within her paradigm of dynamic, infinite, open energy fields integrally interacting in constant change. Other practice methodologies have been developed from the principles of the science of unitary human beings. Barrett's 1988 Rogerian practice method for health patterning is widely accepted as a Rogerian alternative to the nursing process. There are two processes in Barrett's model. The first, pattern manifestation knowing, is the process of becoming familiar with the human and environmental fields. The second process is called voluntary mutual patterning and involves the nurse in helping the client to choose ways to change as part of achieving well-being. Both processes are continuous and simultaneous, not sequential or linear. The outcomes cannot be predicted or controlled (Butcher, 2006).

Scientific advances in quantum mechanics and research based on chaos theory have lent strength to Rogers's ideas. In quantum mechanics, researchers are learning that everything has an impact on everything else, and it is impossible to predict where and how all the influences will come from or what effect they will have. Studies of the electromagnetic field of the brain are revealing how awareness correlates with synchronous firing of neurons, so that the seat of consciousness seems to reside in the patterns of the field (Wheatley, 2006). DNPs will invariably benefit from integrating nursing science with knowledge from a variety of other sciences.

NEUMAN'S SYSTEMS MODEL

In Betty Neuman's model, developed in 1970 and based on systems theory, each individual or group is a client system. Each system, although unique, is composed of common characteristics within a normal range. Environmental stressors disturb a system's stability to various degrees. A system has normal defenses against stressors, but when these are inadequate the client can be negatively or positively affected. Each client has resistance factors that stabilize and move the system toward health. Nursing interventions can affect the client's move toward health on a number of levels. The goal of nursing is to promote the system's stability by assessing the impact of stressors and helping the client adjust to the environment.

The model's three types of prevention—primary, secondary, and tertiary—are interventions that promote wellness. The purpose of primary prevention is to reduce risk factors and prevent identified or suspected stressors before the client experiences a reaction to the stressors, thereby *retaining* wellness. Health promotion is an example of a primary prevention intervention. The aim of secondary prevention is to intervene in ways that strengthen the client's internal resistance to a stressor once a reaction to the stressor has occurred, thereby *attaining* a new state of health. Tertiary prevention is used as an intervention once the client has returned to a stable state after a stressor reaction and secondary prevention have occurred. Tertiary prevention focuses on *maintaining* wellness by supporting the system's strengths and conserving its energy.

Neuman's systems model was first developed for use in nursing education, but it has found wide use in a variety of settings around the world. Nursing administration, psychiatric nursing, case management, gerontological nursing, occupational health nursing, and other specialties have benefited from applying the model in practice (Aylward, 2006).

KING'S INTERACTING SYSTEMS FRAMEWORK AND MIDRANGE THEORY OF GOAL ATTAINMENT

Imogene King's interacting systems framework, introduced in 1971's *Toward a Theory of Nursing*, is grounded in general system theory, a philosophy of science that emphasizes wholeness and the interaction of elements within systems. King sought to identify the essence of nursing and found that this brought her to the nature of human beings, since nurses are humans who give nursing care to other humans. From this abstract conceptualization she derived the middle-range theory of goal attainment. She used concepts of self, perception, communication, interaction, transaction, role, and decision making in her theory. She theorized that the goal of nursing is to help human beings attain, maintain, or regain health and developed a "transaction process model" that she observed in human interactions. In King's transaction model, the nurse and patient interact to set goals they mutually agree upon and then can mutually achieve (King, 2006).

King linked her theory of goal attainment to the nursing process, which strengthened the theory's use and applicability in clinical practice. She considered the nursing process to be a method, and the transaction process model provided theoretical grounding for the method. A nurse uses perception, communication, and interaction to gather the data needed for assessment and the judgment needed to diagnose. When the nurse and patient decide on the goals and the means to achieve them, they are planning and implementing the plan using the transactional process. Evaluation is theoretically based on the feedback loop that often begins the transactional process again (King, 2006).

Other midrange theories have grown from the interacting systems framework. Sieloff devised the theory of departmental power to help explain group power in organizations. Frey used King's framework to develop a theory about chronic illness, families, and children. Brooks and Thomas built a theory of perceptual awareness. The framework has shown broad applicability across the life span and across a variety of systems, including personal, interpersonal, and social. It has been used to address many different client concerns and conditions in multiple nursing specialties and work settings. Several instruments have been developed to measure and test these middle-range theories, such as King's Goal Attainment Scale, Killeen's Nursing Care Survey, the Sieloff-King assessment of group power within organizations, and Rawlins, Rawlins, and Horner's Family Needs Assessment Tool (Sieloff, Frey, & Killeen, 2006).

The interacting systems framework and the midrange theory of goal attainment have a broad scope and have been used to generate a significant amount of nursing knowledge. Sieloff, Frey, and Killeen (2006) noted that King's work provides a theoretical base for research that can be readily applied in nursing practice as part of the continued development of evidence-based nursing.

WATSON'S THEORY OF HUMAN CARING

Jean Watson wrote that her theory of human caring, developed between 1975 and 1979, was an effort to explicate her view that nursing practice, knowledge, and values focus on the patient's own healing processes and personal world of experiences. While complementing the medical practitioner's work, Watson's *carative factors*, as she termed them, also contrasted sharply with medicine's *curative factors* (Watson, 2006). The theory's major concepts include the ten carative factors, the transpersonal caring relationship, the caring moment, and the caring-healing modalities. The ten carative factors are, in brief, the promotion of and/or assistance with the following: (1) a humanistic-altruistic value system, (2) faith-hope, (3) sensitivity to self and others, (4) helping-trusting relationship, (5) expression of feelings, (6) creative problem solving, (7) transpersonal teaching-learning, (8) a supportive environment, (9) need gratification, and (10) existential-phenomenological-spiritual forces (Talento, 1995; Watson, 1979).

The original ten caring factors evolved over time and were transposed by Watson into "clinical caritas processes." These translated factors moved from basic abstractions to open processes, such as (1) a practice of loving kindness, (2) being authentically present, (3) cultivation of spiritual practices, (4) developing a helping-trusting relationship, (5) supporting the expression of feelings, (6) creative use of self in the caring process, (7) engaging in teaching-learning from within another's perspective, (8) creating a healing environment, (9) helping with basic needs with caring consciousness, and (10) opening to spiritual and existential dimensions; soul care for self and others (Watson, 2006).

The transpersonal caring relationship, the second major concept in Watson's theory, describes an intentional attempt to connect with another person through caring. It requires the one providing care to move beyond the self in order to access the spirit of the one being cared for. The third conceptual understanding in the theory is the caring moment, when the nurse and another person interact. Caring-healing modalities, the fourth concept, are the intentional acts, words, behaviors, and various means of communications exercised by the nurse in the process of helping the client heal (Watson, 2006).

The theory of human caring has been used effectively as a framework for studying nursing leadership and management. Anne Liners Kersbergen Brett (1992) studied the caring attributes received or needed by nurse administrators at work, finding that the interpersonal caring attributes were the most needed by nurse managers. Ray (1984) examined the implications of differing definitions of caring in a healthcare organization, developing a classification system of institutional caring. Data from these studies reveal that nurses and nurse administrators greatly value interactional caring, yet perceive that they do not frequently receive the kind of social caring that they need. Ray (1989) developed a middle-range theory of bureaucratic caring for nursing practice as a result of her work within Watson's grand theory.

Nursing leaders who thought caring was being devalued in their highly technology-oriented hospital unit used Watson's theory of human caring to inform their study of caring attributes among nurses and patients. The researchers discovered that the nurses and patients felt there was a high level of relational and contextual caring on the unit, and that caring behaviors were essential to maintain energy and motivate more caring behaviors. The nurse leaders discussed these findings with the unit and identified ways to systematically support caring behaviors and promote a caring culture (Carter, Nelson, Sievers, Dukek, Pipe, & Holland, 2008).

The effects of caring on client outcomes have been tested by research that has shown preliminary linkage between nurse caring behaviors and such outcomes as patient satisfaction, perceived health status, total length of stay, and nursing care costs (Duffy, 1992) and the economic value of caring to healthcare organizations (Issel & Kahn, 1998). Duffy and Hoskins (2003) proposed a model blending caring concepts with an evidence-based practice framework, stating that these apparently diverse paradigms used together might produce the best outcomes for clients and nurses. Nyberg's 1998 model of caring administration is grounded in Watson's theory, as is the attending nurse caring model (ANCM), which was piloted at the Children's Hospital in Denver, Colorado (Watson, 2006). The DNP scholar will find fertile soil for exploration and development of practice modalities from within the theory of human caring.

PATERSON AND ZDERAD'S HUMANISTIC NURSING THEORY

Published in 1976, Josephine Paterson and Loretta Zderad's *Humanistic Nursing* laid out a multidimensional and interactive theory that seeks to bridge theory and practice. Humanistic nursing theory postulates nursing as an existential experience, a shared dialogue between nurse and patient that puts the nurse in the role of nurturing and comforting someone in need. An individual, or group of individuals, generates a call for help with a health-related need, and one or more nurses respond with assistance. Nursing is what happens in the process. The theory is a broad guide for the interactions that occur in this call-and-response model (Kleiman, 2006; Praeger, 1995).

Health, in Paterson and Zderad's theory, is not just the absence of illness. Being healthy means finding meaning in existence and becoming everything one can be within the experiences, relationships, and options of life. The theory speaks of creative relationships characterized by the nurse and patient meeting, relating to each other, and providing an open, receptive presence to each other in a lived dialogue. This process leads to community, and makes it possible for people to find meaning and become healthy through sharing with others (Praeger, 1995).

Paterson and Zderad developed a method of inquiry they called *phenomenologic nursology*. Phenomenology seeks to describe phenomena without explaining or predicting them. Phenomenologic nursology follows a five-step process: (1) the nurse prepares to know something or someone by opening the mind and spirit to the unknown, (2) the nurse gains knowledge of the patient through intuitive impressions and learning about the patient's experiences, (3) the nurse gains scientific knowledge of the patient by analyzing the data, (4) the nurse synthesizes the subjective and objective information to gain perspective on the situation, and (5) the nurse arrives at a new truth, a concept that includes all the information gained, refined into a descriptive construct (Kleiman, 2006; Praeger, 1995).

NEWMAN'S THEORY OF HEALTH AS EXPANDING CONSCIOUSNESS

In her 1978 theory of health as expanding consciousness, Margaret Newman drew from concepts in Martha Rogers's science of unitary human beings, particularly the view that health and illness are a unitary process, manifestations of the greater whole, and are not mutually exclusive states. Within this paradigm, then, the nurse's job is to help people recognize and use their own power to evolve to a higher condition. Health, as defined by Newman, is the expansion of consciousness, and nurses go with their patients and support them in discovering wholeness and meaning. Consciousness is the system's ever-expanding information capability, which is continuously influenced by the forces of time, movement, and space (George, 1995; Pharris, 2006).

Nurses who use Newman's theory in practice do not set goals, predict outcomes, or follow a defined nursing pathway. Rather, nurses enter into partnership with people who have arrived at a point of disruption and uncertainty. Nursing provides a caring relationship in which patients can explore meaning and potential and grow from disorganization to a higher level of organization. Chaos presents an opportunity for transformation, and the nurse joins the patient in the chaos as new patterns develop. The focus is on being with the person who is in turmoil, not on doing things for them. When practicing from this perspective, nurses must focus on what is meaningful to the patient (George, 1995; Pharris, 2006).

PARSE'S HUMAN BECOMING SCHOOL OF THOUGHT

Rosemarie Parse's human becoming school of thought, first presented in 1981, is philosophically rooted in the simultaneity paradigm, which views human beings as unitary and the human–universe process as irreducible and dynamic. Health is an ever-changing state, based on the human being's choices, values, and priorities. Research and practice focus on discerning patterns and improving quality of life. The individual's desires and opinions about his or her health are more important than anyone else's perspectives. This view contrasts with the totality paradigm, used in the medical model, in which the person is seen in bio-logical, psychological, social, and spiritual parts, with health as a state of well-being in the various pieces of the person. Societal norms define health, and research and practice focus on preventing disease and promoting an accept-able state of health. Nurses operating within the totality paradigm use defined goals and treatment regimens to effect change in their patients, whereas nurses who live and work within the simultaneity paradigm are primarily concerned with escorting patients on a journey of discovery (Parse, 2006).

Growing numbers of nurses use Parse's framework to guide practice. For example, the health action model for partnership in community was devel-oped in the 1990s in the Department of Nursing at Augustana College, Sioux Falls, South Dakota. Based on Parse's theory, the model is the result of col-laboration between academia and community nursing practice. The health action model addresses human connections and disconnections, focusing on the importance of the nurse's presence with under-resourced and low-income individuals (Bunkers, Nelson, Leuning, Crane, & Josephson, 1999). Another example is a parish nursing practice model, the congregational health model, first used in the 1990s by the First Presbyterian Church in Sioux Falls, South Dakota. The congregational health model draws parallels between concepts in human becoming theory and the eight beatitudes found in Christian scripture, emphasizing life in community, nursing/human presence, and respect for the choices of others (Bunkers & Putnam, 1995). Both of these models recognize the transformative impact of the nurse interacting with the community and honor the individual's definition of quality of life (Mitchell, Schmidt Bunkers, & Bournes, 2006).

LEININGER'S THEORY OF CULTURE CARE DIVERSITY AND UNIVERSALITY

Grounded in a philosophy of caring, the theory of culture care diversity and universality draws many of its concepts from the discipline of anthropology.

Madeleine Leininger established the following major principles within her theory, first published in 1985: both similarities and differences can be found within cultures, and it is the job of nursing to discover the culturally universal components of care as well as to discern diverse ways of caring; cultural influences of all kinds have a significant impact on healthcare outcomes; and significant differences and similarities exist between professional care and traditional or folk care, and because these can be the source of problems or benefits, they must be identified. The theory of culture care diversity and universality assumes the essentialness of care for health and growth, and emphasizes that culturally congruent care is necessary for well-being (Leininger, 2006).

ANNE BOYKIN AND SAVINA SCHOENHOFER: NURSING AS CARING
Boykin and Schoenhofer postulated in 1993 that need-based models such as the nursing process do not appropriately address what nurses should be doing. Their grand theory of nursing as caring is based on caring in a way that is specific to each nurse, person, and situation, requiring personal knowing of each patient as well as empirical knowledge. All humans are caring, and each person grows in caring by participating in nurturing relationships. Nursing is a discipline, a response to the social call to help others that requires knowing and developing nursing knowledge. Nursing is also a profession, using nursing knowledge to respond to the human needs that arise from the commitment to help. Nursing is a creative process that evolves moment by moment as part of a caring relationship (Boykin & Schoenhofer, 2006; George, 1995).

Nursing as caring proposes that caring is the central value of nursing. Boykin and Schoenhofer warned that if nursing does not focus on being intentionally caring, the profession will lose its unique meaning and place in health care. The nurse who is committed to caring, knowing, and nurturing other people must intentionally express this care in the face of a healthcare environment filled with dehumanizing technology, depersonalizing routines, requirements for measurable outcomes, and an emphasis on financial profits (Boykin & Schoenhofer, 2006; George, 1995).

Core Themes of Nursing Theory
Cradock (1996) said that it is not knowledge alone that makes nurses advanced practitioners: the critical factor is the way nurses use what they

know. DNPs must bring analysis and critical thinking to bear on a variety of client problems, drawing from a broad base of knowledge in multiple scientific disciplines to synthesize the data and make creative inferences to help the client. We are guided in this complex reasoning process by nursing theories that shape and inform our reflections and provide the foundation for our clinical practice (Kenney, 2006).

Early nursing models, such as those proposed by Henderson and Abdellah, were often based on an empirical, reductionistic philosophy, following traditional cause-and-effect scientific thinking. Nursing theories from the late 20th and early 21st centuries tend to come out of the philosophical framework of systems thinking, holism, and continuous unpredictable change unfolding in dynamic, interactive processes. Modern theorists generally center their models on the human or organizational system interacting with its environment, not on the disease. In these models, nurses come alongside the patient to engage in health-promoting processes and achieve the client's goals, whatever those may be. Regardless of the model chosen for a particular situation, theory-based nursing defines the DNP and is at the heart of advanced nursing practice (Benner & Wrubel, 1989; Kenney, 2006).

References

American Association of Colleges of Nursing. (2006). *The essentials of doctoral education for advanced nursing practice.* Washington, DC: Author.

American Nurses Association. (2001). *Code of ethics for nurses with interpretive statements.* Washington, DC: Author.

Aylward, P. D. (2006). Betty Neuman: The Neuman systems model and global applications. In M. E. Parker (Ed.), *Nursing theories and nursing practice* (2nd ed., pp. 281–294). Philadelphia: F. A. Davis.

Backscheider, J. E. (1974). Self-care requirements, self-care capabilities and nursing systems in the diabetic nurse management clinic. *American Journal of Public Health, 64*(12), 1138–1146.

Barrett, E. A. M. (2002). What is nursing science? *Nursing Science Quarterly, 15*(1), 51–60.

Belcher, J. R., & Fish, L. J. (1995). Hildegard E. Peplau. In J. B. George (Ed.), *Nursing theories: The base for professional nursing practice* (4th ed., pp. 33–48). Norwalk, CT: Appleton & Lange.

Benner, P., & Wrubel, J. (1989). *The primacy of caring.* Menlo Park, CA: Addison-Wesley.

Boykin, A., & Schoenhofer, S. O. (2006). Anne Boykin and Savina O. Schoenhofer's nursing as caring theory. In M. E. Parker (Ed.), *Nursing theories and nursing practice* (2nd ed., pp. 334–348). Philadelphia: F. A. Davis.

Bunkers, S. S. (2002). Nursing science as human science: The new world and human becoming. *Nursing Science Quarterly, 15*(1), 25–30.

Bunkers, S. S., Nelson, M. L., Leuning, C. J., Crane, J. K., & Josephson, D. K. (1999). The health action model: Academia's partnership with the community. In E. L. Cohen & V. DeBack (Eds.), *The outcomes mandate: Case management in health care today* (pp. 92–100). St. Louis, MO: Mosby.

Bunkers, S. S., & Putnam, V. (1995). A nursing theory based model of health ministry: Living Parse's theory of human becoming in the parish community. In *Ninth Annual Westberg Parish Nurse Symposium: Parish nursing: Ministering through the arts.* Northbrook, IL: International Parish Nursing Resource Center–Advocate Health Care.

Burns, N., & Grove, S. (2001). *The practice of nursing research: Conduct, critique, and utilization* (4th ed.). Philadelphia: W. B. Saunders.

Butcher, H. K. (2006). Applications of Rogers' science of unitary human beings. In M. E. Parker (Ed.), *Nursing theories and nursing practice* (2nd ed., pp. 167–186). Philadelphia: F. A. Davis.

Carter, L. C., Nelson, J. L., Sievers, B. A., Dukek, S. L., Pipe, T. B., & Holland, D. E. (2008). Exploring a culture of caring. *Nursing Administration Quarterly, 32*(1), 57–63.

Cradock, S. (1996). The expert nurse: Clinical specialist or advanced practitioner? In G. Rolfe (Ed.), *Closing the theory-practice gap: A new paradigm for nursing.* Oxford, UK: Butterworth-Heinemann.

Crews, J. (1972). Nurse-managed cardiac clinics. *Cardio-Vascular Nursing, 8*(4), 15–18.

Duffy, J. (1992). The impact of nurse caring on patient outcomes. In D. Gaut (Ed.), *The presence of caring in nursing* (pp. 113–136). New York: National League for Nursing.

Duffy, J., & Hoskins, L. (2003). The Quality-Caring Model(c): Blending dual paradigms. *Advances in Nursing Science, 26*(1), 77–88.

Dunphy, L. M. H. (2006). Florence Nightingale's legacy of caring and its applications. In M. E. Parker (Ed.), *Nursing theories and nursing practice* (2nd ed., pp. 39–57). Philadelphia: F. A. Davis.

Engebretson, J. (1997). A multiparadigm approach to nursing. *Advances in Nursing Science, 20*(1), 21–23.

Falco, S. M. (1995). Faye Glenn Abdellah. In J. B. George (Ed.), *Nursing theories: The base for professional nursing practice* (4th ed., pp. 143–158). Norwalk, CT: Appleton & Lange.

Falco, S. M., & Lobo, M. L. (1995). Martha E. Rogers. In J. B. George (Ed.), *Nursing theories: The base for professional nursing practice* (4th ed., pp. 229–248). Norwalk, CT: Appleton & Lange.

Fawcett, J. (1997a). Conceptual models of nursing, nursing theories, and nursing practice: Focus on the future. In M. R. Alligood & A. Marriner-Tomey (Eds.), *Nursing theory: Utilization and application* (pp. 211–221). St. Louis, MO: Mosby.

Fawcett, J. (1997b). The structural hierarchy of nursing knowledge: Components and their definitions. In I. M. King & J. Fawcett (Eds.), *The language of nursing theory and metatheory* (pp. 11–17). Indianapolis, IN: Center Nursing Press.

Fawcett, J. (1999). The state of nursing science: Hallmarks of the 20th and 21st centuries. *Nursing Science Quarterly, 12*(4), 311–315.

Fawcett, J. (2000). *Analysis and evaluation of contemporary nursing knowledge: Nursing models and theories.* Philadelphia: F. A. Davis.

Foster, P. C., & Bennett, A. M. (1995). Dorothea E. Orem. In J. B. George (Ed.), *Nursing theories: The base for professional nursing practice* (4th ed., pp. 99–123). Norwalk, CT: Appleton & Lange.

Furukawa, C. Y., & Howe, J. K. (1995). Virginia Henderson. In J. B. George (Ed.), *Nursing theories: The base for professional nursing practice* (4th ed., pp. 67–85). Norwalk, CT: Appleton & Lange.

Galbreath, J. G. (1995). Callista Roy. In J. B. George (Ed.), *Nursing theories: The base for professional nursing practice* (4th ed., pp. 251–279). Norwalk, CT: Appleton & Lange.

George, J. B. (Ed.) (1995). *Nursing theories: The base for professional nursing practice* (4th ed.). Norwalk, CT: Appleton & Lange.

Gesse, T., Dombro, M., Gordon, S. C., & Rittman, M. R. (2006). Wiedenbach, Henderson, and Orlando's theories and their applications. In M. E. Parker (Ed.), *Nursing theories and nursing practice* (2nd ed., pp. 70–78). Philadelphia: F. A. Davis.

Hamric, A. B., & Reigle, J. (2005). Ethical decision making. In A. B. Hamric, J. A. Spross, & C. M. Hanson (Eds.), *Advanced practice nursing: An integrative approach* (3rd ed.). Philadelphia: W. B. Saunders.

Holaday, B. (2006). Dorothy Johnson's behavioral system model and its applications. In M. E. Parker (Ed.), *Nursing theories and nursing practice* (2nd ed., pp. 79–93). Philadelphia: F. A. Davis.

Isenberg, M. A. (2006). Applications of Dorothea Orem's self-care deficit nursing theory. In M. E. Parker (Ed.), *Nursing theories and nursing practice* (2nd ed., pp. 149–159). Philadelphia: F. A. Davis.

Issel, L., & Kahn, D. (1998). The economic value of caring. *Health Care Management Review, 23*(4), 43–53.

Johnson, D. E. (1961). The significance of nursing care. *American Journal of Nursing, 61*(11), 63–66.

Kenney, J. W. (2006). Theory-based advanced nursing practice. In W. K. Cody (Ed.), *Philosophical and theoretical perspectives for advanced nursing practice* (pp. 295–310). Sudbury, MA: Jones and Bartlett.

Kim, H. S. (1997). Terminology in structuring and developing nursing knowledge. In I. M. King & J. Fawcett (Eds.), *The language of nursing theory and metatheory* (pp. 27–36). Indianapolis, IN: Center Nursing Press.

King, I. M. (1990). *A theory for nursing: Systems, concepts, process.* Albany, NY: Delmar.

King, I. M. (2006). Imogene M. King's theory of goal attainment. In M. E. Parker (Ed.), *Nursing theories and nursing practice* (2nd ed., pp. 235–243). Philadelphia: F. A. Davis.

Kleiman, S. (2006). Josephine Paterson and Loretta Zderad's humanistic nursing theory and its applications. In M. E. Parker (Ed.), *Nursing theories and nursing practice* (2nd ed., pp. 125–137). Philadelphia: F. A. Davis.

Leininger, M. M. (2006). Madeleine M. Leininger's theory of culture care diversity and universality. In M. E. Parker (Ed.), *Nursing theories and nursing practice* (2nd ed., pp. 309–333). Philadelphia: F. A. Davis.

Liners Kersbergen Brett, A. (1992). *Caring attributes the nurse administrator needs to receive in order to facilitate a caring environment.* Unpublished manuscript, University of Wisconsin–Oshkosh, Oshkosh, Wisconsin.

Lobo, M. L. (1995). Florence Nightingale. In J. B. George (Ed.), *Nursing theories: The base for professional nursing practice* (4th ed., pp. 33–48). Norwalk, CT: Appleton & Lange.

Malinski, V. M. (2006). Martha E. Rogers' science of unitary human beings. In M. E. Parker (Ed.), *Nursing theories and nursing practice* (2nd ed., pp. 160–166). Philadelphia: F. A. Davis.

McEwen, M., & Wills, E. M. (2006). *Theoretical basis for nursing* (2nd ed.). Philadelphia: Lippincott Williams & Wilkins.

Meleis, A. I. (1997). *Theoretical nursing: Development and progress* (3rd ed.). Philadelphia: Lippincott.

Mitchell, G. J. (1999). Evidence-based practice: Critique and alternative view. *Nursing Science Quarterly, 12*(1), 30–35.

Mitchell, G. J., Schmidt Bunkers, S., & Bournes, D. (2006). Applications of Parse's human becoming school of thought. In M. E. Parker (Ed.), *Nursing theories and nursing practice* (2nd ed., pp. 194–216). Philadelphia: F. A. Davis.

Monti, E. J., & Tingen, M. S. (1999). Multiple paradigms of nursing science. *Annals of Nursing Science, 21*(4), 64–80.

Nyberg, J. J. (1998). *A caring approach in nursing administration.* Boulder, CO: University Press of Colorado.

Orem, D. E. (2006). Dorothea E. Orem's self-care deficit nursing theory. In M. E. Parker (Ed.), *Nursing theories and nursing practice* (2nd ed., pp. 141–149). Philadelphia: F. A. Davis.

Parker, M. E. (2006). Introduction to nursing theory. In M. E. Parker (Ed.), *Nursing theories and nursing practice* (2nd ed., pp. 3–13). Philadelphia: F. A. Davis.

Parse, R. R. (1997). The language of nursing knowledge: Saying what we mean. In I. M. King & J. Fawcett (Eds.), *The language of nursing theory and metatheory* (pp. 73–77). Indianapolis, IN: Center Nursing Press.

Parse, R. R. (1999). The discipline and the profession. *Nursing Science Quarterly, 12*(4), 275.

Parse, R. R. (2006). Rosemarie Rizzo Parse's human becoming school of thought. In M. E. Parker (Ed.), *Nursing theories and nursing practice* (2nd ed., pp. 187–194). Philadelphia: F. A. Davis.

Peden, A. R. (2006). Hildegard E. Peplau's process of practice-based theory development and its applications. In M. E. Parker (Ed.), *Nursing theories and nursing practice* (2nd ed., pp. 58–69). Philadelphia: F. A. Davis.

Pharris, M. D. (2006). Margaret A. Newman's theory of health as expanding consciousness and its applications. In M. E. Parker (Ed.), *Nursing theories and nursing practice* (2nd ed., pp. 217–234). Philadelphia: F. A. Davis.

Phillips, J. R. (1996). What constitutes nursing science? *Nursing Science Quarterly, 9*(2), 48–49.

Praeger, S. G. (1995). Josephine E. Paterson and Loretta T. Zderad. In J. B. George (Ed.), *Nursing theories: The base for professional nursing practice* (4th ed., pp. 301–315). Norwalk, CT: Appleton & Lange.

Ray, M. A. (1984). The development of a classification system of institutional caring. In M. Leininger (Ed.). *Care: The essence of nursing and health* (pp. 95–112). Thorofare, NJ: Slack.

Ray, M. A. (1989). The theory of bureaucratic caring for nursing practice in the organizational culture. *Nursing Administration Quarterly, 13*(2), 31–42.

Reed, P. (1997). Nursing: The ontology of the discipline. *Nursing Science Quarterly, 10(2),* 76–79.

Rogers, M. E. (1970). *The theoretical basis of nursing*. Philadelphia: F. A. Davis.

Rogers, M. E. (1994). The science of unitary human beings. *Nursing Science Quarterly, 7*(1), 33–35.

Roy, C., & Andrews, H. A. (1991). *The Roy adaptation model: The definitive statement*. Norwalk, CT: Appleton & Lange.

Roy, C., & Zhan, L. (2006). Sister Callista Roy's adaptation model and its applications. In M. E. Parker (Ed.), *Nursing theories and nursing practice* (2nd ed., pp. 268–280). Philadelphia: F. A. Davis.

Schaefer, K. M. (2006). Myra Levin's conservation model and its applications. In M. E. Parker (Ed.), *Nursing theories and nursing practice* (2nd ed., pp. 94–112). Philadelphia: F. A. Davis.

Schumacher, K. L., & Gortner, S. R. (1992). (Mis)conceptions and reconceptions about traditional science. *Annals of Nursing Science, 14*(4), 1–11.

Senge, P. M. (1994). *The fifth discipline: The art and practice of the learning organization*. New York: Doubleday Business.

Sieloff, C. L., Frey, M., & Killeen, M. (2006). Application of King's theory of goal attainment. In M. E. Parker (Ed.), *Nursing theories and nursing practice* (2nd ed., pp. 244–267). Philadelphia: F. A. Davis.

Silva, M. C. (1999). The state of nursing science: Reconceptualizing for the 21st century. *Nursing Science Quarterly, 12*(3), 221–226.

Sitzman, K., & Eichelberger, L. W. (2003). *Understanding the work of nurse theorists: A creative beginning*. Sudbury, MA: Jones and Bartlett.

Smith, M. C. (1994). Beyond the threshold: Nursing practice in the next millennium. *Nursing Science Quarterly, 7*(1), 6–7.

Stevenson, J. S., & Woods, N. F. (1986). Nursing science and contemporary science: Emerging paradigms. In G. E. Sorensen (Ed.), *Setting the agenda for the year 2000: Knowledge development in nursing* (pp. 6–20). Kansas City, MO: American Academy of Nursing.

Talento, B. (1995). Jean Watson. In J. B. George (Ed.), *Nursing theories: The base for professional nursing practice* (4th ed., pp. 317–333). Norwalk, CT: Appleton & Lange.

Touhy, T. A., & Birnbach, N. (2006). Lydia Hall: The care, core, and cure model and its applications. In M. E. Parker (Ed.), *Nursing theories and nursing practice* (2nd ed., pp. 113–124). Philadelphia: F. A. Davis.

Watson, J. (1979). *Nursing: The philosophy and science of caring*. Boston: Little, Brown.

Watson, J. (2006). Jean Watson's theory of human caring. In M. E. Parker (Ed.), *Nursing theories and nursing practice* (2nd ed., pp. 295–302). Philadelphia: F. A. Davis.

Wheatley, M. J. (2006). *Leadership and the new science: Discovering order in a chaotic world* (3rd ed.). San Francisco: Berrett-Koehler.

CHAPTER 2

Systems Thinking, Healthcare Organizations, and the Advanced Practice Nurse Leader

Sandra Petersen

The true professional is a person whose action points beyond his or herself to that underlying reality, that hidden wholeness, on which we all can rely.
— PARKER PALMER

Introduction

Health care's bleak outlook necessitates the rapid evolution of advanced practice nursing to a station of independent practice, autonomy, flexibility, and leadership. As the "powers that be" struggle to make sense of a dwindling budget and an ever-expanding deficit coupled with a clamoring for increased access to care for all, the Institute of Medicine (IOM), The Joint Commission, and other authorities, along with the American Association of Colleges of Nursing (AACN), have called for reconceptualizing health professions education and development to meet the needs of the healthcare delivery system while maintaining quality, safety, and ethical practice. Advanced practice nursing is answering that call by moving to prepare transformational leaders to shape evolving practice and the future of health care.

AACN lends credence to this evolution in the second essential of the Doctor of Nursing Practice (DNP):

> DNP graduates must understand principles of practice management, including conceptual and practical strategies for balancing productivity with quality of care. They must be able to assess the impact of practice policies and procedures on meeting the health needs of the patient populations with whom they practice. DNP graduates must be proficient in quality improvement strategies

and in creating and sustaining changes at the organizational and policy levels. Improvements in practice are neither sustainable nor measurable without corresponding changes in organizational arrangements, organizational and professional culture, and the financial structures to support practice. DNP graduates have the ability to evaluate the cost effectiveness of care and use principles of economics and finance to redesign effective and realistic care delivery strategies. In addition, DNP graduates have the ability to organize care to address emerging practice problems and the ethical dilemmas that emerge as new diagnostic and therapeutic technologies evolve. (AACN, 2006)

The advanced practice nurse must be able to discern issues quickly and effectively and contribute to strategic energy and system redesign. This phenomenon is perhaps best described by Senge (1990) in *The Fifth Discipline* when he conveys the development of the *mental model* as "turning the mirror inward; learning to unearth our internal pictures of the world, to bring them to the surface and hold them rigorously to scrutiny." "Learningful" conversations result in intense scrutiny that balances inquiry and advocacy and allows leaders to expose their own thinking effectively and make that thinking open to the influence of others. In 2003, the IOM further described the necessity of such an approach in declaring the following competencies as foundational: patient-centered care; teamwork and collaboration; evidence-based practice; and quality improvement strategies.

Dossey (2008), in her treatise *The Integral Theory of Nursing*, reiterates:

> Our time demands a new paradigm and a new language where we take the best of what we know in the science and art of nursing that includes holistic and human caring theories and modalities. With an integral approach and worldview we are in a better position to share with others the depth of nurses' knowledge, expertise, and critical-thinking capacities and skills for assisting others in creating health and healing. Only an attention to the heart of nursing, for "sacred" and "heart" reflect a common meaning, can we generate the vision, courage, and hope required to unite nurses and nursing in healing. This assists us as we engage in healthcare reform to address the challenges in these troubled times—local to global. This is not a matter of philosophy, but of survival. (p. 10)

Systems Thinking: Dealing with Complexity and Chaos

The AACN essentials statement (2006) further notes, "Advanced nursing practice includes an organizational and systems leadership component that emphasizes practice, ongoing improvement of health outcomes, and ensuring patient safety. In each case, nurses should be prepared with sophisticated expertise in assessing organizations, identifying systems' issues, and facilitating organization-wide changes in practice delivery. In addition, advanced nursing practice requires political skills, systems thinking, and the business and financial acumen needed for the analysis of practice quality and costs."

In his 2002 book *The Ingenuity Gap: Can We Solve the Problems of the Future?* Homer-Dixon presented evidence that the demand for ingenuity arising from the ever-increasing complexity of our world is far outstripping our capacity to supply it. Although in the past we have been able to find solutions—and, in Homer-Dixon's words, "throw huge amounts of energy at our problems"—to keep our ever-expanding complex systems glued together, in the future we will as a result almost certainly find it necessary to accept some large breakdowns in human and natural systems and to develop radical new ways of running things. Homer-Dixon adds, "There are a couple of areas where I sometimes despair about our capacity to deal with what lies ahead. One is our cognitive characteristics and the other is the self-reinforcing nature of our economic system." When Homer-Dixon refers to "cognitive characteristics," he underscores the fact that societies adapt easily to small-scale, incremental change. It is this slow evolution that makes it possible for humanity to face each day and not feel as though our foundations have been shaken. It is part of self-preservation. And yet, Homer-Dixon says, this human capacity is "a real handicap when it comes to dealing with 'slow-creep' problems. We just don't see the change, and the thing about slow-creep problems is they may be slow-creep for a while, but then all of a sudden there's a non-linear shift and we find ourselves in a crisis." How well this describes our current crisis in health care and the need for advanced practice nurses to be well versed in systems thinking and steeped in competency with regard to essential core skills!

Vision and Perspective: Keys to the Future of Advanced Practice

The evolution of the DNP advanced practice role as that of strategic systems thinker and visionary for health care lies largely within the profession's commitment to lifelong learning and the realization that people and organizations do not exist as islands unto themselves, but rather as part of a larger network, web, or matrix of systems that all function more or less independently, yet *inter*dependently. Burns's transformational theory (1978) describes this matrix as a melding of social and spiritual values. He recognized it as a motivational lever that gives people an uplifting sense of being connected to a higher purpose, thus playing to the need for a sense of meaning and identity. Ultimately, one must realize the necessity of developing a dedication to disrupting the system as we know it, while at the same time retaining flexibility, balance, and a sense of social intelligence and responsibility.

Broadly, as we examine the healthcare landscape over the past two decades, common themes emerge. In general, the concern about dwindling access to health care—often linked to cost—that commanded much of the literature around the turn of the century has most recently been eclipsed by a general sense of alarm (perhaps panic) about the rising cost of health care. These observations may have been influenced by rising health insurance rates, the increasing healthcare needs of baby boomers reaching retirement, and by the release of a series of long-range healthcare cost projections. At one extreme are those who hotly contend that Americans have the "best health care system in the world," pointing to the freely available medical technology and state-of-the-art facilities that have become symbolic of the system. At the other extreme, however, are those who strongly criticize the American system as being fragmented and inefficient, pointing to the fact that America spends more on health care than any other country in the world, yet our nation still suffers from rampant lack of insurance, inconsistency in quality, and excessive administrative waste (Casoy, 2008).

The Employee Benefits Research Institute (2005) reported that the erosion of employer-based coverage was offset by increased enrollment in Medicaid, which was initially designed to provide a safety net for the lowest-income Americans. However, as the *Washington Post* noted in late 2008, Medicaid has been the subject of relentless funding cuts by budget-strapped states and Congressional representatives who are ideologically opposed to welfare programs. As the program continues to be slashed, it is certain that Medicaid or other state-funded programs will not be able to offset the losses in employer-based insurance, resulting in more and more uninsured individuals. This brings the insecurity of health care to an all-time high as thousands of people lose their health insurance every day as a result of a sagging job market. Health care is becoming elusive even for affluent Americans. Because any employee is just one pink slip away from becoming uninsured, it becomes clear that some solution in health care is not just important to achieve, but imperative.

Given the recent unrest, it is tempting to believe the notion that the current design of the healthcare system is beyond repair. Yet, a look back reveals the countless metamorphoses of an externally different yet eternally fundamentally flawed entity. Thus, transformational DNPs can drive the avoidance of this abysmal cycle through full dissection and understanding of the underlying structure and root cause(s) of the dysfunction. Is it acceptable to deny people health care based on their ability to pay? Is health care a basic need that should be provided to every American as a matter of course? Or does the solution lie somewhere between the two extremes? Regardless of the answer, we must ensure that the DNP is well armed to overcome the remarkably complex inertia of the American healthcare system and spearhead the effort to create a society in which health care is, at a minimum, cost-effective, of reasonable quality, and readily accessible.

The Advanced Practice Path to Healthcare Solutions

Many of the healthcare problems that plague us today are complex, involving multiple factors that are at least partly the result of past actions taken to alleviate problems. Traditional approaches often attack single factors or problems with little regard to the impact on the whole. Dealing with such problems is notoriously difficult, and the results of conventional solutions are frequently poor enough to create great discouragement about the prospects of ever effectively addressing them. One of the key benefits of the application of systems thinking to such massive, complex concerns is the ability to deal effectively with a variety of problems from a holistic viewpoint. The systems approach helps us raise our thinking to the level at which we create the results we want as individuals and organizations, even in those difficult situations marked by complexity, great numbers of interactions, and the absence or ineffectiveness of immediately apparent solutions (Bass, 1990).

In his book *The Fifth Discipline,* Senge (1990) described the process of systems thinking as "seeing the world anew." He notes, "There is something in all of us that loves to put together a puzzle, that loves to see the image of the whole emerge. The beauty of a person, or a flower, or a poem lies in seeing all of it. It is interesting that the words "whole" and "health" come from the same root as the Old English *hal,* as in 'hale and hearty.' So, it should come as no surprise that the unhealthiness of our world today is in direct proportion to our inability to see it as a whole" (pp. 42–43).

In considering the fragmented state of national health care, the astute DNP can readily see that systems thinking can likely be employed as the much-needed framework for seeing the diversity (and fragmentation) as a "whole." A systems approach provides the framework for seeing interrelationships and patterns of change rather than individual issues. The approach uses a focused sensitivity to the interconnectedness that gives social systems of extreme complexity their unique character.

Systems Thinking and Advanced Practice

Systems thinking has its roots in the field of system dynamics, honed most successfully in 1958 by MIT professor Jay Forrester, who acknowledged the need for a better way of testing new ideas in complex engineering problems and, additionally, realized its value in addressing issues within social systems, such as the provision of health care. Systems thinking allows people to gain an explicit understanding of social systems and improve them in the same way that people can use engineering principles to make explicit and improve their understanding of mechanical systems. Complexity can easily undermine responsibility and creativity and result in feelings of helplessness and hopelessness. To combat this, systems thinking across organizations offers a discipline for understanding the unique structures that undergird complex systems and, through that understanding, a way to effect change that is significant and enduring.

Schyve (2000) notes that systems thinking has already become ubiquitous in health care, largely due to continuous quality improvement initiatives in patient safety. Even ten years ago, the idea of "looking at the whole" (the process) with regard to medical errors, rather than at the individual, might not have been acceptable. The advent of "blameless" cultures within this context provides a much less threatening venue than the former reliance on accusations of error. It is this systems thinking that has enabled many in health care to traverse beyond the old (and extremely ineffective) "name, blame, and shame" approach to patient safety to a more effective focus on human factors engineering and the systems within which doctors, nurses, pharmacists, and other healthcare professionals function. If systems thinking can successfully be applied to this one critical aspect of patient safety, could not the transformational advanced practice nurse leader consider an application of this strategy to the whole?

ADOPTING A SYSTEMS PERSPECTIVE

Transformational leadership in advanced practice roles involves a willingness to take reasonable risks based on empirical data, a commitment to action, reflection of core values, and a drive for excellence at all levels. As leaders seek to hone their skills in their enthusiasm for creating the future, systems thinking must be an integral part of problem solving. Bass (1990) notes that more charismatic transformational leaders may achieve this alignment with systems thinking through evoking strong emotions that result in the identification of followers with the leader, perhaps through stirring appeals. Others may achieve the same result through quieter methods such as coaching and mentoring.

Nevertheless, the approach to any complex situation must begin with the deep insight that the problems and the hopes for improvement are inextricably tied to how the problem solvers think. Learning about a problem of great complexity requires a conceptual framework of "structural" or systems thinking to facilitate the ability to discover the underlying structural causes of poor performance (Wheatley, 2002). Lyman and Chermack (2006), in their theory of responsible leadership for performance (RLP), suggest a general, integrative theoretical framework of leadership that addresses the nature and challenges of leadership that is both responsible and focused on performance. Two core premises govern the framework. The first is that leadership is itself a system consisting of purposeful, integrated inputs, processes, outputs, feedback, and boundaries. The second is that leadership takes place within a performance system, that is, a system of joint, coordinated, and purposeful action. Leadership can therefore be conceived of as a system of interacting inputs, processes, outputs, and feedback that derives meaning, direction, and purpose from the larger performance system and environment within which it occurs. From this perspective, leadership is defined as a focused system of interacting inputs, process, outputs, and feedback wherein individuals or groups influence or act on behalf of specific individuals or groups of individuals to achieve shared goals and commonly desired performance outcomes, within a specific performance system and environment.

As leaders come to understand the structures within systems that cause patterns of behaviors or patterns within relationships that result in problems (inputs), they see more clearly how to effect change and adopt mechanisms that will work successfully on a larger scale (outputs). Ouchi's (1981) "Theory Z" (sometimes called participative theory or "Japanese management") also speaks of an organizational performance-driven culture that mirrors the Japanese culture, in which workers are participative and capable of performing many and varied tasks. Theory Z emphasizes things such as broadening of skills, generalization versus specialization, and the need for continuous training of workers to address this need for redesign. Redesigning the way one addresses decisions or behaviors (throughputs) through careful analysis of as many problem patterns as possible on a small scale inherently leads to redesign of the larger system structure. Then, and only then, can consumers of the system provide feedback to validate the effectiveness of the changes.

The Essence of Problem Solving

Senge (1990) noted that there are multiple levels of explanation in any complex situation. These include reactive, responsive, and generative explanations. As leaders begin to look for patterns within relationships, it is critical that these investigations remain focused on structure and patterns rather than on specific events.

Event explanations "lay blame" or result in a *reactive* stance to problems. To further explore this concept, let's take the example of the patient who has a fall. A reactive stance might be to immediately restrain the patient in response to that event. We assume in this instance that because the patient could move and has fallen, we must keep him from moving in the future. As one can quickly see, the reactive stance leaves no room for discussions about why the fall occurred or what could be done to improve the patient's fall risk, if one even exists. There are no discussions regarding quality of life for the patient, and, certainly, there are no explorations of root cause or how falls might affect other patients. This type of explanation is tied to a single event and is the most likely type to reinforce the flaws within a reactive system, maintaining the status quo. Little room is left for problem solving or quality improvement.

Approaching this same scenario from a *responsive* stance, we might look at patterns of behavior, asking whether the patient had incurred falls in the past. If he had multiple falls, at what times did the falls occur? We might also look at fall risk and prevention for this patient and, ultimately, for other patients within the system, tracking and trending in response. The responsive approach focuses on explaining patterns of behavior and envisioning long-term results and trends that can benefit the larger system. The responsive approach allows for quality improvement in response to data gathered through tracking and trending within a system, thus breaking the hold of reactivity and the "short-term fix."

Generative explanation, the most powerful of the three, focuses on finding the root cause(s) for patterns of behavior. In the case of the falling patient, for example, we might look at the types of situations in which the falls occur. We could ask, "Under what circumstances did the falls occur?" We could consider falls occurring during transfers; perhaps staff are not using appropriate transfer techniques or appropriate equipment. Perhaps there are critical steps missing from transfer procedures that result in the failure of the process. It is at this level of explanation that patterns of behavior can be changed—not just reacted to or responded to, but actually *changed*.

Ultimately, the systems perspective tells advanced practice leaders that we must look beyond individual mistakes, karma, or unrelenting bad luck to understand important issues. We must also look beyond personalities, politics, and events to observe and explain the structures that result in individual actions and use this knowledge to discern processes whereby certain types of events become more likely. Senge (1990) quotes Donella Meadows, who said: "A truly profound and different insight is the way you begin to see that the system causes its own behavior" (p. 68).

Systems Thinking, Advanced Practice, and the Learning Organization

"Experience is the best teacher" is a phrase that has been a mantra within the healthcare environment for many years. "See one, do one, teach one" has long been a part of nursing and medical education. We learn through taking an action and observing the consequences of that action; then we adjust and take a new and different action. Thus, learning is woven throughout the fabric of life and, indeed, throughout complex healthcare organizations—at least the ones that are successful. Lack of learning within an organization often results in its demise or in very poor performance.

In a large, complex organization, however, the primary consequences of our actions may well be in the distant future or in a distant, but interrelated, part of a larger system in which we operate. For this reason, we are often puzzled by the underlying causes of current problems within our organizations. We are unable to look at underlying structures or patterns of behavior that may have resulted in less than stellar outcomes. Instead, we are very likely to fixate on events and on "working harder" to try to resolve or troubleshoot current issues.

Early in 1992, Jeanie Duck of the Boston Consulting Group wrote about the "reductionist" approach to managing an organization and ferreting out issues. The reductionist management model has long been popular in the United States as a means of explaining and quickly addressing issues. Duck noted that the premise of reductionism is that to understand something, you reduce it to its simplest components and analyze the components in great detail. At the outset, the reductionist approach makes complex tasks (or problems) more manageable. However, the disadvantage to this approach is that the organization is no longer able to see the consequences of actions or decisions, and the connection to the larger system is lost. Learning organizations must successfully abandon reductionism. Once that occurs, leaders and employees within the organization can then continually expand their capacity to create results. New and expansive patterns of thinking that foster interconnectedness within the organization are encouraged.

As the role of nursing leadership continues to expand, the advanced practice leader will no doubt be called upon to foster the development of learning organizations and to function as a change agent to facilitate organizational functioning within larger complex systems. Adopting a sustained culture of learning enables an organization to maintain a competitive advantage in times of change and to inspire its workforce to achieve greater results and improved quality. Furthermore, organizations can draw on a learning culture to encourage innovation or manage change.

David Garvin, of Harvard Business School and QualityGurus.com fame, defines a learning organization as an organization "skilled at creating, acquiring, and transferring knowledge, and at modifying its behavior to reflect new knowledge and insights" (Garvin & Gray, 2009). This is best accomplished by first assessing the organization's culture, leadership, and tolerance for change. The organization must be open to developing a conceptual framework for systems thinking and a shared vision to make patterns clearer and effectively initiate change.

Advanced practice leaders have the responsibility for instilling the ideas of personal mastery in all employees as a basis for shared vision and connection throughout the organization. As a basis for change, personal mastery (Senge, 1990) is the discipline of continually clarifying and deepening one's personal vision, of focusing one's energies, of developing patience, and of seeing reality objectively and letting go of mental models (ingrained ideas) from the past. An organization's commitment to and capacity for learning can be no greater than that of its employees. The roots of this idea are detailed in both Eastern and Western spiritual traditions, as well as in some secular traditions. More and more healthcare organizations are tapping into this idea as healthcare entities around the country are now developing leadership residencies aimed at personal leadership growth as a valuable resource within the organization. The learning organization grows and changes as its people learn and develop personal mastery. Thus, becoming a learning organization can be viewed as a continual process involving employees at all levels.

As organizations focus on personal mastery for employees, the organization progresses to team learning and a free flow of information and ideas that eventually, if carefully guided, leads to a shared vision for the organization and, ultimately, a more effective organization. James P. Lewis (2001) noted the impact of team learning and the shared vision in his book *Project Planning, Scheduling and Control*. He cited the example of a non–learning organization that decided to implement an electronic charting system based on executive input only. Final decisions were based upon the huge financial outlay already made, choice of product, and scope of implementation. Contract negotiations were completed at a high level without the involvement of clinicians. Not involving those on the front line (clinicians) in the early stages cost the organization financially and functionally when the unwieldy system caused patient care to be more difficult than before the implementation.

Senge (1990) notes, "To practice a discipline is to be a lifelong learner. You 'never arrive'; you spend your life mastering disciplines. You can never say, 'We are a learning organization,' any more than you can say, 'I am an enlightened person.' The more you learn, the more acutely aware you become of your ignorance" (p. 43). A learning organization is one that constantly provides its employees timely access to relevant, practical information that inspires innovation. It involves creating a culture in which learning is embedded and in which it is communicated to and understood by all that there are many places to seek information. As Margaret Wheatley (1992) expounded, "Innovation is fostered by information gathered from new connections; from insights gained by journeys into other disciplines or places; from active, collegial networks and fluid, open boundaries. Innovation arises from ongoing circles of exchange, where information is not just accumulated or stored, but created. Knowledge is generated anew from connections that weren't there before" (p. 113).

The Downside to Systems Thinking

Systems thinking has a proven track record as a means of addressing problems within complex systems and has been successfully applied in healthcare venues. However, the principles of systems thinking are not typically conveyed in basic healthcare education. Although the DNP competencies clearly proclaim these principles as essential, nurses at the undergraduate level are generally educated in the personal mastery of knowledge, skills, and abilities to provide assistance to sick, often frail and vulnerable, individuals or populations. The individual ethical creed to "do no harm" pertains primarily to the nurse as an individual assisting individuals, not to systems and processes.

Given this perspective, a systems thinking approach to healthcare reform presents challenges for the advanced practice leader. The general understanding is that a system is perfectly designed to produce what it produces; or, conversely, whatever we get from a system is what the system is designed to produce, whether the design of the system was planned or unplanned, and whether the results were intended or unintended. Different individuals within the same structure tend to produce similar results. Therefore, when performance is poor or expectations unmet, it is relatively easy to find someone or something to blame. The paradigm shift of interrelationships and interrelatedness reinforces the fact that systems may cause their own crises. Such crises are not the fault of individuals nor the result of external factors but inherent within the system or processes that fall short.

According to Lyman and Chermack (2006), systems are composed of many related components: people, equipment, processes, and data. Each component directly or indirectly has the potential to affect not only the function of the system, but also the functions of other components within the system. Traditional nursing leaders tend to consider structure as an external constraint based on the performance of individual components; however, in human systems, it is the basic *interrelationships* among components, not structural constraint, that control behaviors. As a result, the purpose of a system then becomes to maximize the output of the system, not the output of each of its components. The silos of leadership that exist throughout health care generally focus only on their own decisions and may ignore how their decisions affect others, creating instability within the system as a result. Senge (1990) illustrated this concept in the example of the engineer who noted that one could build a car from the then "best" engine, drive train, suspension, and tires, but it would be unlikely to run. Every system, including those in health care, must *optimize*—rather than *maximize*—the performance of each of its components in order to maximize the system's production.

As noted in the IOM competencies, the production (output) of a healthcare system has multiple dimensions. The dimensions of safety, effectiveness, patient centeredness, timeliness, efficiency, and equity are often used to describe the output of the system (IOM, 2003). It is uncommon for the system to *maximize* the level of each of the multiple dimensions of its output; rather, the system must *optimize* the level of each dimension. This optimization, however, is a value judgment by those who design and manage the system, and, to some degree, those who use the output of the system. These stakeholders in the healthcare system do not always agree on the relative priorities for the dimensions of the system's output, thus presenting a problem, but also an opportunity for compromise that must be recognized by the astute leader.

Multifaceted, multilayered healthcare systems are all at significant risk of producing unintended consequences. Even apparently "inconsequential" changes in healthcare systems at any level will almost always produce unintended consequences. It is predictable that unintended consequences will likely emerge, but what those consequences will be, and whether they will be beneficial or destructive, is often unpredictable. At worst, well-intentioned changes could result in unintended harm. Margaret Wheatley (1992) espoused an interesting perspective on unintended consequences, seeing them as unintended opportunities to find new ways of looking at things and to redesign poor processes. In her book *Turning to One Another: Simple Conversations to Restore Hope to the Future*, written in 2002, Wheatley notes that failures within organizations are the signal that more connections need to be made within the organization; she contends that the solution lies within untapped conversations and undiscovered connections.

A Challenge to Advanced Practice Leaders: Operationalizing Systems Thinking

The evolution of the advanced practice leader is the by-product of concerted effort to align personal behavior with values and to learn how to listen and to appreciate others' talents, abilities, and insights. Without this diligent effort dedicated to the development of the capacity to lead, a lack of personal charisma, personal mastery, information sharing, and mental mastery would render us ineffective in the pursuit of the shared vision and the transformational leadership so vital to the survival of health care in the future (Ouichi, 1981).

Once personal mastery is achieved, however, one must transcend the traditional activity of management as most of us know it and focus on wielding power within a system. This endeavor not only encompasses the balancing of structures within an organization or system, but also the embodiment of shared vision and empowerment, while inducing people and resources to migrate from the current state to the desired state while seeking their own personal mastery (Senge, 2006). Although this sounds very noble, the reality is that, as the current state approaches the desired state, promotion of the activity and motivation typically decline; this goes on until someone takes notice and raises the red flag of organizational panic and urges reactive decision making (which rarely produces good results). Therefore, the task of the leader becomes sustaining the effort long enough to close the gap between what *was* and the present while avoiding panic, reactivity, and, ultimately, disaster.

The Learning Organization and the Inquiring Mind: Sustaining the Effort

In *The Fifth Discipline*, Peter Senge (1990) describes five basic disciplines that support shared vision and empowerment, but places systems thinking in the primary position. He calls it "the fifth discipline" because it is the conceptual cornerstone that underlies all of the other learning disciplines. As he points out, all are concerned with a shift of mind from seeing parts to seeing wholes, from seeing people as helpless reactors to seeing them as active participants in shaping their reality, from reacting to the present to creating the future.

When it comes to operationalizing and applying systems thinking concepts within the learning organization or across many organizations, C. West Churchman (1913–2004), a pragmatic philosopher with a deep concern for the welfare of humanity, laid the groundwork for the most practical approach to creatively shaping the future. In the 1950s he worked with R. L. Ackoff and E. L. Arnoff to develop and describe the philosophical and methodological aspects of operations research, designed as an interdisciplinary approach to "real-world problem solving" (Ulrich, 2004, p. 6).

Early in 1971, Churchman adapted the design of what he called "inquiring systems"—systems capable of facilitating learning and organizational change.

The purpose of these inquiring systems is to create knowledge, thereby "creating the capability of choosing the right means for one's desired ends" (Churchman, 1971, p. 200). Churchman's model for the design of inquiring systems provides the basis for sustaining evolving organizations. Churchman's theoretical work was driven by his unrelenting interest in determining whether it is "possible to secure improvement in the human condition by means of the human intellect" (Ulrich, 2004, p. 7). One of his significant contributions to the development of systems theory was his recognition that "problem solving often appears to produce improvement, but the so-called 'solution' often makes matters worse in the larger system" (Churchman, 1982, p. 19n). He argued that "simple, direct, head-on attempts to 'solve' system problems don't work and, indeed, often turn out to be downright dangerous" (Churchman, 1979, p. 4). No problem exists in isolation; rather, problems are inextricably linked to each other and to the environment, thus requiring an approach to the whole.

UNDERLYING CONCEPTS OF CHURCHMAN'S SYSTEMS MODEL

Churchman's inquiry systems model is centered on the *client* as the "complex of persons whose interests ought to be served" (Churchman, 1971, p. 48). Clients can be described by their value structure. Each client has a set of possible futures (i.e., goals or objectives) and a preference for one future over others. Clients have trade-off principles that reveal how much of one objective they would relinquish in order to achieve or increase another objective, establishing a means of "balancing" a given system.

Within Churchman's model, the *environment* is limitless. It consists of all things outside the system that may, in some direct, indirect, or even barely comprehensible way, affect—or be affected by—what happens within the system. Also within the model, a *decision maker* controls system resources. He or she "*co-produces* the future along with the environment, which he [or she] does not control" (Churchman, 1971, p. 47). The decision maker's preferred future may not be identical to that of other stakeholders (clients), and his or her trade-off principle may not be the same.

The system *planner* is the person who should at all times strive toward improvement in the human condition. Churchman (1971, 1979) envisions a planner who seeks to identify the client's underlying principles and trade-off principles, to create measures of performance based on those principles, and to trace out all potential consequences of any given action. The planner's intentions are presumed to be "always good with respect to the client"

(Churchman, 1971, p. 47), and the planner assumes the role of trying to ensure that the decision makers' value structure also supports those of the client.

The *measure of performance* is, in simple form, the degree of attainment of a stated goal, purpose, or objective, sometimes measured by the probability or amount of attainment and sometimes by evaluating benefits and costs (Churchman, 1979).

Agents and factors both within and without the system may be said to *co-produce* the measures of performance. By their influence, co-producers may either assist to actualize or prevent the achievement of the client's objectives. Following the work of Edgar A. Singer, Churchman states that "[s]omething is a producer of an event if at least one description of the event would be different were the producer not there" (1979, p. 87). Churchman goes on to note that "in the case of organizational decision making, the co-producers are many but often operate in subtle and non-formalized manners." Indeed, "part of an organization's 'unconscious' is the existence of co-producers who block the implementation of 'good' ideas, but are never mentioned" (Churchman, 1979, p. 87).

The aforementioned roles belie Churchman's dedication to creating learning systems within organizations. Foremost in these systems is the recognition that decision makers must be as open-minded and creative as possible, so that their problem-identifications and proposed solutions reflect not merely the concerns of interest to the decision makers, but also the implications of the problem and its solutions for the whole system—indeed, for the environment itself (Ulrich, 2004).

To create a learning system, leaders, acting as planners, must move away from focusing on the obvious (e.g., data, hard facts). For planners who focus on the obvious—*goal planners*— "reality stops at the boundaries of the problem" (Churchman, 1979, p. 108). In contrast, *objective planners* attempt to reframe the obvious within the context of a larger problem. For the objective planner, "reality stops at the boundaries set by feasibility and to some extent by responsibility" (Churchman, 1979, p. 106). Although this larger perspective moves the system in the direction of learning, Churchman ponders another level: *ideal planning*. Whereas goals are deemed short term and objectives long term, ideals are considered to stretch indefinitely into the future and to approach the essential question of how to improve the human condition. The ideal planner moves past the feasible and the realistic and attempts to define purposes that could hold if these restraints were removed. In the ideal system, planners and decision makers work not with the obvious and the tangible, but with limitless imagination (Churchman, 1979).

Because the bounds of creativity can never fully be known, Churchman's model (1979) for inquiring systems is one constructed not of answers, but of many questions. Inquiry—and its corollary, decision making—is conducted in a learning system through a process of unfolding questions. As each new aspect of the environment is considered, more layers of influence (co-production) or impact are discovered and must be addressed in turn. Churchman lays out a dialectical framework within which the questions are posed, stakeholders' interests are considered, the environment is limitless, and the ethics are those of the whole system. The inquiry model begins with the questions in Table 2-1 and can be readily applied in problem solving (Churchman, 1979, pp. 79–80).

Within any human service organization dedicated to benevolent purposes, the DNP leader can readily see how Churchman's model could be used to provide organizational assessment and a blueprint for a holistic systems approach to problem solving. The complexities of healthcare issues lend themselves to the use of Churchman's design of inquiring systems and provide the transformational leader with a solid, methodical approach that promotes engagement by all parts of the organization.

If we consider the example of an organization providing primary family care, the construction of a simple spreadsheet could readily identify key stakeholders whose purposes and counterpurposes the organization must consider in addressing problems. The spreadsheet might list each stakeholder as a *client* with particular needs and objectives—purposes—relating to optimal health care. For example, geriatric clients served by the practice might be identified as having several purposes, including a desire for fulfilling quality of life, for the attention of a cost-effective skilled medical provider, and for the cost-effective provision of medication. In Churchman's model, client purposes are both those things the client desires (e.g., fulfilling quality of life) and those things the client *should* have (e.g., safe, cost-effective care and medications).

Continuing with the example, a stakeholder may be represented by more than one client category. Young adult clients of the primary care practice, for example, may have purposes both as "parents"—concerned about their children's health—and as "patrons" who may themselves access

■ **Table 2-1   Churchman's Problem-Solving Model**

The Client
- What is his or her purpose(s)?
- What should be his or her purpose(s)?
- How is the variety of his or her purposes unified under a measure of performance?
- How should the variety of his or her purposes be unified under a measure of performance?

The Decision Maker
- What is the decision maker able to use as resources?
- What should the decision maker be able to use as resources?
- What can the decision maker not control, which nonetheless matters—the environment?
- What should the decision maker not control, which nonetheless matters—the environment?

The Planner
- How is the planner able to implement his or her plans?
- How should the planner be able to implement his or her plans?
- [Ideally] What is the guarantor that his or her planning will succeed, that is, will secure improvement in the human condition?
- [Ideally] What should be the guarantor that his or her planning will succeed, that is, will secure improvement in the human condition?

Source: Churchman, C. W. (1979). *The Design of Inquiring Systems.* New York: Basic Books (pp. 79–80).

the healthcare system. In addition, every stakeholder has the potential to act as a *co-producer* of the solution to the problem posed. They may do so by assisting the decision maker or by placing obstacles in the decision maker's path. It is important to note that the decision makers are also clients, in that they too have purposes to be served.

MAXIMIZING THE EFFORTS OF INQUIRY

As one completes the inquiry just described, it becomes easier to observe patterns within the desires and needs of clients at all levels of the system. These patterns become the basis for the understanding of the overall system; leaders, as a result, can then target innovation (change) efforts more effectively. This is where the approach of systems thinking is fundamentally different from that of traditional methods of analysis. Instead of isolating smaller parts of a system (e.g., individual clients), systems thinking looks at the whole, considering larger numbers (patterns) of interactions to gain understanding.

If we continue our consideration of the primary care clinic described earlier, we might, for instance, through traditional analysis, make a change in practice that would benefit one group of clients but work to the detriment of another. Let's say that we decide to see all pediatric sick cases in the morning to accommodate working mothers and move geriatric chronic cases to the afternoon. We find, however, in examining feedback from the geriatric clients, that they are only able to get public transportation to appointments in the morning, with the latest senior bus picking up at 11:30 A.M. If the senior clients catch the earlier buses to make an afternoon appointment, they have a long wait time *and* they are exposed to the sick children. Over time, if we continued with this plan (sans the feedback), we would see that the benefits of this innovation would begin to quickly evaporate and our organization and patients would suffer.

Avoiding this global failure is a key advantage of systems thinking. By closely examining all the interactions created by a decision, potential backfires within the system can be detected and, it is hoped, avoided (see Figure 2-1). In the example case, a compromise of selected days for pediatric morning appointments might achieve a balance of the needs of all patients accessing the system. Examination of feedback leads to innovation that is a better fit for the big picture and to results that create substantial, lasting benefits.

The arrows in a causal loop diagram are usually labeled with an "S" or an "O." "S" means that when the first variable changes, the second one changes in the same direction (for example, as you schedule more pediatric appointments in the mornings, the number of moms desiring to make these appointments goes up too). "O" means that the first variable causes a change in the opposite direction in the second variable (for example, the more pediatric appointments scheduled in the morning, the fewer geriatric appointments occur in the afternoon because of exposure to sick children and long wait times for transportation).

In causal diagrams, the arrows join to form loops, with each loop labeled with an "R" or a "B." "R" means reinforcing and refers to causal relationships within the loop creating exponential growth or collapse. (For instance, the more appointments made in the morning, the happier working moms become; because the moms are happier, they tell their friends, and more and more pediatric appointments are made, and so on, in an upward spiral). By the same

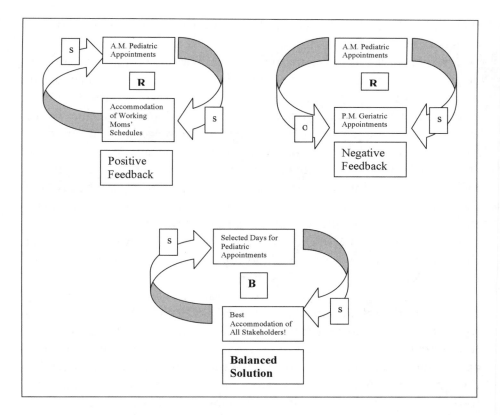

■ Figure 2-1   Feedback, Causal Loop Diagrams, and Business Decisions

Causal loop diagrams provide a unique systems thinking tool that can be helpful in avoiding system backfires by using arrows to connect variables (things or situations that change over time) in a way that shows how one variable affects another. This figure shows some examples of how the family clinic might use feedback loops to examine process.

token, as more pediatric appointments are made, fewer geriatric appointments are made overall. Pediatric patients are taking up the morning slots, so there are few morning appointments available for older patients. The geriatric patients don't like the afternoon slots because of long transportation wait times and exposure to sick children. This could cause a downward spiral in the business and a dire decrease in revenue for the practice. The "B" means balancing and refers to factors in the loop that could keep things in equilibrium. (For example, if only selected mornings—one or two per week—are reserved for pediatric patients with working moms, geriatric patients can continue to be accommodated at times they prefer.) The result is a sustainable process that would be supported by both groups of patients (stakeholders).

Causal loop diagrams can be very complex and contain many different "R" and "B" loops, all connected with arrows. The use of these diagrams can offer leaders and their teams valuable perspectives on what is happening within an organization. This type of systems thinking helps avoid reactive decisions and explores the possibilities of negative outcomes for the business before they happen. For example, by understanding the relationship between morning pediatric appointments and the exposure of frail elderly clients to long wait times, a poor business decision can be avoided.

Summary: The DNP Systems Thinker

Advanced practice leadership must acknowledge the healthcare system as an open system, affected by and, to some degree, dependent upon larger systems of which it is a part. We have learned the value of studying and changing the microsystems of health care—the people, equipment, and data at the level of direct patient care. But these microsystems are subsystems within macrosystems such as hospitals, nursing homes, and clinics. These macrosystems, in turn, are part of the megasystem of American health care, which itself is a component of the even larger economic, political, and social metasystems of society as a whole and, ultimately, a part of global systems.

Employing a systems approach to seeking solutions in health care will ultimately alter the role of the various disciplines within health care. This reconsideration of roles will become the purview of advanced practice leaders at all levels. These advanced systems thinkers will ultimately lead the way as we seek to begin the inquiries expressed by the following questions: What are the human vulnerabilities with respect to our capacity to keep up with new knowledge, to remember, or to analyze large amounts of data? How might the principles of distributed cognition (interaction and feedback) and information-sharing technology protect us from these vulnerabilities? How might system redesign as a result of a shared vision protect us from making fatal design errors? What are the human vulnerabilities with respect to our thinking, emotions, and actions?

The challenges ahead require that the advanced practice leader be well prepared in the application of systems thinking to the healthcare environment. Through careful analysis of the structure of both microsystems and macrosystems, how their performance is best measured, and how they interrelate, one can make a determination of their vulnerabilities and strengths within the context of a structural explanation. Detection of behavioral patterns in underlying structure may assist in optimizing system components to maximize results of the system. Systems thinking may further provide the tools for identifying and monitoring for unintended consequences and illuminate the possible interventions to prevent harm from such consequences.

References

American Association of Colleges of Nursing. (2006). *The essentials of doctoral education for advanced nursing practice.* Retrieved from http://www.aacn.nche.edu/DNP/pdf/Essentials.pdf

Bass, B. (1990). *Bass and Stogdill's handbook of leadership: Theory, research, and managerial applications* (3rd ed.). New York: Free Press.

Burns, J. M. (1978). *Leadership.* New York: Harper & Row.

Casoy, F. (2008). The case of universal healthcare. Written statement for the American Medical Student Association. *The Washington Post,* December 26, 2008. Retrieved from www.residentandstaff.com/press_release.asp?id=10165122

Churchman, C. W. (1971, 1979, 1982). *The design of inquiring systems: Basic Concept of Systems and Organizations.* New York: Basic Books.

Dossey, B. M. (2008). Integral and holistic nursing: Local to global. In B. M. Dossey & L. Keegan (Eds.), *Holistic Nursing: A Handbook for Practice* (5th ed.). Sudbury, MA: Jones and Bartlett.

Duck, J. (1992). *The seduction of reductionist thinking.* Boston: The Boston Consulting Group.

Employee Benefits Research Institute. (2005). Uninsured unchanged in 2004, but employment-based health coverage declined. *EBRI Notes, 25*(5). Retrieved from www.ebri.org.

Forrester, J. (1958). Industrial dynamics: A major breakthrough for decision makers. *Harvard Business Review, 36*(4), 37–66.

Garvin, D., & Gary, L. (2009). What makes for an authentic learning organization: An interview with David Garvin. Retrieved from http://harvardbusiness.org/product/what-makes-for-an-authentic-learning-organization-/an/U9706C-PDF-ENG

Homer-Dixon, T. (2002). *The ingenuity gap: Can we solve the problems of the future?* New York: Vintage Books.

Institute of Medicine. (2003). *Health professions education: A bridge to quality.* Washington, DC: National Academies Press.

Lewis, J. (2001). *Project planning, scheduling, and control: A hands-on guide to bringing projects in on time and on budget.* New York: McGraw-Hill.

Lyman, S., & Chermack, T. J. (2006). Responsible leadership for performance: A theoretical model and hypotheses. *Journal of Leadership and Organizational Studies.*

Ouichi, W. (1981). *Theory Z: How American business can meet the Japanese challenge.* Reading, MA: Addison-Wesley.

Schyve, P. M. (2000, September). *Testimony of Paul M. Schyve, Panel 5: State coalitions and public policy advocates*. Written Statement. National Summit on Medical Errors and Patient Safety Research. Retrieved from http://www.quic.gov/summit/wschyve.htm

Senge, P. (1990, 2006). *The fifth discipline: The art and practice of the learning organization*. New York: Doubleday.

Ulrich, W. (2004). *An appreciation of C. West Churchman* (rev. version, 26 March 2009). Retrieved from http://www.wulrich.com/cwc_appreciation.html (Originally published 1988 as "C. West Churchman—75 years," *Systems Practice, 1*(4), 341–350).

Wheatley, M. (1992). *Leadership and the new science: Discovering order in a chaotic world*. San Francisco: Berrett-Koehler.

Wheatley, M. (2002). *Turning to one another: Simple conversations to restore hope to the future*. San Francisco: Berrett-Koehler.

CHAPTER 3

Clinical Scholarship and Evidence-Based Practice

Catherine Tymkow

True scholarship consists in knowing not what things exist, but what they mean; it is not memory but judgment.

—JAMES RUSSELL LOWELL

Any discussion of scholarship and evidence-based practice and the doctor of nursing practice (DNP) role must first begin with some essential questions. These include questions as basic as the following: What is scholarship? Are evidence-based practice and clinical scholarship the same thing? How does clinical scholarship differ from the traditional definition of scholarship? Why do we need nursing scholars in practice settings? What is the role of the DNP in clinical scholarship? What are the knowledge resources, tools, and methods necessary to implement and support clinical scholarship and evidence-based practice?

These questions are important ones to consider as healthcare organizations and schools of nursing redefine and expand nurses' roles. If nursing is to maintain a full partnership with medicine in the delivery of health care, the education of nurse leaders and nurses in advanced practice roles must be at a comparable level with other doctorally prepared healthcare practitioners such as MDs, PharmDs, and PsyDs. The merging of nursing leadership skills, evidence-based decision making, and expert clinical care will ensure that nursing has a strong and credible presence in an ever-changing and complex healthcare system.

The Doctor of Nursing Practice degree is a terminal practice degree and is now considered by many healthcare organizations as the preferred degree for nursing leaders involved in the delivery and organization of clinical care and healthcare systems. The DNP's academic preparation, with a strong curricular base in advanced practice principles, experiential learning, intra/interprofessional collaboration, and application of the best clinical research evidence, can best fulfill nursing's goals for leadership in practice and clinical education. In addition, clinical scholarship, including critical inquiry, analysis, synthesis, creativity, and research, must be a distinguishing feature of the DNP's role and expertise.

The purpose of this chapter is to define and explore the meaning of clinical scholarship, to distinguish evidence-based practice from other forms of scholarly activity, to describe the unique role of the DNP in scholarship, and to provide an overview of the language, methodological tools, strategies, and thought processes that are necessary to ensure that nursing's scholarship is useful, significant, and of the highest quality. Entire books are dedicated to research processes, methodologies, and evidence-based practice. This is not the intent of this chapter; rather, it is to explore the concepts, provide resources, and whet the reader's appetite for more in-depth information on the topic.

What Is Clinical Scholarship?

In Sigma Theta Tau International's (1999) *Clinical Scholarship Resource Paper*, Melanie Dreher, chair of the task force, wrote that "clinical scholarship is about inquiry and implies a willingness to scrutinize our practice" (Dreher, 1999, p. 26). Also, "clinical scholarship is not clinical proficiency, . . . unless we are questioning the reason for its use in the first place . . . ; and neither is it clinical research, although it is informed by and inspires research" (p. 26). Finally, she notes that "clinical scholarship is an intellectual process. . . . It includes challenging traditional nursing interventions, testing our ideas, predicting outcomes, and explaining both patterns and exceptions. In addition to observation, analysis, and synthesis, clinical scholarship includes application and dissemination, all of which result in a new understanding of nursing phenomena and the development of new knowledge" (p. 26).

The American Association of Colleges of Nursing's (AACN) *Position Statement on Defining Scholarship for the Discipline of Nursing* (1999) defines scholarship as "those activities that systematically advance the teaching, research, and practice of nursing through rigorous inquiry that: 1) is significant to the profession, 2) is creative, 3) can be documented, 4) can be replicated or elaborated, and 5) can be peer-reviewed through various methods" (p. 1). Citing the work of Schulman (1993), the National Organization of Nurse Practitioner Faculties (2005) notes further that *practice*, in order to be considered scholarship, "must be public, susceptible to critical review and evaluation, and accessible for exchange and use of other members of one's scholarly community" (p. 6).

These definitions are congruent with the evolving definition of scholarship in academia since Boyer's (1990, 1997) groundbreaking work *Scholarship Reconsidered: Priorities of the Professoriate*. Ernest L. Boyer was an American educator, chancellor, and president of the Carnegie Foundation for the Advancement of Teaching (Carnegie Foundation for the Advancement of Teaching, 1996). Since the publication of *Scholarship Reconsidered* (1990), a new and expanded role for scholarship has emerged in academia that makes the previously mentioned definitions of scholarship more compatible with the goals and processes of practice disciplines. The traditional definition of scholarship in academia did not account for the nuances and rigors of clinical practice knowledge and its application for problem solving and interactive, human engagement (AACN, 2006). Boyer's model (1990, 1997), however, is well suited to scholarship in nursing practice. In Boyer's view, scholarship is not linear; rather, there is a constant, reciprocal, iterative relationship between each of its four aspects. It embraces the concepts of discovery (building new knowledge through research and careful inquiry in order to refine existing knowledge), integration (interpreting knowledge through dissemination in various forms), application (using knowledge for problem solving, service, and growth), and teaching (developing and testing instructional materials to advance learning, including the formation and sustaining of an engaging environment for learning between teacher and student (Boyer, 1990, 1997; Stull & Lanz, 2005).

The AACN's *Essentials of Doctoral Education for Advanced Nursing Practice* (2006) embodies much of Boyer's criteria in the specification of the eight core essentials and specialty focused competencies as the basic underpinnings to be integrated into the Doctor of Nursing Practice curriculum (AACN, 2006). Essential 3 of the core elements is "clinical scholarship and analytic methods for evidence-based practice" (AACN, 2006). In this document the authors state that "scholarship and research are core elements of doctoral education" (AACN, 2006), and, further, that "research doctorates are designed to prepare graduates with the research skills necessary to discover new knowledge in the discipline. However, DNPs engaged in advanced nursing practice provide leadership for evidence-based practice. This requires competence in knowledge development activities such as the translation of research in practice, the evaluation of practice, activities aimed at improving the reliability of health care practice and outcomes, and participation in collaborative research" (DePalma & McGuire, 2005). Therefore, DNP programs focus on the translation of new science, its application, and its evaluation. In addition, DNP graduates generate evidence to guide practice.

More recently, the idea that only those with research doctorates (PhD, DNS, and DNSc) should conduct "discovery" research for generating new knowledge has been challenged (Ironside, 2006; Reed & Shear, 2004; Webber, 2008). Webber (2008) asserts that level-appropriate research should be promoted from the baccalaureate through doctoral level because "everyday practice involves daily interaction with an informed public, interpreting the most updated research that is available with the click of a mouse, and identifying phenomena unique to the practice. The only missing piece is the skills necessary to investigate the phenomenon" (p. 468).

As DNP programs have proliferated, the curriculum has evolved to include more focus on research and evidence-based practice. An Internet review of the curricula from several national DNP programs makes it clear that growing numbers of schools are adding courses such as Theory, Research Methods, Discovery and Utilization of Evidence-Based Care, and Translating Evidence into Practice so that graduates have the skills needed to participate in whatever level of research is appropriate to their setting and scholarship goals.

Evidence-Based Practice and Clinical Scholarship: Are They the Same?

Scholarship is an evolutionary process that raises the level of the profession through participation in the generation of new knowledge and through scientific and social exchange. "The difference between evidence based nursing practice and scholarship or applied nursing research is that evidence based practice is practice driven" (French, 1999, p. 77). Whereas scholarship was often viewed by many practicing professionals as an add-on, optional activity, evidence-based practice has become a necessity in our current information-based technological age. Computers have given everyone access to both good and bad information. The defining feature of evidence-based practice is the linking of current research findings with patients' conditions, values, and circumstances. In addition, it involves "the conscientious, explicit, and judicious use of current best evidence for making decisions about the care of individuals" (Sackett, Richardson, Rosenberg, & Haynes, 1997, p. 2). Nursing's unique addition to this process must offer a more holistic approach that adds artful practice and ethical standards to the empirics of evidence (Fawcett, Watson, Neuman, Hinton Walker, & Fitzpatrick, 2001).

The work of clinical scholars has increased during the past two decades. A review of published nursing articles from 1986 to 2008 in the Cumulative Index to Nursing and Allied Health Literature (CINAHL) database resulted in 81 published articles with clinical scholarship as the focus. When "evidence-based practice" was added to the search terms, an additional 7 articles were found. When "evidence-based practice" alone was used as the search term, the search returned 3,835 articles published between the years 1993 and 2009. Although not all of the latter were nursing articles, 1,729 articles, or nearly half, were nursing-focused articles.

Holleman, Eliens, van Vliet, and van Acterburg (2006) extensively reviewed six databases, including CINAHL, PubMed, Scirus, Invert, Google, and the Cochrane databases, focusing on the years between 1993 and 2004. In their meta-analysis of the literature on promotion of evidence-based practice (EBP) and professional nursing associations, the authors found 179 articles that addressed EBP activities. Of the 179 articles, 47 dealt with EBP as structural measures (policy, role, quality indicators), 103 as competence- and attitude-oriented (journals, conferences, workshops, research committees, etc.), and only 29 as behavior-oriented (care models, guidelines). The increase in EBP articles shows the growing interest and use of evidence to guide practice. Despite this progress, there remain significant gaps in nursing science discovery and application or implementation in practice. The Doctor of Nursing Practice is intended to bridge this gap (McCloskey, 2008).

The principles of EBP were an outgrowth of the work of Dr. Archie Cochrane, a British epidemiologist who criticized the medical profession for not using evidence from randomized clinical trials as a basis for clinical care. He believed that the evidence from these trials should be systematically reviewed and constantly updated to afford patients the best-quality care (Cochrane Collaboration, 2004). Evidence-based practice includes an emphasis on the efficacy of treatments or interventions based on the results of experimental comparison between untreated control groups, treatments, or both. The core principles include (1) formulating the clinical question; (2) identifying the most relevant articles, research, and other best evidence; (3) critically evaluating the evidence; (4) integrating and applying the evidence; and (5) reevaluating the application of evidence and making necessary changes. Table 3-1 presents the hierarchy of evidence for practice.

That the definition of "evidence-based practice" has been adapted to include provisions for the provider's experience and patient's values in making the ultimate clinical care decisions is in keeping with James Russell Lowell's (1819–1891) definition of scholarship: "True scholarship consists in knowing not what things exist, but what they mean; it is not memory, but judgment." Although Lowell was not a healthcare professional, his definition is applicable to advanced nursing practice. It is through the incorporation of intuition, observation, theory, research, intelligent analysis, and judgment based on the data that nurses provide care that is truly individualized, reflective, and evidence based. With an increased knowledge of the theory and the tools necessary to critique and translate research into practice, the DNP is in a prime position to affect the delivery of care and to aggregate and translate evidence that can be disseminated to improve overall care and outcomes in a myriad of clinical areas. The translation and dissemination of clinical knowledge is the core of clinical scholarship.

■ Table 3-1   Hierarchy for Evaluating Evidence for Practice

Level 1 (strongest)	Systematic reviews/meta-analysis of all randomized controlled trials (RCTs); clinical practice guidelines based on RCT data
Level 2	Evidence from one or more RCTs
Level 3	Evidence from a controlled trial; no randomization
Level 4	Case control or cohort studies
Level 5	Systematic reviews of descriptive/qualitative studies
Level 6	Single descriptive or qualitative study
Level 7 (weakest)	Opinions of authorities/experts

Note: All levels assume a well-designed study.

What Is the Role of the Doctor of Nursing Practice in Clinical Scholarship?

In advanced practice, scholarship should be integrated with practice as a purposeful, systematic, and conscious endeavor. The emphasis is on inquiry, outcomes, and evidence to support practice (Sigma Theta Tau International Clinical Scholarship Task Force, 1999). Because of their education, advanced practice nurses, particularly DNPs, are expected to have mastery of essential information so that the teaching of staff, patients, and communities becomes a key function of the role. The dynamic nature of health care requires that DNPs be up to date on new information, and that they be able to discern nuances in research findings so as to translate those findings in understandable ways that improve care and practice. This requires constant critique and integration and synthesis of new information from various sources into formats that can be disseminated to patients, colleagues, and others.

What distinguishes the role of the DNP from other advanced practice degree holders? The answer is not a simple one; the difference is, in fact, a combination of knowledge, expert skill, and the integration of *best* research to advance the practice and the profession. This skill comes from additional formal education, experience, and the translation, application, and evaluation of research in practice. Although most practicing nurses are exposed to "research" and "evidence" in practice, the DNP must not only embrace the process but also implement the findings in ways that ultimately change or, at least, improve practice and outcomes. Scholarship is the dissemination of those findings in publications, presentations, and Internet offerings that can be used by others. As envisioned in the *Essentials of Doctoral Education for Advanced Practice Nursing* (AACN, 2006), the DNP program prepares graduates to:

1. Use analytical methods to critically appraise existing literature and other evidence relevant to practice.
2. Lead the evaluation of evidence (existing literature, research findings, and other data) to determine and implement the best evidence for practice.
3. Design and implement processes to evaluate outcomes of practice and systems of care.
4. Design, direct, and evaluate quality improvement initiatives to promote safe, timely, effective, efficient, equitable, and patient-centered care.
5. Evaluate practice patterns against national benchmarks to determine variances in clinical outcomes and population trends.

6. Apply relevant findings to develop practice guidelines and improve practice and the practice environment.

7. Inform and guide the design of databases that generate meaningful evidence for nursing practice.

8. Use information technology and research methods appropriately to:
   ■ collect appropriate and accurate data to generate evidence for nursing practice
   ■ analyze data from clinical practice
   ■ design evidence-based interventions
   ■ predict and analyze outcomes
   ■ examine patterns of behavior and outcomes
   ■ identify gaps in evidence for practice

9. Function as a practice specialist/consultant in collaborative knowledge-generating research.

10. Disseminate findings from evidence-based practice to improve healthcare outcomes.

These objectives encompass the essential skills, tools, and methods necessary to implement and support clinical scholarship and evidence-based practice. They can be distilled into six categories: (1) translating research in practice, (2) quality improvement and patient-centered care, (3) evaluation of practice, (4) research methods and technology, (5) participation in collaborative research, and (6) disseminating findings from evidence-based practice. Each of these areas is discussed in the following sections.

Translating Research in Practice

The use of evidence to support clinical practice is not a new phenomenon. Medical professionals have relied on data from science, empirical observation, case reviews, and other means for centuries (Monico, Moore, & Calise, 2005). However, as electronic access to sources of data has increased, the amount of evidence now available as a basis for clinical practice is often overwhelming. The key to making best-practice decisions is in using the best-quality evidence, evidence that is scientifically based and that has been replicated with success in repeated research and application. Although critical appraisal of research for use in practice is an important aspect of evidence-based practice, it is not the only criterion. Unfortunately, many lack the knowledge and skills on which to base their practice decisions (Pravikoff, Tanner, & Pierce,

2005). Melnyk and Fineout-Overholt (2005) specify three primary knowledge sources for EBP: valid research evidence, clinical expertise, and patient choice. Currently, evidence generated from large-scale randomized controlled trials is considered the gold standard for application in interventions (Fawcett & Garrity, 2009). Depending on the clinical situation and the patient's personal preference, other sources of evidence may be appropriate, including meta-analyses of all relevant randomized controlled trials; EBP guidelines from systematic reviews of randomized controlled trials, case control, or cohort studies; expert opinion; and nursing theory (Fawcett & Garrity, 2009; Melnyk & Fineout-Overholt, 2005).

To understand research evidence that may be used in practice, the following sections on qualitative and quantitative research offer a brief description of the processes and questions to be considered in the evaluation of such research. Exhaustive coverage of every research method is beyond the scope of this chapter. However, the definitions, discussion, and examples are meant to illustrate how different types of research might be applied or used in practice, and how their rigor and adequacy as evidence for practice should be evaluated.

Understanding, Distinguishing, and Evaluating Types of Research Evidence

QUALITATIVE RESEARCH EVIDENCE

Qualitative research is based on four levels of understanding:

1. What is the nature of reality? (Ontology)
2. What constitutes knowledge? (Epistemology)
3. How can we understand reality? (Methodology)
4. How can we collect the evidence? (Methods)

(Porter, 1996, as cited in Maggs-Rapport, 2001)

Types of Qualitative Research Studies

There are several kinds of qualitative research studies, including critical social theory, ethnographic studies, grounded theory research, historical research, phenomenological studies, and philosophical inquiry. Each of these methods is discussed briefly so as to provide an overview of the scope and potential uses of qualitative evidence and to provide a basis for evaluating the use of qualitative studies as a basis for changes in practice.

Critical Social Theory *Critical social theory* uses multiple research methods as a basis for promoting change in areas where power imbalances exist (Burns & Grove, 2009). Based on the ideas of Horkheimer (1895–1973), Marcuse (1898–1979), Adorno (1903–1969), and Habermas (1929–), critical social theory is based on the belief that individuals should seek freedom from domination (Maggs-Rapport, 2001). Habermas, particularly, believed that people must understand the nature of "constraining circumstances" before they could be liberated from them (Maggs-Rapport, 2001). Another critical social theorist, Giddens (1982, as cited in Maggs-Rapport, 2001), believed that we can understand why people act in certain ways only if we can appreciate the meanings of their actions.

The DNP might use data from critical social theory to identify meaning or patterns of concern where certain societal cultural norms exist in the form of barriers that affect particularly vulnerable populations such as the elderly, the incarcerated, abused women, and the chronically ill. Analysis would necessarily include an examination of the underlying conditions, a critique of the social phenomena, and the discovery and revelation of the social and political injustices embedded in the experience of the population in question that could lead toward removal of barriers (Maggs-Rapport, 2001).

Ethnographic Research *Ethnographic research* is used to describe the nature or characteristics of a culture in order to gain insight into the lifeways or behaviors of a group. Distinguishing features are immersion in the participant's way of life (Polit & Hungler, 1997) and the fact that the information gathered speaks for itself, rather than being interpreted or explored for additional meanings (Maggs-Rapport, 2001).

In one ethnographic study, Kovarsky (2008) compared clients' and families' personal experiences of outcomes and interventions with written professional discourse, technical reports, and other conceptualizations of evidence in practice. Unfortunately, the author notes, "the dismissal of subjective, phenomenally oriented information has functioned to marginalize and silence voices . . . of clients when constituting proof of effectiveness," and further, "the current version of EBP needs to be reformulated to include subjective voices from the life-worlds of clients as a form of evidence" (Kovarsky, 2008, p. 47). As one example of an ethnographic approach, Kovarksy proposed the personal experience narrative as a measure of qualitative outcomes and intervention analysis (Kovarsky, 2008, p. 48). Citing a study by Simmons-Mackie and Damico (2001), Kovarksy describes an ethnographic interview with a patient experiencing post-stroke aphasia.

When asked to comment on life before her stroke, K. [the patient] said: "Before teacher . . . now I don't know . . . .what." and "uh . . . uh . . . always, always . . . uh . . . busy, busy, busy, . . . teachin . . . teachin . . . always, I love it. . . . it's me . . . But now . . . here (points to mouth) talk, not uh . . . teaching." When asked about a typical day, she shrugged and said "nothing . . . here (points to television)" and later added "eat . . . and (points to newspaper) and shows (points to television)." (Simmons-Mackie & Damico, 2001, as cited in Kovarsky, 2008, p. 51)

These statements support an altered level of life activity that cannot totally be accounted for or appreciated in objective technical descriptions of outcomes of disease processes and their sequelae.

The ethnographic narrative is a method of subjective evidence gathering that can enhance the specificity and richness of other research methodologies, including evidence gained from logical positivist approaches such as randomized controlled trials. In particular, DNPs in public health or community health could use this method in conjunction with other, more traditional, forms of evidence to gain a better real-world understanding of the populations they serve.

Grounded Theory Research *Grounded theory research* is focused on the influence of interactional processes (identification, description, and explanation) between individuals, families, or groups within a social context (Strauss & Corbin, 1994). It is an observational method that is used to study problems in social settings that are "grounded" in the data obtained from those observations (Burns & Grove, 2009; Glasser & Strauss, 1967). In this regard, grounded theory is an applicable framework for study of a myriad of contexts, situations, and settings.

For example, a study of the implementation of evidence-based nursing in Iran (Adib-Hajbaghery, 2007) sought to distinguish factors influencing the implementation of evidence-based practice in Eastern countries (versus Western countries), particularly Iran. A brief description of this study using the grounded theory approach is presented here. Data collection consisted of purposive sampling of 21 nurses (nine staff and six head nurses in differing clinical settings) with experience in nursing greater than five years. An interview questionnaire consisted of open-ended questions, such as "What is the basis of care you give your patients?" (p. 568), "In your opinion, what is the basis of evidence based nursing?" (p. 568), and "Can you describe some instances in which you used scientific evidence in nursing?" (p. 568). "Issues were clarified and interviews were audiotaped, transcribed verbatim and analyzed consecutively" (Adib-Hajbaghery, 2007, p. 568). Thirty-six hours of observations and interviews were carried out concurrently and involved observations of those interviewed and others working on the units. According to the procedure identified by Strauss and Corbin (1998), each interview was analyzed before the subsequent interview took place, and the results were coded in three ways: open coding (breaking down, examining, comparing, conceptualizing, and categorizing), axial coding (putting data back together in new ways by linking codes to contexts, consequences, and patterns of interactions), and selective coding (identifying core categories and systematically relating and validating relationships) (Adib-Hajbaghery, 2007). To confirm the credibility of the data, participants were given a full transcript of their responses and a list of codes and themes to determine whether the codes and themes matched their responses. To establish validity, two peer researchers also checked codes and themes using the same procedure as the researcher. The results were that two main categories emerged from the research: (1) the meaning of evidence-based nursing (EBN) and (2) factors in implementation of EBN, including the following themes: possessing professional knowledge and experience, having opportunity and time, becoming accustomed, self-confidence, the process of nursing education, and the work environment and its expectations (Adib-Hajbaghery, 2007).

The process and results of grounded theory research and analysis provide rich data for application in practice when paired with evidence from other sources. This is especially true when there is little clinical trial evidence to support the affective dimension of care or practice.

Historical Research *Historical research* is a description or analysis of events that have shaped a discipline. Although historical research may not be used directly in practice, it provides the foundation for examination of the discipline and for providing future directions (Burns & Grove; 2009; Fitzpatrick & Munhall, 2001). Often history is handed down in written documents. The Library of Congress's (n.d.) American Memory Collection has original writings, newspaper clippings, photos, and other documents that provide a realistic account of the influence and actions of famous women in history, including nursing leaders. Pictures and other documents showcase the original early work of early nurse leaders such as Lavinia Dock (1858–1956), Margaret Sanger (1879–1966), Clara Barton (1821–1912), and Mary Breckinridge (1881–1965), which provide a basis for advanced nursing practice and can be used by DNPs in education to provide a historical perspective for practice.

Another source of historical research is oral history. Decker and Iphofen (2005) describe a method of oral history research to discover knowledge about, and change within, a profession, particularly as it relates to evidence-based practice. Tropello (2000) used oral history technique in her dissertation, "Origins of the Nurse Practitioner Movement: An Oral History." The purpose was to gain a better understanding of current advanced nursing practice roles through an exploration of the original movement. Eight participants in the original movement were the primary sources, and the information obtained and transcribed from taped interviews was enhanced by supportive papers, correspondence, and other documents, including secondary sources. One conclusion of the study was that the politics of the 1960s, which emphasized greater freedoms for women and a focus on social programs, helped alleviate healthcare manpower shortages (Tropello, 2000). This movement has paved the way for additional professionalization in nursing, including the evolution of the Doctor of Nursing Practice curriculum. Started as a research project, it became part of the core curriculum under the continuing education division of the School of Nursing at the University of Colorado. The program used a nursing–physician team approach to aid families with limited access to primary providers (Tropello, 2000).

Another oral history intervention project was that of Taft, Stolder, Knutson, Tamke, Platt, and Bowles (2004), who recorded the oral histories of World War II veterans in nursing homes. Themes of patriotism, loss, tense moments, makeshift living, self-sufficiency, and uncertainty were uncovered. The authors' conclusions were that "oral histories, listening[,] and valuing supports, involves, and validates elders" (Taft et al., 2004, p. 38.). The National League for Nursing (NLN) provides audio and videotapes of nurse theorists whose original work and theory development continue to provide frameworks for advancing nursing practice (Moccia, 1987). In order for DNPs to prescribe their future, they must have a clear understanding and appreciation for their history so that they can build on and shape evidence-based practice in ways that preserve the essence of nursing.

Phenomenological Research The aim of a *phenomenological (hermeneutic) study* is to understand a phenomenon through the recognition of its meaning.

Researchers explore an experience as it is lived by the participants in the study. The phenomenon of interest may include any number of experiences, such as death, divorce, pain, or cancer. The researcher collects data and interprets the experiences as they are lived (Burns & Groves, 2009). Phenomenology focuses on the subjective and particular experiences to discern the real truths of any phenomena (Hallet, 1995, as cited in Yegdich, 1999). One example of a phenomenological study by Marineau (2005) was that of perceptions of telehealth support by an advanced practice nurse for patients discharged from the hospital with acute infections. Because empirical data were insufficient in patients who had previously been enrolled in a quantitative pilot study of telehealth, eidetic phenomenology was used to capture patients' lived experiences after discharge. Theme categories were as follows: initial response, engaging in care, and experiencing the downside. Of the ten participants in the trial, only one had a negative experience. The study was seen as useful in adding to the understanding of the transitional process of care (Marineau, 2005).

In another phenomenological approach, Maggs-Rapport (2001) used van Manen's (1990) social scientific approach to look at women's immediate response to the phenomenon of egg sharing (donation of one woman's eggs to another woman) after consultation with a clinician and their lived experiences of egg sharing in return for free fertility treatment. The in-depth, open-ended interviews of this technique established a conversational relationship about the meaning of the experience and produced a narrative that "enriches the understanding of the phenomena" (Maggs-Rapport, 2001). Before each description can by transformed into phenomenological language, meaning units must be made of each description (Giorgi, 2000). However, only a small number of descriptions are necessary before the nature of the phenomenon becomes apparent (van Manen, 1990; Giorgi, 2000).

Other studies that utilized the phenomenological approach in advanced practice include studies about the needs of patients and families living with severe brain injury (Bond, Draeger, Mandleco, & Donnelly, 2003); high risk perinatal experience (Harvey, 1993); the meaning of U.S. childbirth for Mexican immigrant women (Imberg, 2008); the meaning of desire for euthanasia (Mak, 2003); and perimenopausal mental disorders (Rasgon, Shelton, & Halbreich, 2005). Phenomenological techniques with a strong nursing orientation include those of Crotty (1996); Diekelmann, Allen, and Tanner (1989); and Munhall (1994, 2007). Phenomenological studies contribute to the evidence base by enhancing our understanding of the true meaning of patients' experiences and the broader dimensions of a problem, thus aiding in a more holistic perspective in practice.

Philosophical Inquiry *Philosophical inquiry* is used to explore the nature of knowledge, values, meaning, and ethical factors related to a question of interest. Although philosophical inquiry is related to theory, it is not the same as theory, which is more specific and concrete (Pesut & Johnson, 2007). Citing Edwards (2001), Pesut and Johnson (2007) describe three "strands" that compose philosophical inquiry: (1) philosophical presupposition, which involves identifying and analyzing presuppositions in nursing (an example might be a concept analysis of nursing practice or advanced practice); (2) philosophical problems, such as what constitutes knowing in a particular situation, or ethical analyses, such as the ethics of caring in situations where nurses' and patients' values conflict; and (3) scholarship, in which nurse theorists' works are examined from a philosophical perspective. In this case, as noted by Burns and Grove (2009), the researcher would "conduct an extensive search of the literature, examine conceptual meaning, pose questions and propose answers including the implications for those answers" (p. 26).

In a practical application of philosophical inquiry, Dorn (2004) described a model, caring-healing inquiry for holistic nursing practice, to guide nursing research and quality improvement in a tertiary hospital. The model, which integrated the values of the hospital, provided the basis for nurses to describe their contributions to care through research and practice improvement. In a partnership between a hospital and university nursing program, a nursing research committee was formed, composed mostly of advanced practice nurses. The group served as an advisory group for program planning and development. The nurse-researcher faculty member facilitated the work of the committee and provided staff development in research and clinical innovation. Knowledge about the process of philosophical inquiry and a focus on value analysis, as demonstrated in these examples, provides DNPs with a basis for facilitating ethical decision making in practice.

Evaluating Qualitative Research Evidence

What are the evaluative questions? Regardless of the type of research design, the general criteria for evaluation of qualitative studies are as follows (Gifford, Davies, Edwards, Griffin, & Lybanon, 2007; Patton, 1990; Russell & Gregory, 2003):

1. *Question, purpose, and context:* Is the research question clear, the primary purpose and the focus of the study stated, and the context described?
2. *Design:* Was the design appropriate, were the units of analysis and sampling strategy described, and the sampling criteria clear?
3. *Data collection:* What types of data were collected? Were data collection processes systematic and adequately described? How were logistical issues addressed?
4. *Data analysis:* Was data analysis systematic and rigorous? What controls were in place? What analytical approach or approaches were used? How were validity and confidence in the findings established?
5. *Results:* Were results surprising, interesting, or suspect? Were conclusions supported by data and explanation (theory)? Were the authors' positions clearly stated?
6. *Ethical issues:* How were ethical issues and confidentiality addressed?
7. *Implications:* What is the worth/relevance to knowledge and practice?

Context Matters In her discussion of evidence-based nursing and qualitative research, Zuzelo (2007) notes that critical appraisal skills are among the most important aspects of the evidence-based movement in health care. Also, the associated terms *relevance* and *best*, when applied to practice, are value-laden terms that must be fully explored within the context of nursing practice, so that the unique contribution of nursing is not subsumed into the disease-based medical model of clinical decision making. Additionally, she proposes that "nursing[,] as both a science and an art, needs to assure that qualitative research is as much a part of the considered evidence as quantitative evidence is" (Zuzelo, 2007, p. 484). This is important because qualitative research questions provide an avenue for truly knowing, connecting with patients, and considering individual differences when making clinical decisions. These are the hallmarks of nursing that nurses at every level must retain and that DNPs must foster as role models to ensure that "best practice" does not exclude the best of nursing's perspective.

QUANTITATIVE RESEARCH EVIDENCE
Steps in the Quantitative Research Process
The important aspect of any quantitative research project is that the project builds on prior results or evidence and that it provides a basis for future research and discovery (Burns & Grove, 2009). Figure 3-1 shows the steps in the quantitative research process.

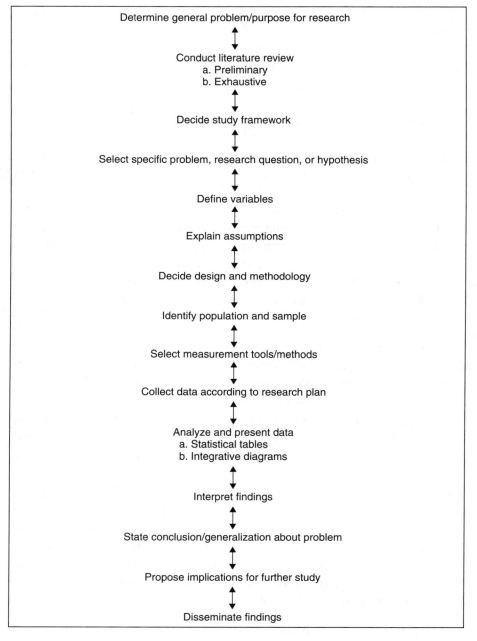

■ Figure 3-1   The Quantitative Research Process

Source: Burns, N., & Grove, S. K. (2009). *The practice of nursing research, appraisal, synthesis, and generation of evidence* (6th ed.). St. Louis, MO: Elsevier Saunders, p. 37. Reprinted with permission.

The *research problem* is often derived because there is a gap in knowledge that needs to be addressed or described. Research problems or questions often arise from direct observations made in practice. The *purpose* of the study is to address the problem. To better understand the problem, an extensive *literature review* must be done in order to develop an understanding of the nature and scope of the problem and to determine what research has already been done. A framework, map, or theoretical base made up of concepts is developed to provide structure and help the researcher make sense of the findings. The *research objectives, questions, or hypotheses* set the study limits, in terms of who will be studied, what question(s) will be addressed, and what relationships among variables exist.

The remaining steps are to define the variables in conceptual terms (theoretical meaning) and operational terms (how the variables will be measured or manipulated), explain assumptions (those things we take for granted to be true, whether proven or not), and identify study limitations (any issue within the study that serves to limit a study's generalizability beyond the population or sample studied). Limitations may be weaknesses in the study itself or in the theoretical basis.

Categories and Selection of a Design

Quantitative research may be categorized as experimental, quasi-experimental, or nonexperimental (descriptive or correlational). Quantitative research may be either basic research (as in laboratory studies) or applied (as in clinical research). In an experimental or quasi-experimental study, the researcher actively manipulates the independent variable (treatment or intervention) to see the effect on the dependent variable. In an experimental study, the variables and the setting are highly controlled. In a nonexperimental design, the researcher may simply want to describe or explain a phenomenon or predict a relationship (Burns & Grove, 2009).

Quantitative designs may also be retrospective (the proposed cause and effect have already occurred), prospective (the cause, but not the effect, has occurred), cross sectional (examines groups in various stages of development), or longitudinal (the same subjects are studied over a period of time). None of the categories are mutually exclusive (Schmidt & Brown, 2009).

The Population and Sample

The *population* is everyone or everything that meets the criteria for inclusion. The criteria for inclusion may be narrow or broad, depending on the size and scope of the study and the specific research question to be addressed. The *sample* is a subset of the population and the process for how the subset will be selected. This may be random (all have a better than zero chance of selection), nonrandom (convenience), cross sectional (groups studied over time), or stratified (divided to ensure representation from groups when some variables are known). Often the population and the sample are determined by the method and how accessible the population is to the researcher (Burns & Grove, 2009).

Measurement Instruments

Measurement instruments are tools used by the researcher to answer the operational questions posed in research studies. These tools may be questionnaires, tests, indicators of health status, and a variety of other measurement techniques.

Data Collection, Analysis, and Interpretation

Most data collected in quantitative research studies are coded numerically so that they can be systematically analyzed and interpreted through the use of statistics. A plan for data collection and analysis is an important part of the research process and is crucial to meaningful interpretation of results. Interpretation involves "1) examining the results from data, 2) exploring the significance of findings, 3) forming conclusions, 4) generalizing the data, 5) considering the implications for further study, and 6) suggesting further studies" (Burns & Grove, p. 45). Once interpreted, the researcher synthesizes and reports implications for further study or practice, or both.

This cursory overview of the research process provides the basis for evaluating evidence from research. The reader is referred to a research text for a complete discussion of definitions and the various designs, analyses, and implementation processes.

Evaluating Quantitative Evidence

When a quantitative study is appraised for use in practice, three questions are generally considered: Is the study valid? Is the study reliable? and Is the study applicable in the identified case?

Is the Study Valid? Specifically, were the methods used scientifically sound? Are the independent (manipulated variable) and dependent variables (observed result) clearly identified? Is the study free from bias or confounding variables?

Bias is a standard point of view or personal prejudice, especially when there is a tendency "to affect unduly or unfairly, or to impose a steady negative potential upon" (*Funk & Wagnalls*, 2003, p. 135). It is an influence or action that distorts or "slants findings away from the expected" (Burns & Grove, 2009, p. 220). In research, bias may occur when participants' characteristics specifically differ from those of the population (Burns & Grove, 2005). This is always possible because volunteers are used for samples. It is less likely to occur, however, if the sampling strategy is well planned and followed and there is random assignment to groups. Bias may also occur if the instruments or measurement tools are faulty, or the data or statistics are inaccurate.

Selection Bias If a researcher decides to prospectively compare two types of strategies for educating nursing students, such as online instruction and traditional classroom instruction, selection bias may occur if the students are allowed to select which group they enter. Students who select online teaching may be very different from those who choose the traditional classroom experience. Random assignment to the groups minimizes the risk of selection bias. ■

Gender Bias Another form of bias is *gender bias*. Gender bias occurs in research when one gender, more than the other, is used to study research interventions. Timmerman (1999) outlined a procedure for ensuring that research decisions avoid gender bias. The procedure includes critically analyzing the literature, testing gender-specific differences, and identifying researchers' personal biases. The following example of binge-eating behaviors between men and women illustrates the point. Timmerman (1999), citing Hawkins & Clement (1984) and Spitzer et al. (1992), states "we know that men tend to binge less frequently, consume less during binges and are less distressed by their binge eating behavior than women." And, "in this case, the literature provides justification for either separately studying binge eating behavior in men and women, or, if the sample has both men and women, analyzing the data separately for men and women" (Timmerman, 1999, p. 642). Table 3-2 lists some gender-based studies. Additional gender-based studies can be found online through the Office on Women's Health of the U.S. Department of Health and Human Services.

Confounding Variables *Confounding* occurs when a third variable, either known or unknown, produces the relationship with the outcome instead of the research intervention itself. Or, stated differently, confounding may

■ Table 3-2   Gender-Based Studies

Authors and Date of Publication	Title
Bernarde, Keogh, & Lima (2007)	Bridging the gap between pain and gender research
Bushnell, Hurn, Colton, Miller, del Zoppo, Elkind, et al. (2007)	Advancing the study of stroke in women: Summary and recommendations for future research
Doster, Pardum, Martin, Goven, & Moorefield (2009)	Gender differences, anger expression, and cardiovascular risk
Luttik, Jaarsma, Lesman, Sanderman, & Hagedoorn (2009)	Quality of life in partners of people with congestive heart failure: Gender and involvement in care
Masharani, Goldfine, & Youngren (2009)	Influence of gender on the relationship between insulin sensitivity, adiposity and plasma lipids in lean nondiabetic patients
McCollum, Hansen, Lu, & Sullivan (2005)	Self-care differences in men and women with diabetes
Reeves, Fonarow, Zhao, Smith, & Schwamm (2009)	Quality of care in women with ischemic stroke in the GWTG program

occur when comparing two groups that may be different in additional ways from the treatment being studied (Leedy & Ormrod, 2010). Randomizing participants to either the intervention or study group helps to eliminate the possibility of confusion because there is an equal chance that extraneous variables will appear equally in both groups, thus minimizing the confounding effect.

One type of confounder is the effect of *history*. The history effect occurs when an event outside the researcher's control occurs at the same time as, or during, the period of the intervention. For example, in a study of patients with hypertension, a researcher was interested in the impact of a low-salt diet on hypertension levels. A baseline blood pressure was taken; patients were then started on the low-salt diet. However, during the study period, some of these same patients also began a rigorous exercise routine, whereas others did not. In this case, the intervening exercise program would make it difficult to attribute the outcome solely to the effect of the intervention.

Adding a control group using low-salt diet with exercise, or using statistical tests to control for this confounding variable, would minimize the threat to validity in this study.

In another example of confounding, a researcher was interested in comparing lung cancer and smoking incidence in various regions of the country. In this study, a particular region was seen to have a significantly higher rate of lung cancer death among smokers (15 times higher) than other regions of the country. The confounding factor was the fact that these smokers had also worked in asbestos coal mines for many years. When the researchers controlled for the variable of working with asbestos by removing the confounder, the rate of cancer due to smoking was nearly the same as that in other regions of the country. Figure 3-2 shows the relationship among the independent variable (smoking) and confounding variable (working in an asbestos coal mine) in relationship to the dependent variable (lung cancer) (International Development Research Center, 2009).

Is the Study Reliable? The *reliability* of a study is based on questions such as the following: Does the instrument or test measure what it is supposed to measure? Does it do this consistently? Do the items on the instrument consistently measure the same characteristic? How much consistency is there between raters? (Burns & Grove, 2009; Fain, 2009). Reliability is measured through the use of a reliability coefficient (r) and ranges from 00.0 (lowest) to 1.00 (highest). Therefore, the closer a reliability score is to 1.00,

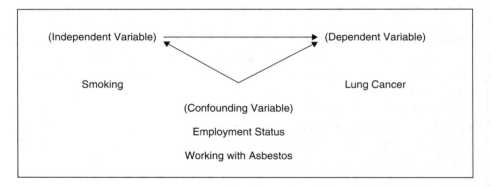

■ Figure 3-2   Interrelationships Among Smoking, Working in an Asbestos Coal Mine, and Risk for Lung Cancer in a Cohort/Case Control Study

Source: International Development Research Center. (2009). Figure 26.1. http://www.idrc.ca/en/ev-56459-201-1-DO_TOPIC.html. Used with permission of IDRC Canada, www.irdc.ca.

the higher the reliability. In most cases a coefficient of 0.80 or higher is considered acceptable if the instrument has already been tested and has been used frequently. If an instrument is new, a reliability coefficient of 0.70 may be acceptable (Griffin-Sobel, 2003, as cited in Schmidt & Brown, 2009). Reliability also focuses on stability (test–retest reliability—whether an instrument yields the same results for the same two people on two different occasions), homogeneity (internal consistency—the extent to which all of the items within a single instrument yield similar results), and equivalence (interrater reliability—the extent to which two or more individuals evaluating the same product or performance give identical judgments) (Fain, 2009; Leedy & Ormrod, 2010).

A simple example of reliability is seen in the selection of timing devices used in sports events. Timing devices must work consistently each and every time so that competitors are ensured an equal chance of winning. An example of interrater reliability is that of a classroom situation in which two evaluators are trained to use the same tool with a Likert scale to measure student performance on oral presentations.

Are the Results of the Study Applicable in the Identified Case? Once the science of a study has been appraised and the reliability of results assessed, the next important questions are, Do the results apply to the case of interest? Are the populations in the study and in the proposed population for application similar? If the populations studied are not similar, the significance of results in the study has little value for real-life implementation in a given clinical situation.

Is the effect size sufficient so that application of the study intervention will make a significant difference? The *effect size* is calculated by determining the mean difference between two groups (intervention and control) and dividing by the standard deviation. It is not the same as the statistical significance, but rather is the size of the difference between two groups. The effect size is often used in meta-analysis for combining and comparing estimates from different studies in order to determine the effectiveness of an intervention. "An effect size is exactly equivalent to the Z-score of a normal standard deviation. For example an effect size of 0.8 means that the score of the average person in the experimental group is 0.8 standard deviations above the average person in the control group, and hence exceeds the scores of 79% of the control group" (Coe, 2002, p. 2.). Thus,

$$\text{Effect size} = \frac{\text{Mean of experimental group} - \text{Mean of control group}}{\text{Standard deviation}}$$

Generally, in evaluating any quantitative study, additional questions include the following: Why was the study done? How was the sample size decided? How were the data analyzed? Were there any surprises or unexpected events that occurred during the study? How do the results of this study compare with others? (Melnyk & Fineout-Overholt, 2005).

The standard of care for practice is increasingly based on scientific evidence. Finding the most current research based on well-conducted clinical trials is an important first step. But how do we evaluate that evidence in practice? Several statistical measures help in the evaluation of study results. Table 3-3 briefly describes some commonly used statistical tests. An excellent guide to biostatistics is also available from MedPageToday (n.d.).

What happens if the evidence conflicts with patients' values and preferences? What if our own experience conflicts with the evidence? The key is that the evidence must be relevant to the problem and tested through application. In addition, some scholars (Fawcett et al., 2001; Kitson, Harvey, & McCormack, 1998; Rycroft-Malone, Seers, Titchen, Harvey, Kitson, & McCormack, 2004) insist that evidence as defined by medicine is too narrowly focused and does not recognize the complexities of nursing practice. They recommend that the definition include the influence of context in the application of evidence (Scott-Findley & Pollack, 2004). This would include findings from qualitative research.

Regardless of the definition, however, once evidence is implemented, the results must be evaluated. Did the evidence support better decision making? Was the patient's care improved? In what way was care or outcomes improved? If they were not improved, why not? (Melnyk & Fineout-Overholt, 2005).

Determining and Implementing the Best Evidence for Practice

A distinguishing feature of evidence-based nursing is that nurses treat and work *with* patients rather than "work on them" (McSherry, 2002). In addition, nursing's approach is more holistic, so that "effectiveness of treatment" is but one indicator; cost effectiveness and patient acceptability also matter (McSherry, 2002). According to the Agency for Healthcare Quality and Research (AHQR, 2002, as cited in Melnyk & Fineout-Overholt, 2005), three benchmark domains must be considered when evaluating evidence: quality, quantity, and consistency. *Quality* refers to the absence of biases due to errors in selection, measurement, and confounding biases (internal validity). *Quantity* refers to the number of relevant, related studies; total sample size across

■ Table 3-3   Clinical Statistical Measures

Clinical Statistic	Description
Odds ratio (OR)	The odds of risk for a person in the experimental group having an adverse outcome compared with a person in the control group. An odds ratio of 1 means the event is equally likely in both groups. An odds ratio greater than 1 means the event is more likely in the intervention group than the control group. An odds ratio less than 1 means the event is less likely in the intervention group than the control group. Used most in case control and retrospective studies.
Relative risk ratio (RR)	The risk of an outcome in the intervention/treatment group (Y) compared to the control group (X). RR = Y/X. A relative risk of 1 means there is no difference between the two groups. A relative risk of less than 1 means a smaller potential for the effect to occur in the intervention group than in the control group. Used most in randomized controlled trials and cohort studies.
Relative risk reduction (RRR)	The percentage of reduction in the treatment group (Y) compared with the control group (X). RRR = $1 - Y/X$? 100%.
Absolute risk reduction (ARR)	The difference in risk between the control group (X) and the intervention group (Y). ARR = $X - Y$.
Number needed to treat (NNT)	The number of patients that must be treated over a given period of time to prevent one adverse outcome. NNT = $1/(X - Y)$.

Source: Long, C. O. (2009).Weighing in on the evidence. In N. A. Schmidt & J. M. Brown (Eds.), *Evidence-based practice for nurses*. Sudbury, MA: Jones and Bartlett, p. 323. Modified with permission.

studies; size of the treatment effect; and relative risk or odds ratio strength (causality). *Consistency* refers to the similarity of findings across multiple studies regardless of differences in study design. These considerations make it essential that all types of evidence be considered when delivering individual care and implementing systems of care. Based on these domains of evidence,

a critical appraisal of types of studies can be facilitated and evaluated to determine the best approach for practice.

Quality Improvement and Patient-Centered Care

In patient care, a process that facilitates continuous improvement is central
to an environment that produces changes in practice that are patient centered
and focused on care that is both evidence based and of high quality. The
process must be based on a commitment by all those involved to change
practice, and this commitment must be made in advance so that the research
findings are applied early on in the process (French, 1999). As changes are
made, they must be continuously evaluated for their impact on care and care
systems. The EBP process is consistent with total quality improvement, and
often the same resources can be used for both processes.

The steps in the quality management, monitoring, and evaluation
processes are based on the work of William Edwards Deming, an American
author, professor, statistician, and consultant best known for his work in
improving manufacturing production efficiency during World War II.
Deming believed that quality is based on continuous improvement of
processes and that when work is focused on quality, costs decrease over time
(Deming, 1986).

As an advanced practice nurse, the DNP must be constantly attuned and
knowledgeable about changes in practice to ensure that current best practice is
maintained within the context of empirical evidence and patients' preferences.

Conceptual Frameworks for Evidence and Practice Change

Two conceptual frameworks that help in the promotion and translation of
evidence into practice are the PARIHS (promoting action on research implementation in health services) model (Rycroft-Malone et al., 2002) and the
AGREE (appraisal of guidelines for research and evaluation) model (AGREE
Collaboration, 2001). The PARIHS model, which is based on the work of
Kitson, Harvey, and McCormack (1998), suggests that the integration of evidence is based on three factors: the nature of the evidence, the context of
the desired change, and the mechanism of facilitating change. This evidence,
and its translation for practice, includes practice guidelines and other forms
of evidence specific to patient outcomes. The use of randomized controlled
trials was central to implementation of this model. The model was revised

by Rycroft-Malone et al. (2002) to include research information, clinical experience, and patient choice. In the new conceptualization, which involves continuous improvement of patient care through evidence-based nursing, there was recognition of a need for different types of evidence to answer some clinical questions. Evidence based on one's "professional craft" or experience was part of the evidence contribution (Rycroft-Malone et al., 2004).

Further work by Doran and Sidani (2007) identified gaps in the PARIHS model that led to an intervention framework that specifically addressed indicators for evaluating nursing services, systems, performance measures, and feedback to design and evaluate practice change. The intervention framework incorporates the work of Batalden and Stoltz (1993) and Batalden, Nelson, and Roberts (1994), which identified four categories of information in making care improvements. This information included "clinical (e.g. signs and symptoms), functional (e.g. activities of daily living), satisfaction (e.g. perceived benefit of care) and cost (i.e. both direct and indirect cost to the health care system and the patient)" (Doran & Sidani, 2007, p. 5). Figure 3-3 depicts Doran and Sidhani's (2007) outcomes-focused knowledge translation intervention framework.

The purpose of the AGREE instrument, as defined by the collaborators, "is to provide a framework for assessing the quality of clinical practice guidelines" (AGREE Collaboration, 2001, p. 2). Further, "by quality . . . we mean the confidence that the potential biases of guideline development have been addressed adequately and that the recommendations are both internally and externally valid, and are feasible for practice. This process involves taking into account the benefits, harms and costs of the recommendations, as well as the practical issues attached to them. Therefore, the assessment includes the judgments about the methods used for developing the guidelines, the content of the final recommendations, and the factors linked to their uptake" (p. 2). The AGREE instrument consists of 23 items organized in six domains: scope and purpose (items 1–3), stakeholder involvement (items 4–7), rigor of development (items 8–14), clarity and presentation (items 15–18), applicability (items 19–21), and editorial independence (items 22–23). The complete instrument and user guide are available for downloading from the Internet.

The nursing faculty at one family nurse practitioner program, the Lienhard School of Nursing at Pace University, used the AGREE instrument to teach family nurse practitioner students how to critically appraise clinical practice guidelines (Singleton & Levin, 2008). In this program, students

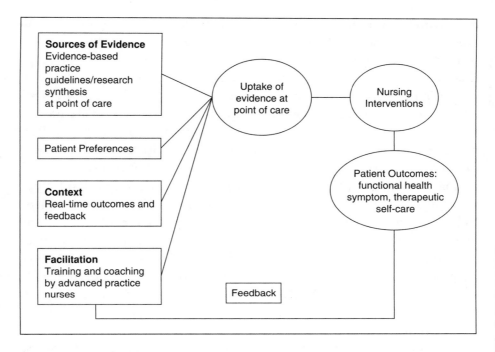

■ **Figure 3-3 Outcomes-Focused Knowledge Translation Intervention Framework**

Source: Doran, D. M., & Sidani, S. (2007). Outcomes-focused knowledge translation: A framework for knowledge translation and patient outcomes improvement. *Worldviews on Evidence-Based Nursing, 4*(1), 3–13. Reproduced with permission from Blackwell Publishing, Ltd.

practice critiquing single studies, systematic reviews, and clinical practice guidelines. Tables 3-4 and 3-5 present an exemplar of a learning activity using the AGREE instrument.

The Johns Hopkins model is another evidence-based model, which was developed as a collaborative effort between Johns Hopkins Hospital and the Johns Hopkins School of Nursing. The model is explained in six sections. Section I introduces the concept, the evolution of EBP, and the role of critical thinking in EBP. Section II describes the components of the model. The model uses the PET process (practice question, evidence, and translation). Section III further explores the PET process in developing EBP projects. Section IV describes the environment necessary for the success of EBP. Section V provides examples of EBP projects. Section VI contains tools used for EBP at Johns Hopkins. A table of contents and sample, including levels of evidence

■ Table 3-4   Learning Activity for the Critical Appraisal of Clinical Practice Guidelines

Steps

1. Preparatory reading:
   Slutsky, J. (2005). Using evidence-based practice guidelines: Tools for improving practice. In B. M. Melnyk & E. Fineout-Overholt (Eds.), *Evidence-based practice in nursing and healthcare: A guide to best practice* (pp. 221–227). Philadelphia: Lippincott Williams & Wilkins.
2. Focus for assignment:
   Academy of Breastfeeding Medicine. (2004). *Breastfeeding the near term infant (35–37 weeks gestation)*. New Rochelle, NY: Academy of Breastfeeding Medicine.
3. Work in teams.
4. Obtain the guideline.
5. Use the AGREE instrument to critically appraise the guideline.
6. Report back.

Source: Singleton, J., and Levin, R. (2008). Strategies for learning evidence-based practice: Critically appraising clinical practice guidelines. *Journal of Nursing Education, 47*(8), 380–383. Modified with permission.

■ Table 3-5   Sample Domain and Items from the AGREE Instrument for Critical Appraisal of Clinical Practice Guidelines, with Rating Scale

Scope and Purpose

The overall objective(s) of the guideline is (are) specifically described.

The clinical question(s) covered by the guideline is (are) specifically described.

The patients to whom the guideline(s) is (are) meant to apply are specifically described.

Rating Scale

Strongly agree	4	3	2	1	Strongly disagree	

Source: Singleton, J., and Levin, R. (2008). Strategies for learning evidence-based practice: Critically appraising clinical practice guidelines. *Journal of Nursing Education, 47*(8), 380–383. Modified with permission.

from the model and guidelines, can be downloaded from the Nursing Knowledge International website.

The model and guidelines have "leveled objectives" for baccalaureate-, graduate-, and doctoral-level nursing students. At the doctoral level, the focus is on reviewing, rating, synthesizing, evaluating, and translating evidence at an advanced level (Newhouse, Dearholt, Poe, Pugh, & White, 2008). An example of one evidence-based project, developed by the Neuroscience Nursing Practice Committee, is a question related to the correct procedure for establishing nasogastric tube placement in adult patients. Using the PICO (patient, intervention, comparison, and outcomes) format and levels of evidence, the existing protocol that required insufflations of air was discontinued. A table of the process and levels of evidence is shown in the Johns Hopkins model instructor's guide (Newhouse et al., 2008), available on the Internet.

Designing and Implementing Processes to Evaluate Outcomes of Practice and Systems of Care

As nursing moves practice decisions from those based on tradition to those based on empirical evidence, the advanced practice nurse, particularly the DNP, is in the best position to effect and assess change within the clinical setting. Why? Evidence-based practice and quality management are both practice-driven processes (French, 1999). Each is informed by experience and outcomes that can be directly seen and measured. In most cases, the observations and questions that arise during daily practice provide the basis for the questions, which can be empirically tested and their results implemented and evaluated. The findings of previous research studies can be replicated in a variety of settings with resources that are already in place.

The curriculum of Doctor of Nursing Practice programs includes specialty-focused competencies delineated by specialty nursing organizations, and the core essentials include courses and application experiences in research methods and statistical analysis (AACN, 2006). This education, coupled with advanced clinical knowledge, provides the DNP with the requisites necessary to design and collaborate in studies that can make a practical difference in the delivery of clinical care (French, 1999; Reavy & Tavernier, 2008). Table 3-6 lists some examples of clinical studies concerning advanced practice nursing interventions and outcomes, as well as studies or interventions designed by DNPs.

The *Essentials of Doctoral Education for Advanced Practice Nursing* (AACN, 2006) states that "DNP graduates must understand principles of practice management, including conceptual and practice strategies for balancing productivity and quality care" (p. 4). In addition, "they must be able to assess the impact of clinical policies and procedures on meeting the health needs

■ Table 3-6   Selected Studies of Advanced Practice Nursing
Interventions and Outcomes

Author and Date of Publication	Design, Sample, and Setting	Interventions	Outcome Variables	Findings
	Advanced Practice Nursing (APN) Interventions and Outcomes			
Scarbrough & Landis (1997)[a]	Descriptive. 431 patients on three units (FNPs); 821 patients on three units (MDs & RNs). Community hospital; 3-month study.	Evaluated two methods of implementing a hospital-based immunization program. Determined interest, obtained informed consent, administered vaccine, provided education, documented care.	Documentation on patient medication administration record	69 of 431 patients received vaccines in FNP group; 10 of 821 pts. received vaccine in MD/RN group. Conclusion: FNPs administered vaccine at a higher rate.
Naylor et al. (1999)[a]	Randomized controlled trial. Hospitalized adults older than 65 years at discharge. Intervention group (*n* = 177); control group (*n* = 186). Data at 2, 6, 12, and 24 weeks postdischarge at two urban academically affiliated medical centers.	APNs administered standardized discharge protocol for elders at risk for readmission. Included APN visits within 48 hours of admission, every 48 hours during admission, and two home visits within 48 hours of discharge and as needed. On-call availability 24 hours and weekly phone calls.	Readmissions; time to readmission; acute care visits after discharge; functional status; patient satisfaction; cost	Intervention-group patients had fewer hospital days per patient; time to first readmission was prolonged to 24 weeks. Medicare reimbursement was $0.6 million for intervention group vs. $1.2 million for control group. No significant differences in acute care visits, functional status, depression, or patient satisfaction. Conclusion: APN-centered discharge plan and home care intervention for

(continues)

■ Table 3-6   Selected Studies of Advanced Practice Nursing
Interventions and Outcomes (CONTINUED)

Author and Date of Publication	Design, Sample, and Setting	Interventions	Outcome Variables	Findings
		Advanced Practice Nursing (APN) Interventions and Outcomes		
				at-risk hospitalized older adults promotes positive outcomes and decreases cost.
Burns & Earven (2002)[a]	Descriptive. Patients requiring long-term ventilation in medical intensive care unit (MICU). N = 669 patients in 6-year period. Large university medical center.	APNs provided interventions based on pathways from scientific evidence. APNs worked on monitoring patient progress, prevention of complications, and coordinating care.	Length of stay (LOS); duration of ventilation; extubation status; reintubation; complications; discharge placement; cost	Decrease in the mean number of ventilator days; decreased mean LOS; decreased mean MICU LOS; decreased cost. Researchers concluded that APNs were effective in improving a number of outcomes in this population of highly complex patients.
		Studies by Doctors of Nursing Practice (DNPs)		
Andrews (2008)	Case study. Rare disease diagnosis: pheochromocytoma genetics, 40-year-old African American man with refractory hypertension presenting to ER.	Holistic evidence-based approach to clinical history taking and evaluation for correct diagnosis.	Lab tests; assessment of diagnostic clues and probability characteristics; genetic pedigree analysis; BP management; surgical intervention; genetic testing	Advanced practice nurses' well-honed evidence-based approach and interview skills allowed them to play a pivotal role in the exploration, diagnosis, and management of this type of complex situation.

■ Table 3-6 Selected Studies of Advanced Practice Nursing Interventions and Outcomes (CONTINUED)

Author and Date of Publication	Design, Sample, and Setting	Interventions	Outcome Variables	Findings
Studies by Doctors of Nursing Practice (DNPs)				
Doyle-Lindrud (2008)	Case study. Gestational breast cancer; 33-year-old Asian woman with breast lump and positive pregnancy test. Outpatient cancer center.	Health history and examination; health promotion; anticipatory guidance; collaborative approach to care; chronic disease management.	Lab tests; radiology; long-term follow-up care; psychosocial care; chronic care management	The DNP elements of doctoral competency were illustrated in the evaluation, collaboration, anticipatory planning, and management of care in this complex situation.
Dohrn (2008)	Case study. HIV treatment for pregnant women in rural Eastern Cape, South Africa, an area with 30–35% HIV prevalence and less than half of facilities providing prevention interventions. Pregnant women enter antenatal care after 24 weeks.	Design of midwifery model of care; interviews; observations; self-assessment of skills and capacity to deliver HIV care.	Voluntary testing and counseling; mother-to-child prevention intervention; antiretroviral treatment; peer counseling; community worker outreach; fast-tracking for antiretroviral therapy; maternity nurse training; anticipatory counseling; early postpartum care/education; midwife training; nurse mentoring; communication between nurses/MDs; strengthening community worker role.	Study resulted in consensus on model of care for HIV-infected women that included HIV prevention, testing, and management that has the potential to affect qualitatively and quantitatively the health of South Africans by decreasing the number of infants born with HIV, decreasing maternal mortality and the number of AIDS orphans, and improving quality of life.

aFrom Cunningham, R. S. (2004). Advanced practice nursing outcomes: A review of selected empirical literature. *Oncology Nursing Forum, 21*(2), 219–230.

of the patient populations with whom they practice" (p. 4). Also, "they must be proficient in quality improvement strategies and in creating and sustaining changes at the organizational and policy levels" (p. 4).

Quality Improvement Initiatives to Promote Safe, Timely, Effective, Efficient, Equitable, and Patient-Centered Care

The design of quality improvement initiatives must be empirically based and dependent on sources of knowledge that include research evidence, clinical experience, reasoning, authority, quality improvement data, and the patient's situation, values, and experience (Brown, 2005). These are the tools that can help the DNP decide whether the clinical guidelines and scientific evidence are consistent with the context, values, and desires of the patient (Glanville, Schirm, & Wineman, 2000).

For the past century, most outcome measurement has been focused on the outcomes of medical care, particularly negative outcomes. However, in the past several years there has been a greater focus on positive indicators of nursing care delivery (Melnyk & Fineout-Overholt, 2005). The development of nurse-sensitive patient outcomes (NSPOs) was an outgrowth of public demand for greater accountability by healthcare providers.

Some examples of nurse-sensitive indicators of quality include health-promoting behaviors (Mitchell, Ferketich, & Jennings, 1998), compliance/adherence (Ingersoll, McIntosh, & Williams, 2000), quality of life (Ingersoll et al., 2000), support systems available to assist with caregiver burden (Craft-Rosenburg, Krajicek, & Shin, 2002), trust in care provider (Ingersoll et al., 2000), and length of stay (Hodge, Asch, Olson, Kravitz, & Sauve, 2002). Table 3-7 presents additional examples of evidence-based outcome indicators.

The success of evidence-based practice depends on asking the right questions at the right time, critically analyzing results of other studies for fit in a given situation, observing for differences in responses, and evaluating. In this regard, quality improvement evaluation is important in advanced practice to ascertain the impact of interventions and their effect on cost-effective care. DNP and advanced practice nurse (APN) interventions are appropriately evaluated on the basis of physiological, psychosocial, functional, behavioral, and knowledge-focused effectiveness (Glanville et al., 2000). The evaluation process involves the selection of appropriate measurement instruments. Glanville et al. (2000) make the point that instruments that measure effec-

■ Table 3-7   Selected Evidence-Based Outcome Indicators for Advanced Practice Nursing

Outcomes	Examples and Indicators
Patient satisfaction	Ambulatory care: Survey
Risk	Morbidity and mortality: Summary Patient falls: Reports Medication errors: Medication administration records (MARs); comprehensiveness of exams
Knowledge	Blood pressure medication: Blood pressure control
Condition specific	Postoperative pain: Pain management scale Diabetes management: Blood glucose levels
Infection control	Surgical procedures: Hand washing; nosocomial infection rates
Compliance	Fluid restriction: Daily weights Prenatal and postpartum visits

tiveness in care processes are not the same as those that measure outcomes. For example, a tool that measures risk for patient infections is not the same tool as one that actually tracks infection rates in a group of postsurgical patients. Similarly, in process management the focus is on which components produce or contribute to practice variations that may ultimately affect, but are not the same as, outcomes (Ingersoll, 2005).

Some basic provisions for an effective outcomes model are to keep the outcomes as short as possible; to use outcomes, not activities or processes; and to use singular, not compound, outcomes (Duignan, 2006). Components of an effective outcomes management model include the following:

1) identification of the problem, 2) scanning the existing evidence and standards of care, 3) identification of benchmark targets, 4) determination and selection of outcomes measuring and monitoring tools, 5) development of specific guidelines to drive care delivery processes, 6) assessment of existing processes, 7) measurement and monitoring of processes and outcomes of care, 8) reporting findings to key stakeholders and decision makers, and 9) refining care delivery processes and data collection techniques based on findings. (Ingersoll, 2005, pp. 314–315)

A significant time commitment is required for designing systems for promoting safe, timely, patient-centered care. However, the benefits are efficiency and effectiveness. Since the Institute of Medicine (IOM) studies, patient safety has been a primary focus of quality improvement initiatives. Safety issues are of concern in every care setting—primary, secondary, and tertiary. A review of the literature from 1995 to 2009 in the Medline and CINAHL databases produced 136 (Medline) and 51 (CINAHL) nursing studies that involved quality improvement projects with safety as a focus. Only 4 studies included the word *evidence* in the title. Topics included studies on drug errors, environment, technology, acute care, pediatrics, critical care, culture, intravenous infusions, long-term care and home health, rural health, legislation and oversight, policy, diabetes, anesthesia, health education, chemotherapy, childhood vaccines, blood and HIV, neuroscience issues, food and drug issues, nurse injury, radiation, emergency services, and behavioral health. In addition to safety issues, a number of studies dealt with issues of timely (24 studies in CINAHL), effective (13,000 studies in CINAHL), and equitable care (467 studies in CINAHL), which are also important dimensions of quality and need to be addressed, especially as they affect safety and quality outcomes. Patient-centered care was addressed in 6,100 CINAHL studies. Direct care providers, including DNPs, must take a lead role in continuing the effort to improve care delivery systems that benefit patients, families, and providers of care.

Using Practice Guidelines to Improve Practice and the Practice Environment

As Goolsby, Meyers, Johnson, Klardie, and McNaughton (2004) have noted, "clinical practice guidelines are protocol-driven, step-wise recommendations for diagnosing, and treating specific conditions, or patient populations" (p. 178). Clinical decision making is grounded in the use of clinical research, expert opinion, and clinical practice guidelines. Further, clinical practice guidelines "minimize differences in practice patterns and the risk of misdiagnosis or treatment failures" (Goolsby, Meyers, et al., 2004, p. 178). Unfortunately, practice guidelines are not always used, for a variety of reasons. Time, communication, involvement, resources, patient expectations, and perceived priority are all facilitators or barriers to the implementation of evidence-based practice guidelines (DiCenso, Cullum, & Ciliska, 1998; Gagan

& Hewitt-Taylor, 2004; Lopez-Bushnell, 2002; McCaughan, Thompson, Cullum, Sheldon, & Thompson, 2002; Rutledge & Bookbinder, 2002).

One way to eliminate some of the barriers is through the use of "linkage agents." As described by Cooke et al. (2004), advanced practice nurses (particularly DNPs) are in an excellent position to propose scientifically based recommendations to reduce cost and improve quality, documentation, and outcomes. In developing an institutional change model to promote evidence-based practice with cancer patients, the linking agents from the nursing research department at one hospital functioned as rotating consultants three to four hours per month. The linking agent consultants rotated to clinical units for one hour of monthly case presentation and analysis to assist clinical nurses in translating research into practice. The theoretical framework used was a quality of life model with four domains: psychological, social, physical, and spiritual (Padilla, Ferrell, Grant, & Rhiner, 1990). Each month one or more topics related to the four domains was discussed relevant to a case study. A brief five-minute lecture was presented on EBP principles at the beginning of the session. The program started as a research outreach program and evolved into an EBP program that linked a case study format with critical thinking and practical application. This approach could be modified and used in a variety of clinical practice settings.

Evaluation of Practice

He who every morning plans the transaction of the day and follows out that plan, carries a thread that will guide him through the maze of the most busy life. But where no plan is laid, where the disposal of time is surrendered merely to the chance of incidence, chaos will soon reign.

—VICTOR HUGO

Evaluating practice and changes in practice are essential to the successful implementation of any quality improvement or evidence-based practice initiative. Evaluation is an ongoing process that must start early in a project and be continual. Planning for evaluation is as important as the change itself and must be a systematic process. Classification schemes allow an organized approach to evaluating outcomes. Outcomes may be classified according to population served (e.g., pediatric, adult, geriatric), time (long term, medium term, or short term), or type (care related, patient related, or performance related) (Schmidt & Brown, 2009).

Using Benchmarks to Evaluate Clinical Outcomes and Trends

One method of evaluating practice is to evaluate practice patterns against national benchmarks to determine variances in clinical outcomes and population trends. Benchmarking is "the continual process of measuring services and practices against the toughest competitors in the industry" (Hebda & Czar, 2009). Organizations that regularly collect data on outcomes in health care are state boards of health and the Centers of Medicare and Medicaid Services (CMS). The Joint Commission on Accreditation of Hospitals (JCAHO) and the Magnet Recognition Program (American Nurses Credentialing Center, 2005) also have performance measurement standards that are based on quality indicators. In addition to these organizations, many hospitals and healthcare facilities have memberships in organizations that benchmark indicators of quality in specialty services (Schmidt & Brown, 2009).

Nursing services are an important aspect of outcome evaluation and reporting at any healthcare institution because nurses make up such a large part of the healthcare workforce. Effectiveness of nursing care is determined by nurse-sensitive indicators. Nursing administrators are responsible for maintaining evaluation systems and reporting nurse-sensitive outcomes. As leaders in clinical care and outcome evaluation, DNPs must be in the forefront of designing outcome evaluation plans for advanced practice.

DNPs in advanced practice roles are also included in medical outcome working groups within their scope of practice. The American Medical Association–Physician Consortium for Performance Improvement (AMA-PCPI) has performance measures available for 31 topics or conditions (Gallagher, 2009). The general approach to measurement includes six steps: "1) identifying the opportunities for improvement, 2) involving representation from medical specialties and other care disciplines, 3) linking measures to an evidence base, 4) supporting clinical judgment and patient preferences, 5) testing measures, and 6) promoting a single set of measures for widespread use and multiple purpose" (Gallagher, 2009, p. 185). Table 3-8 contains a brief listing of websites for healthcare outcomes and data.

Guiding Database Design to Generate Meaningful Evidence for Nursing Practice

A systematic process for patient care and practice data is essential to guide practice. This requires the development of standardized databases to guide

■ Table 3-8   Websites for Healthcare Outcome Information

Organization	Website
AcademyHealth	http://www.academyhealth.org
Agency for Healthcare Research and Quality	http://www.ahrq.gov/clinic/outcome.htm
Centers for Medicare and Medicaid Services	http://www.cns.hhs.gov/home/rsds.asp
Health Care Excel	http://hce.org
Institute for Healthcare Improvement	http://www.ihi.org
The Joint Commission	http://www.jointcommission.org
National Cancer Institute	http://outcomes.cancer.gov
National Committee for Quality Assurance	http://www.ncqa.org
National Quality Forum	http://www.qualityforum.org
University of Iowa College of Nursing	http://www.nursing.uiowa.edu/excellence/ nursing_knowledge/clinical_effectiveness/ nocoverview.htm

Source: Rich, K. A. (2009). Evaluating outcomes of innovations. In N. A. Schmidt & J. M. Brown (Eds.), Evidence-based practice for nurses. Sudbury, MA: Jones and Bartlett, p. 388. Modified with permission.

outcomes research for practice. Clinical databases from computerized medical records and disease registries exist as the result of documentation of care or research protocols. Outcome data are also available from birth logs, death records, discharge summaries, and clinical pathways. Most important, the outcome must be measurable and the data must relate to the care processes or interventions (Arthur, Marfell, & Ulrich, 2009).

Another useful resource for evidence based on outcomes is the National Guideline Clearinghouse (NGC), an initiative of the Agency for Healthcare Quality and Research (AHRQ), the American Medical Association, and America's Health Insurance Plans (AHIP). Users can subscribe to the NGC weekly e-mail update service. The site provides information about new and updated guidelines from the Centers for Disease Control and Prevention (CDC), the National Institute for Clinical Excellence (NICE), the Program for

Evidence-Based Care (PEBC), and others. Conference information is also available, as well as food and drug advisory information.

The Cochrane Collaboration Review is another source that provides reprints online of the newest intervention reviews. The *Review* lists authors and their affiliations; an abstract including background, objectives, search strategies, selection criteria, data collection, and analysis; authors' conclusions; and a plain-language summary. The library contains sections for clinicians, researchers, patients, and policy makers. The Cochrane Library, a collection of medical and healthcare databases, is available online through Wiley Inter-Science. Podcasts are also available.

These and other evidence-based resources are effective tools to aid in the efficient delivery of evidence-based care. Table 3-9 provides a brief description of other available databases. The use of these resources is valuable when combined with the best empirical knowledge and judgment. The true measure of their effectiveness is in the evaluation of the outcomes of management and care decisions and delivery processes.

As nursing takes on larger, more autonomous roles in the delivery of health care through advanced practice, the need for accountability will continue to increase. DNPs, with their knowledge of clinical practice, research, and informatics, can best represent advanced practice nursing by participating in and guiding the development of databases that are relevant to the care that DNPs and advanced practice nurses provide. Becoming involved in professional organizations that have quality initiatives is an excellent way for DNPs to become knowledgeable in research that contributes to quality care and the profession. The ANA and specialty organizations such as the Oncology Nursing Society, the Advanced Practice Registered Nurses' Research Network, and the Midwest Nursing Centers Consortium Research Network, a practice-based research network funded by the AHRQ, provide avenues for collaboration and dissemination of information on quality and outcomes (Burns & Grove, 2009).

The Use of Information Technology and Research Methods

Computers have changed the face of clinical care, making them a necessary tool for research and evidence-based practice. They provide efficiency in the inputting of statistical data and the retrieval of the most current information on relevant clinical trial outcomes, supportive research, and accepted

■ Table 3-9   Evidence Databases

Source	Content
ACP Journal Club	Articles reporting original studies and systematic reviews.
Agency for Healthcare Quality and Research (AHRQ)	Produces guidelines and technology assessments on selected topics from 12 evidence-based practice centers.
AIDSLINE	Indexes the published literature on HIV and AIDS. The index includes journal articles, monographs, meeting abstracts and papers, newsletters, and government reports (Fain, 2009).
Bandolier	Reviews literature; offers subjects by medical specialty.
CANCERLIT	Includes cancer literature from journal articles, government reports, technical reports, meeting abstracts and papers, and monographs.
CDC Sexually Transmitted Disease Treatment Guidelines	Includes Web-browseable source with crosslinks.
Cochrane Database of Systematic Reviews	"[R]eviews individual clinical trials and summarizes systematic reviews from over 100 medical journals" (Fain, 2009, p. 277).
DynaMed	Point-of-care resource to support clinical decision making.
EPPI	Evidence for Policy and Practice Information and Coordinating Center, Institute of Education, University of London.
Essential Evidence Plus (Formerly InfoPOEMS)	Includes reviews and commentary of recently published articles by the Journal of Family Practice.
Evidence Based Practice at the University of Iowa (http://www.uihealthcare.com/depts/nursing/rqom/evidencebasedpractice/index.html)	Includes an evidence-based practice toolkit, information about recent evidence-based practice projects, and an evidence-based practice model and resources.
HealthLinks: Evidence Based Practice (http://healthlinks.washington.edu/ebp)	Includes metasearch engines and links to peer-reviewed journals, a DNP toolkit, and other publications.

(continues)

■ Table 3-9   **Evidence Databases** (CONTINUED)

Source	Content
HealthSTAR	Indexes materials from books, book chapters, government documents, newspaper articles, and technical reports. The focus is the clinical and nonclinical aspects of healthcare delivery.
HSTAT	Health Services Technology Assessment Text; full-text guidelines.
Joanna Briggs Institute	International institute that provides resources for evidence-based practice for healthcare professionals in nursing, medicine, midwifery, and allied health.
Johns Hopkins Evidence-Based Practice Center Projects	Includes systematic reviews of evidence.
MD Consult	Includes full-text access to journal articles, textbooks, practice guidelines, patient education handouts, and drug awareness information. MD Consult is a good, quick source for background information on a topic.
MEDLINE	A compilation of information from Index Medicus, Index to Dental Literature, and the International Nursing Index. It includes published research in allied health, biological sciences, information sciences, physical sciences, and the humanities.
MedPage Today	Includes daily research updates, news by specialty, policy news, CMEs, and surveys. Includes an excellent tool, The MedPage Guide to Biostatistics, that can be used as a reference guide when reading research articles.
National Guideline Clearinghouse	Provides nonintegrated evidence-based practice clinical guidelines and recommendations on selected topics from a number of organizations.
Prescriber's Letter	Includes evidence-based information on new drug developments, with links to articles and continuing education offerings.
PubMed	Provides source for queries and evidence-based filters for Medline.

■ Table 3-9   Evidence Databases (CONTINUED)

Source	Content
ScHarr	School of Health and Related Research; comprehensive, up-to-date evidence on the Web.
TRIPCeRes	British meta-search engine. Covers 58 different resources for evidence.
University of Minnesota (http://evidence.abc.umn.edu/ebn.htm)	Links and EBP tutorial with case scenarios.

Source: Fain, J. A. (2009). *Understanding evidence-based practice. Reading, understanding and applying nursing research* (3rd ed.). Philadelphia: F. A. Davis, pp. 276–278. Modified with permission.

practice protocols. It is essential to pay attention to the kind of data that is retrieved and how it is used to make clinical decisions and evaluate practice. Please see Chapter 4 for further discussion of the use of technology in advanced practice nursing.

Collecting Appropriate and Accurate Data

Data and observations from practice can be augmented and strengthened through evidence from clinical trials. There are several electronic databases that provide access to clinical trial data and other peer-reviewed research and outcome data. However, clinical trial data and data from other aggregate sources do not always address the outcomes that can be uniquely attributed to APN/DNP practice. In order for APN/DNPs to assess and demonstrate their effectiveness, data are needed that reflect what they do. Although the primary goal of outcome data and analysis is to improve care, DNPs in direct practice may be asked to justify their roles in terms of factors such as cost, time, patient outcomes, and revenue generation, among other indicators (Burns, 2009).

Most institutions rely on aggregated data to determine nursing outcomes. Unfortunately, most aggregated data do not show the APN/DNP's specific contribution to the outcomes (Burns, 2009). For this reason it is important that measures be selected that truly reflect the APN/DNP role. This means developing role-sensitive indicators and collecting data that are specific to those indicators in a systematic way. Indicators such as satisfaction with APN/DNP care related to a particular program or procedure that the APN/DNP initiates, controls, or coordinates are better than trying to extrapolate the APN/DNP's role in a multidisciplinary effort. Time savings or clinical outcomes related to a change in practice coordinated by the APN/DNP may also be role sensitive.

A well-designed assessment plan uses a model that considers organizational factors, employee behavior, patient characteristics, patient experience, and outcomes (Minnick & Roberts, 1991, Figure 4.1, as cited in Minnick, 2009). Instruments for measuring outcomes are also a necessary component in the assessment process. A systematic search of the databases mentioned in Table 3-9, such as AHRQ, PubMed, CancerLit, CINAHL, and PsycINFO, may be helpful as a starting place for appropriate measurement tools.

Analyzing Data from Clinical Practice

Data from practice are rich and can be analyzed in a number of ways, depending on the nature of the research question. Computer-based statistical tools such as absolute risk (AR) and absolute risk reduction (ARR) calculations, relative risk (RR) and relative risk reduction (RRR) calculations, number needed to treat (NNT), survival curves, hazard ratios, and sensitivity and specificity are helpful measures for assessing risk of disease in studies of different cohort groups and in aiding clinical decision making. In an excellent article in the *Journal of the American Academy of Nurse Practitioners,* Goolsby, Klardie, Johnson, McNaughton, and Meyers (2004) analyzed the implementation of clinical practice guidelines (CPGs) and their outcomes in a hypothetical patient situation. The analysis includes a review of commonly used statistical concepts, including some of those just mentioned, with examples of their application in interpreting and reporting research. Johnston (2005) also provides a detailed section on statistical measures and their meaning in a chapter entitled "Critically Appraising Quantitative Evidence."

Designing Evidence-Based Interventions

Selecting and defining the problem is one of the most critical steps in the design of any evidence-based intervention. The problem statement provides the direction for the study design and is usually stated at the beginning. Essential to good design is adequate background information that includes a rationale for pursuing an intervention, evidence from research that has already been done on the topic, and the goals to be achieved (Fain, 2009). Depending on the problem to be addressed, evidence-based interventions may be generated from quantitative research, qualitative research, outcome studies, patient concerns and choices, or clinical judgment.

Models serve as good frameworks for design. Several models that were originally designed for research utilization were the historical precursors to evidence-based practice. Three well-known models for research utilization and evidence-based practice include the conduct and utilization of research in nursing (CURN) model (Horsely, Crane, & Bingle, 1978), the Kitson model (Kitson, Harvey, & McCormack, 1998), the Stetler/Marram model (Stetler, 1994; Stetler & Marram, 1976), and the Iowa model of research utilization (Titler et al., 1994). As evidence-based practice has evolved, these models have been adapted, and other models have been developed. Some later models include the ARCC model (Melnyk & Fineout-Overholt, 2002), the Rosswurm and Larrabee model (1999), the Iowa model of evidence-based practice to promote quality care (Titler, 2002), and the Johns Hopkins model (Newhouse et al., 2005). Each of these models has been successful in disseminating research or in facilitating change toward evidence-based practice. Figure 3-4 shows a schematic of the Iowa model.

It is beyond the scope of this chapter to detail the specifics of each model. However, although there are nuances and structural differences, all of the models support some form of practice change through the systematic review of research and other evidence, such as clinical practice guidelines, to create a culture of research conduct and research utilization. Certainly, the first step in the design of any practice intervention is to define the clinical practice questions. Once that is accomplished, critical questions include the following: What patients will be affected? What treatment or intervention or practice change is involved? What old practice would need to be discontinued? What outcomes are expected? (Collins et al., 2008). The next step is to review the evidence, basing the analysis on the hierarchy of evidence (see Table 3-1) and a search of all relevant databases (e.g., Cochrane, CINAHL, National Guideline Clearing House). Once the evidence has been verified, assessing applicability to the population and environment is crucial. Questions to be considered may include the following: Will implementing this practice increase patient safety? Are there ethical or legal considerations? Will other departments or providers be affected? How will the change affect practitioner time? How will patients react to the change? The next step is to develop a plan for the change. Who are the key stakeholders? How will they be apprised and included? Who has final sign-off authority? Is a pilot study indicated before full-scale implementation? Finally, determine the methods of education and communication. How much time, cost, and personnel resources will be needed?

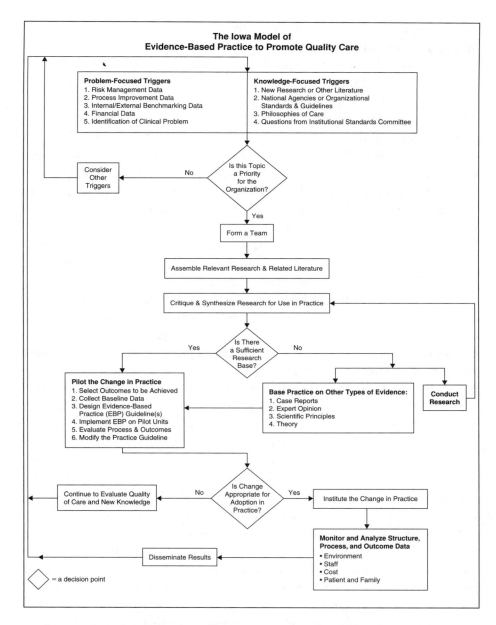

■ Figure 3-4   The Iowa Model of Evidence-Based Practice to Promote Quality Care

Source: Titler, M. G., Kleiber, C., Steelman, V. J., Rakel, B. A., Budreau, G., Everett, L. Q., et al. (2001). The Iowa model of evidence-based practice to promote quality care. *Critical Care Nursing Clinics of North America, 13*(4), 497–509. Reproduced with permission.

When implementing the plan, the following questions should be considered: Who is responsible for coordinating the effort? What contingency plans are in place in the event a change must be made? Who is managing issues that may arise? Evaluate the implementation on an ongoing basis. How will feedback be generated? Who will conduct the evaluation? What is the method of analysis? What are the measurement tools? How will results of the evaluation be presented? (Collins et al., 2008). Some specific strategies to promote guideline implementation are outlined by Carey, Buchan, and Sanson-Fisher (2009). Table 3-10 summarizes their recommendations.

Predicting and Analyzing Outcomes

Often in clinical practice the occurrence of one event in time may be the basis for predicting a future event. In such instances a predictive relationship is established. In this case, the practitioner or researcher is looking for a correlation between the two events that may predict the outcome of a future intervention or occurrence that could be designed to affect or influence the independent variable. Although correlational prediction is not the same as cause and effect, it is stronger than a purely descriptive study (Melnyk & Cole, 2005). This type of study would be appropriate if, for example, the DNP were interested in how a person's initial attitude toward insulin affected compliance with the regimen 3, 6, or 12 months after the therapy began.

Correlation statistics would be used to measure the relationship between the two variables. The results of the correlation could later be used to design interventions, such as educational strategies or follow-up programs, that would help those with negative attitudes toward therapy learn, adapt, and achieve more positive outcomes. Correlational statistics are also used to measure the strength of relationship between two variables. A direct correlation is seen in correlation coefficients between the values of 0 (no correlation) and 1 (large positive correlation) and means that when there is a large change in the value of one predictor, there is a large change in the value of the other predictor; likewise, a small change in one predictor is accompanied by a small change in the other predictor. A relationship that has a correlation coefficient of 0.5 is stronger than 0, but less than 1.0. Conversely, in a negative correlation—between 0 (no correlation) and –1 (large negative correlation)—large changes in the value of one predictor would be accompanied by small changes in the other, or small changes in one would be accompanied by large changes

■ Table 3-10   Strategies to Promote Guideline Implementation:
Theoretical Constructs and Examples of Application

Strategy	Relevant Constructs	Key Illustrative Examples
	Phase 1	
Concrete and specific recommendations	Knowledge, executability, decidability	Concrete and specific recommendations were more likely to be adopted by general practitioners (GPs) than vague, nonspecific recommendations. Observational study. (Grol et al., 1998)
Identify priorities	Goal setting, action planning	Of 228 primary care patients with cardiovascular disease risk factors who made an action plan to identify behavioral change goals, 53% also reported making behavioral change related to their action plan. Descriptive study. (Handley et al., 2006)
Set targets for implementation	Goal setting	
Present a rationale	Beliefs, attitudes, perceived relative advantage	Recommendations compatible with current values were more likely to be adopted by GPs than those perceived as controversial or incompatible with values. Observational study. (Grol et al., 1998)
Highlight clinical norms	Normative beliefs, attitudes, modeling/verbal persuasion	An intervention to improve myocardial infarction care that involved using local medical opinion leaders to influence peers through small-group discussions, informal consultation, and revisions of clinical protocols was compared with performance feedback alone. Hospitals in both groups improved from baseline to follow-up on indicators of quality; however, the improvement was greatest for those allocated to the peer intervention. Randomized controlled trial. (Soumerai et al., 1998)
Orient to the need of the end user	Complexity	Among the guideline characteristics most commonly endorsed to promote use by GPs was "clarity, simplicity and availability of a short format." Descriptive study of 391 GPs. (Watkins et al., 1999)

■ Table 3-10 Strategies to Promote Guideline Implementation:
Theoretical Constructs and Examples of Application (CONTINUED)

Strategy	Relevant Constructs	Key Illustrative Examples
		Phase 2
Skills training	Skills, knowledge, self-efficacy	Continuing medical education (CME) improves knowledge, skills, attitudes, and patient outcomes. CME that is interactive, uses multimedia, live media, and involves multiple exposures is more effective than other types. Systematic review. (Marinopoulos et al., 2007)
Social influences	Normative beliefs, attitudes, modeling, verbal persuasion	The use of local opinion leaders in hospital settings can be effective in promoting evidence-based practice. Systematic review of 12 studies. (Doumitt et al., 2007)
Environmental influences	Cues to action, environmental triggers	Guideline adherence improved due to the implementation of a computerized clinical decision aid that gave clinicians real-time recommendations for venous thromboembolism prophylaxis. Time series study. (Durieux et al., 2000)
Patient-mediated	Knowledge, skills, and attitudes of patients	Patient request for a new drug and patient acceptability were cited as contributing to decisions to prescribe a new drug in approximately 20% of cases. Descriptive study. (Prosser, Almond, & Walley, 2003)
Feedback	Positive/negative reinforcement; goal setting; skill development	Audit and feedback are effective strategies for improving care, particularly when baseline adherence to the recommended practice is low. Systematic review of 118 studies. (Jamtvedt et al., 2006)
Incentives	Positive/negative reinforcement	Five of six studies examining physician-level incentives, and seven of nine studies examining provider group–level incentives demonstrated partial or positive effects on quality indicators. Systematic review. (Peterson et al., 2006)

(continues)

■ Table 3-10   Strategies to Promote Guideline Implementation:
Theoretical Constructs and Examples of Application (CONTINUED)

Strategy	Relevant Constructs	Key Illustrative Examples
		Phase 3
Pilot testing with iterative refinement of implementation strategies	Perceived advantages; beliefs; trialability	Breakthrough collaborative model intervention that involved a series of iterative plan-do-study-act cycles was found to be effective in improving care for chronic heart failure. Quasi-experimental, controlled study. (Asch et al., 2005)

Source: Carey, M., Buchan, H., & Sanson-Fisher, R. (2009). The cycle of change: Implementing the best evidence clinical practice. *The International Journal for Quality in Health Care, 21*(1), 37–43. Reproduced with permission.

in the other. Therefore, a negative correlation coefficient of –0.6 shows a stronger negative relationship between two variables than a coefficient of 0, but not as strong as a coefficient of –1.0 (Lanthier, 2009).

An example of this kind of analysis is shown in a correlation study on salary and income levels. Table 3-11 shows salary levels and corresponding years of education. Figure 3-5 shows an example of a correlation scatter plot, with years of education on the y axis and income on the x axis. Each point on the plot shows one person's answers to the questions regarding years of education and income. In a positive correlation such as this, the line is always in the upward direction. In another example, Table 3-12 and Figure 3-6 show a negative relationship between grade point average (GPA) and number of hours watching television. The scatter plot (Figure 3-6) shows the direction of the line when the correlation is negative. In these cases, the researcher is measuring conditions that already exist and looking for relationships—either positive or negative.

EXAMINING PATTERNS OF BEHAVIOR AND OUTCOMES

Although much of the research and evidence for practice is focused on cause and effect, patterns of behavior, dispositions, and attitudes are also outcomes that require examination. Behavioral theories can be classified as intrapersonal (individual), interpersonal (relational), and community based. The stages of change model (Prochaska & DiClemente, 1986), the health belief model

■ Table 3-11   Salary and Years of Education

Participant	Income	Years of Education
#1	125,000	19
#2	100,000	20
#3	40,000	16
#4	35,000	16
#5	41,000	18
#6	29,000	12
#7	35,000	14
#8	24,000	12
#9	50,000	16
#10	60,000	17

Source: Lanthier, E. (2002). *Correlation*. http://www.nvcc.edu/home/elanthier/methods/correlations-samples.htm. Copyright 2002 by Elizabeth Lanthier, PhD. Reproduced with permission.

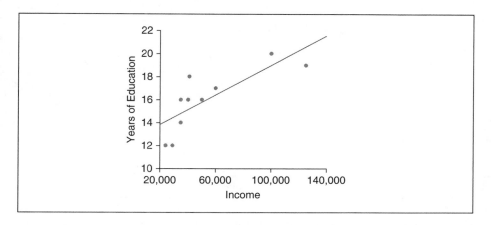

■ Figure 3-5   Regression Scatter Plot, Salary, and Education in Years

Source: Lanthier, E. (2002). *Correlation*. http://www.nvcc.edu/home/elanthier/methods/correlations-samples.htm. Copyright 2002 by Elizabeth Lanthier, PhD. Reproduced with permission.

■ Table 3-12   Grade Point Average and TV Use

Participant	GPA	TV Use (hr/wk)
#1	3.1	14
#2	2.4	10
#3	2.0	20
#4	3.8	7
#5	2.2	25
#6	3.4	9
#7	2.9	15
#8	3.2	13
#9	3.7	4
#10	3.5	21

Source: Lanthier, E. (2002). *Correlation.* http://www.nvcc.edu/home/elanthier/methods/correlations-samples.htm. Copyright 2002 by Elizabeth Lanthier, PhD. Reproduced with permission.

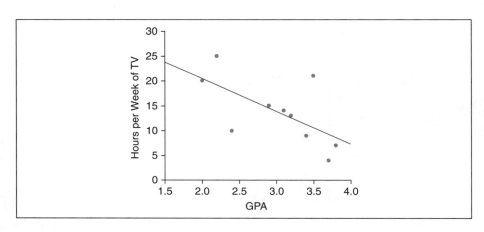

■ Figure 3-6   Regression Scatter Plot, Hours of Television Use, and Grade Point Average

Source: Lanthier, E. (2002). *Correlation.* http://www.nvcc.edu/home/elanthier/methods/correlations-samples.htm. Copyright 2002 by Elizabeth Lanthier, PhD. Reproduced with permission.

(Rosenstock, 1966), and the theory of reasoned action (Fishbein & Ajzen, 1980) are useful in examining behaviors and their relationship to outcomes.

One way of examining data is through the use of aggregated data derived from large data sets. Organizations such as AHRQ, the CDC, the National Institute for Child Health and Development (NICHD), and the National Institutes of Health (NIH) have large national data sets from various sources, such as quality of life surveys, hospital discharge data, and infection control data. The data sets can be accessed or purchased to allow researchers to develop clinical, behavioral, or interventional outcome questions that can be statistically analyzed. The advantage of this kind of analysis is that the data sets are large enough to provide an adequate sample and effect size from which to generalize intervention effects. AHRQ also maintains a database of comparative effectiveness reviews that synthesizes information from the most current studies on numerous diseases through the Evidence-Based Practice Centers (AHRQ, 2009).

In addition to aggregated evidence, clinical trial data, and comparative effectiveness reviews, some innovative healthcare systems are bringing "'practice-based evidence' to the bedside or work setting in aggregate form so that providers have the most up-to-date information available on outcomes *before* evidence based interventions are begun" (Lambert & Burlingame, 2009, p. 1). As an example, this kind of decision support has been trialed in the Mental Health Services Centers for the state of Utah. The state partnered with an outcomes measurement vendor (OQ, LLC) to provide aggregated evidence from clinical trials and laboratory research that resulted in a five-minute self-report outcome measurement for patients in any setting—outpatient, inpatient, or residential. Adult patients use a handheld personal digital assistant (PDA), computer kiosk, or paper survey to report information to clinicians based on the domains of symptomatic distress, interpersonal relations, and functional ability. Adolescents and parent/guardians provide information on age-normed questionnaires. The scoring is derived from empirically tested software that alerts the provider that a patient is at risk for a less than optimal outcome from treatment and gives the care provider options for consideration using a clinical decision support tree. According to the designers, the advantage of this kind of tracking is that the system provides immediate evidence-based support for direct patient care. Furthermore, it provides a method for storing data for future review, evaluation, and benchmarking (Lambert & Burlingame, 2009). Use and expansion of this kind of system to document and support clinical practice and scholarship would be an easy transition for nurses who are familiar with the use of PDAs "to support the application of current standards, and knowledge for clinical decision making" (Stroud, Erkel, & Smith, 2005).

IDENTIFYING GAPS IN EVIDENCE FOR PRACTICE

In a systematic analysis of reviews published by the Joanna Briggs Institute between 1998 and 2002, high-quality evidence to support nursing interventions was not evident (Averis & Pearson, 2003). Further, the report identified considerable gaps in the evidence base available for nurses in relation to 22 discrete areas of practice that were examined in the analysis. However, the impetus to improve patient safety generated by the IOM reports *To Err Is Human* (Kohn, Corrigan, & Donaldson, 2000), *Crossing the Quality Chasm* (IOM, 2001), and *Health Professions Education: A Bridge to Quality* (IOM, 2003) and the availability of support for EBP through educational restructuring and systems support are increasing.

Nevertheless, gaps in the evidence remain. Research by nurses and family physicians suggests that a translational model to fill the gaps is necessary (Armson et al., 2007; Gumei, Tiedje, & Oweis, 2007). One such model, developed in Canada, uses a small, self-formed group-discussion format within local communities. The impetus for this model was the need to stay competent in view of the vast amount of medical information currently available. In these groups a facilitator guides physicians' discussion using sample patient cases and prepared modules on selected clinical topics. The groups have been ongoing for 15 years and have attracted international interest (Armson et al., 2007; Kelly, Cunningham, McCalister, Cassidy, & MacVicar, 2007). Nurses engage in similar forums in hospital grand rounds, within their professional specialty organizations, and at regional and national conferences. However, collaborative engagement needs to be broader and more systematic. DNPs are in an excellent position to initiate this kind of practice-based dialogue in community-based practice settings.

The American Nurses Association, the American Association of Colleges of Nursing, the National Organization of Nurse Practitioner Faculties, and professional nursing organizations in each specialty all have agendas for advancing research and evidence for practice in their respective areas. As examples, the American Academy of Nurse Practitioners, Nurse Practitioner Associates for Continuing Education (NPACE), and the Practicing Clinicians Exchange provide excellent forums for translating current research into practice and for networking with peers about research and clinical outcome information.

The JCAHO, the National Database of Nursing Quality Indicators, and individual hospital report cards may be used as sources of research or outcome analysis to identify gaps in care delivery or in patient or staff education in particular institutions or practice groups. Examples include adverse events, smoking cessation, rates of adherence to best practice, blood glucose control, patient satisfaction rates, time spent with patients, tests ordered, and number of consultations (care related); knowledge, functional status, and access to care (patient related); and collaboration, technical quality, exam comprehensiveness, and adherence to guidelines (performance related) (Kleinpell, 2009). Within these and other categories, the gaps may be identified through the development of a specific plan based on target areas of APN practice. Planning questions should include the following: What exactly can be measured? How can it be measured? What will be done with the information? When should it be done? (Kleinpell, 2007). Figure 3-7 shows a sample timeline for outcome assessment.

As advanced practice nursing evolves into the DNP role, it will be imperative that direct care providers, senior-level nurse executives, and doctorally prepared nurse educators take lead roles in quality improvement to positively affect patient safety (O'Grady, 2008). Identifying, testing, and disseminating information about nurse-sensitive quality indicators is essential to close the gap in quality care delivery. All advanced practice nurses prepared at the clinical doctorate level must be involved in this effort.

Participation in Collaborative Research

It is a credit to the profession of nursing and its leaders that there are several evidence-based practice centers in the United States: the American Nurses Association National Center for Nursing Quality, Sigma Theta Tau International, the National Institute of Nursing Research (NINR) at the NIH, and centers at many of the major university schools of nursing. However, as O'Grady (2008) notes, turf battles have limited collaboration. On the macro level, "APN organizations along with governmental and private research enterprise must come together to develop a research plan that identifies the most critical research questions" (O'Grady, 2008, p. 12). On the micro and macro levels, APNs individually and as a group must "demonstrate specific clinical performance and patient outcomes" (O'Grady, 2008, p. 12). This

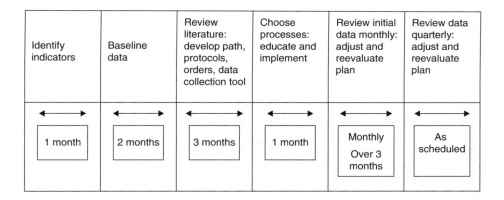

Identify indicators	Baseline data	Review literature: develop path, protocols, orders, data collection tool	Choose processes: educate and implement	Review initial data monthly: adjust and reevaluate plan	Review data quarterly: adjust and reevaluate plan
◄──►	◄──►	◄──►	◄──►	◄──►	◄──►
1 month	2 months	3 months	1 month	Monthly Over 3 months	As scheduled

■ Figure 3-7   Timeline for Outcome Assessment of APN Practice

Source: Kleinpell, R. M. (2007, May). APNs invisible champions? *Nursing Management,* 18–22. Adapted with permission.

means "clearly distinguishing APN's in the context of interdisciplinary practice" (O'Grady, 2008, p. 12). Individual studies can demonstrate gaps in care in smaller samples, but the time has come for a more comprehensive and collaborative agenda for research that focuses on such issues as roles, function, outcomes, access improvements for vulnerable populations, interdisciplinary collaboration impacts, cost effectiveness, safety, and other indicators. In order to discover gaps in care that are of concern to APNs/DNPs, nurses must have representatives from their ranks on research decision-making bodies. The AHRQ is positioned to take the lead in outcomes research, whereas the NIH focuses on biomedical aspects of disease management (O'Grady, 2008). To have their voices heard and their studies funded and disseminated, DNPs must use the power of their professional organizations to garner positions on national and international research collaboratives.

Participating in collaborative research is an excellent way for advanced practice nurses to resolve clinical dilemmas and highlight their expertise through well-constructed questions that interest scientists and engage professional peers within and outside nursing. The dynamic nature of scientific evidence and the speed with which it is now possible to generate new knowledge through the use of technology demand that all care providers combine their expertise to interpret, plan, and evaluate the outcomes of interventions based on these new discoveries. Collaboration "implies collective action toward a common goal in a spirit of trust and harmony"

(D'Amour, Ferrada-Videla, San Martin-Rodriquez, & Beaulieu, 2005). Even within nursing, specialization demands collaboration between peers and patients to resolve complex clinical dilemmas if patients are to be treated holistically instead of as a collection of organ systems. In fact, as Nolan (2005) notes, patients must be included as "shapers of knowledge and action" (p. 329).

Nursing now has a body of knowledge, separate and unique from that of medicine, that provides the basis for unique contributions to science and to the care of individuals. At the same time, "nursing scholarship remains contextual and contingently situated" (Fairman, 2008). Nurses have shown in practice that they are creative and capable of managing changing circumstances and dynamic cultural milieus, thus ensuring that advanced practice nurses with both research and clinical skills are in a prime position to function as practice consultants in collaborative knowledge-generating research (AACN, 2006). This role is illustrated in the following example.

A DNP was a voluntary member of an advisory board of a suburban primary healthcare network that provided care to uninsured patients. The members of the board were very interested in ascertaining information about the effectiveness of the organization and its efforts to provide cost-effective, timely primary care. A question of particular interest was, Are emergency department visits decreased by the offering of this service? If they are, how much cost is actually saved? The DNP collaborated with the organization's administrator and developed an initial research question and a preliminary plan for presentation to a grant funding agency. The DNP researched the literature and took the preliminary plan to her institution's research group; with the help of a colleague from the college's health administration program, the DNP designed a study that was submitted to a grant funding agency that specialized in grants to medical centers and community health agencies. The agency did not fund the grant that year. However, the following year the original proposal was reframed as a cohort study, "Emergency Room Usage Among Uninsured Patients with Access to a Primary Care Provider" (Tymkow, Shen, and MacMullen, 2006), and resubmitted as a subproject of a much larger NIH grant that was funded. A primary aim of the larger National Center on Minority Health and Health Disparities (NCMHD) grant was to build capacity for research in healthcare disparities through mentoring by senior-level researchers (Samson, 2006). The DNP who was a mentee became the primary investigator, working with two co-investigators on this project. At this writing, the data collection has been completed and the results are being analyzed and will be presented to the agency. Although this was a small pilot study, the researchers hope to use the data gathered from the pilot for a larger study involving additional primary providers of care to uninsured patients. In this case the DNP is functioning as a member of a collaborative multidisciplinary research team.

In another example of collaborative research, Oman, Duran, and Fink (2008) describe a collaborative EBP project to institute evidence-based policy and procedure development at the University of Colorado Hospital using the hospital's evidence-based multidisciplinary practice model. The model established the evidence base through valid and current research and through other forms of evidence or benchmark data, including cost-effectiveness analysis; pathophysiology; retrospective or concurrent chart review; quality improvement and risk data; international, national, and local standards; infection control data; patient preferences; and clinical expertise. The more sources that are added to the research core, the stronger the evidence. However, all sources are contributory to the evidence.

The Evidence-Based Practice Council used the levels of evidence of Stetler (1994) to guide the process of gathering evidence. As described by Oman et al., since there was nothing addressing policy and procedure in the literature, the members identified steps and created an algorithm to describe the process. Once developed, the algorithm was piloted on the units using six nurse champions, mentored by a researcher. The champions and researcher reviewed an orthostatic vital sign policy that was scheduled for update. After obtaining 12 research-based articles, eight clinical articles, one national guideline, and anecdotal recommendations, the group was divided into subgroups, and each person was assigned two reports to review using a standardized critique form. Each nurse was responsible for reading the articles, completing the critique form (with levels of evidence), and presenting the findings at a journal club. The policy being reviewed was checked for references and levels of evidence by the research scientist. A comparison of agreement between the policy author and reviewers was then determined, and the percentage of agreement between reviewer and author tabulated. Only clinically based policies were reviewed. This process is a good example of how collaboration between practice and education could be merged in any number of areas.

Whether collaboration involves clinical research or quality improvement, DNPs in clinical and leadership roles are key stakeholders in the process. As identified in the IOM report *Crossing the Quality Chasm* (IOM, 2001), communication and collaboration are requisites to the achievement of quality systems and patient outcomes. These skills are also a necessary part of a culture of collaboration that begins in educational programs and continues in the professional work setting. Collaborative efforts may include small, unit-based or practice-based efforts or large, systemwide initiatives. These efforts have been driven by consumer demand for excellence, accountability, and transparency in quality care, patient safety, and patient satisfaction (Freshman, Rubino, & Chassiakos, 2010). In any collaborative initiative, three levels of expertise are required: system leadership, including the authority to implement change; clinical technical expertise (guidance and know-how); and day-to-day leadership (details of the system) (Baker, Reising, Johnson, Stewart, & Baker, 1997, cited in Freshman, Rubino, & Chassiakos, 2010).

Disseminating Findings from Evidence-Based Practice

A primary reason for disseminating research is to use the findings to improve practice and improve health outcomes. Communicating the results of research and evidence-based practice trials is the culminating step of the research and research utilization processes. It is one of, if not *the*, most important steps in research and the application of research in practice because it is the communication of research findings that provides the basis for meaningful critique, development of new questions, and testing of research evidence in practice (Lyder & Fain, 2009).

The methods used to communicate evidence from practice trials are similar to those used for communicating research findings: journal publications, podium or poster presentations, Internet webinar sessions, media communications, journal clubs, and community presentations. However, the forums for dissemination may be broader because the audience of interest may be more diverse, including those with practice, research, and community development interests. In addition, the choice of method for communicating information depends on a number of important factors. For example, a journal publication may be personally advantageous to the author, but the time from submission to actual publication and dissemination may delay utilization of important evidence-based treatments in practice. Oral reports at national conferences may facilitate timelier dissemination. Webinars may be the fastest way to disseminate information, but may not reach all the desired audiences. Journal clubs are useful forums for discussions of research findings in academic settings. Reports of community-based studies to advisory boards or media venues may also become the basis for further research and political support that help nonprofit and other community organizations. Nevertheless, because theory, research, and practice must be constantly intertwined, the circular and reciprocal relationship among these elements must be apparent regardless of where the research is presented (McEwen &Wills, 2007).

Preparing a Journal Publication

Preparing a journal article for publication is time consuming and at times tedious, but the rewards of feeling that you have made a contribution and seeing your work in print are worth the effort. Once the topic for an article has been established, the next step is that of selecting the journal. Peer-reviewed journals have the most rigorous review criteria. Therefore, publication in one of these journals is considered to be more credible. The actual content will be determined by the editorial guidelines of the journal, which may be found in the "Information for Authors" section of the journal. In most cases, the guidelines may also be obtained from the journal's website. Generally, the submission requirements cover technical details such as page length, margins, font style and size, reference format, use of graphics and figures, and method of submission. It is very important to follow the submission requirements because many journals will not review articles that are not submitted in the correct format.

Once submitted, articles in peer-reviewed journals are blind (anonymously) reviewed by several reviewers. It is not uncommon for the review process to last several weeks or months, and articles may be rejected, accepted with revisions, or accepted. It is common to have articles returned for revision. The key to success is to be persistent, correct those things that can be corrected, give an explanation for those that cannot, and return the submission in the agreed-upon time frame.

Preparing a Research Presentation

Regardless of where or how evidence is reported, the essential element is that it combines the knowledge and values of the study patients or population with practitioner expertise and the best in available and current research evidence. Reporting evidence also requires knowledge of the audience and their needs. Specifically, the presenter must ask: What is the specific content to be addressed? How will the audience use the information? What is the knowledge level of those who are to receive the information? What is the time allowed for the presentation? What audiovisual resources are available for the presentation? Once these questions have been answered, specific learning objectives should be developed in order to guide and organize the presentation.

Table 3-13 shows an outline for presentation of research study findings. Important points of each aspect of the study can be displayed as a PowerPoint presentation to aid in maintaining the presentation within the designated time frame and keep the audience focused on the important elements of the presentation. Table 3-14 lists some useful websites concerning PowerPoint presentations.

Preparing a Poster Presentation

Disseminating information from scholarship—original research, practice innovations, clinical projects—through poster presentations has become an accepted medium for the exchange of ideas in a more personal and less

---

■ **Table 3-13   Outline for Research Presentation**

   I. Introduction
  II. Purpose of the study
 III. Theoretical framework
 IV. Hypothesis
  V. Design
     A. What kind of study
     B. Intervention
     C. Sample
       1. Population
       2. Inclusion/Exclusion criteria
     D. Instruments
 VI. Analysis
     A. Method
     B. Types of statistical tests used
 VII. Findings
VIII. Discussion
 IX. Implications
     A. Research
     B. Clinical practice

■ Table 3-14 Resources and Websites for Developing Multimedia and PowerPoint Presentations

Vanderbilt University	http://www.vanderbilt.edu/cft/resources/teaching_resources/technology/presentation
University of Wisconsin	http://www.cew.wisc.edu/accessibility/tutorials/pptmain.htm
University of South Florida	http://etc.usf.edu/presentations/web
WebAim	http://www.webaim.org/techniques/powerpoint/alternatives.php

formal environment than the podium presentation. It is both efficient and effective. Presenters and participants have the freedom to engage in a dialogue that allows for education, clarification, and networking. Posters also allow for the formatting of data in creative ways. As Berg (2005) notes, "imagery can be substituted for words and this is a powerful way to convey information" (p. 245). Like any presentation, posters require preparation. The following steps are essential.

PLAN AHEAD

A good poster presentation takes considerable time. The planning stage is a most important step. In this stage, considerable thought should be given to the message you are trying to convey. What is the purpose? The format for a research presentation will be different from that of a practice innovation. Is the conference only for nurses, only for advanced practice nurses, or for a multidisciplinary audience? How much background information or detail do you need to include? Is the audience generally familiar with the topic or not? If they are, don't include familiar details, but if they aren't, don't make the information so specific that those who are not familiar with the topic will be put off. Avoid using abbreviations that only a select audience will understand. These and other considerations specific to the venue should be thought about during the planning stage (Berg, 2005; Hardicre, Devitt, & Coad, 2007).

DECIDE ON LAYOUT AND FORMAT

Most people read top to bottom, and left to right. This is the usual sequence for poster layout. Generally, the layout for a research poster presentation is as follows: title, abstract, introduction, methods, results, discussion, and acknowledgments. If the presentation is a practice innovation, the layout will be different. The innovation is usually in the center, with explanatory text at the periphery or below the diagram or explanation of the protocol or change (Hardicre et al., 2007). References are also included, as in the research poster. "The poster should be easy to read from a distance of up to 6 feet. Section heads should be at least 40 pt. and supporting text 32 pt." (Halligan, 2005, p. 49). Titles should be short, with letters two to three inches high (Berg, 2005).

DETERMINE THE CONTENT

If the purpose of the poster is to display a research project, it will not be the same as one that is designed to describe a clinical innovation. The content of the research poster should follow the guidelines established by the conference guidelines. If the study is funded by an outside or government agency, some grant-funded studies require specific wording of the acknowledgment; this should be determined during the poster planning. If an abstract is required, it should include the main purpose of the study, be clearly worded, and be succinct. A key component is to keep it simple because posters "show," they do not "tell" (Miracle, 2008).

Clinical project content will vary according to the specific topic and scope. The title for either a research study or clinical innovation should be creative, but, most important, it should accurately reflect the content of the project. The title banner should also include authors and affiliations in order of authorship and/or contribution to the effort. In many instances the organizational logo will be included as well (Hardicre et al., 2007).

PREPARE A BRIEF PRESENTATION

"The poster is a story board of information" (Jackson & Sheldon, 1998, as cited in Hardicre et al., 2007, p. 398). However, it also gives the presenters an opportunity to present themselves. As with any kind of communication, you want to convey confidence and knowledge. Preparing a short presentation script or handouts for participants allows you to organize your thoughts and prepare for possible questions. The handouts are always welcomed by participants, who are inundated with information during a conference. Be sure to include your name and contact number or attach a business card so that participants may contact you with questions. This is a very effective networking tool (Miracle, 2008).

Media Communications

Communicating with large audiences is often facilitated through professional media communications. This kind of communication is essential when there is a major event or change, such as a policy to be initiated. It is usually best to engage the resources of a professional organization to make the preliminary contact and to aid in constructing the message.

Journal Club Presentations

Another way to facilitate the communication of evidence-based research is through journal club presentations. Journal clubs are not new, especially in academic and many professional settings. However, using them to facilitate evidence-based practice is a more recent development, especially as a forum for clinical guideline development (Kirchoff & Beck, 1995, as cited in McQueen, Miller, Nivison, & Husband, 2006). In a small survey study of the use of journal clubs to determine changes in practice, McQueen et al. (2006) found that journal clubs were effective in "1) focusing staff on clinical evidence in discussions, 2) increasing confidence as they became more aware of evidence, and, 3) bridging the evidence-practice gap" (p. 315). Additionally, with the aid of the Internet, evidence-based articles or studies can be posted in advance and facilitated online, thus increasing the possibility of wider participation. In one pilot study of this format, nurses in New Zealand branded the journal club's website and the articles for discussion. An article is posted for one month and removed on the Friday before the following month's posting (Trim, 2008). Table 3-15 presents an outline of a journal club.

Whether live or Internet-based, journal clubs provide a mechanism for promoting professional debate, increasing confidence, and, most important, improving practice and quality care (Sheratt, 2005, as cited in McQueen et al., 2006). With their educational background and advanced skills, DNPs are in an excellent position to implement this kind of strategy in a collaborative, interdisciplinary format. Please see Chapter 11 for further discussion of dissemination of findings from evidence-based practice.

Summary

Scholarship and evidence-based practice are not the same, but each has elements that support the other. Scholarship involves research and application, as does evidence-based practice. Whereas scholarship may be a joint or

■ Table 3-15   Online Journal Club

Outline of the Journal Club

1. A specific clinical question is chosen.

2. All evidence-based literature related to the question is derived from online databases.

3. A reference list of all literature for review is generated.

4. High-level-evidence RTCs and systematic reviews are critiqued and given more weight than quasi-experimental case studies and opinions.

5. Participants critically appraise the relevant literature before attending the journal club.

6. Journal club discussions center on the critical appraisal of evidence found for clinical interventions.

7. Implications for practice and further research are discussed, with key findings recorded in minutes.

8. A resource folder that includes a reference list of resource critiques, guidelines for practice, treatment resources, standardized assessments, disease management strategies, and gaps in evidence is created.

9. A system for ongoing evaluation of outcomes and changes in practice is developed and communicated.

Source: McQueen, J., Miller, C., Nivison, C., & Husband, V. (2006). An investigation into the use of a journal club for evidence-based practice. *International Journal of Therapy and Rehabilitation, 13*(7), p. 313. Modified with permission.

singular effort, evidence-based practice requires teamwork and collaboration. The outcome of scholarship is a scholarly product, a new way of thinking, or a change in awareness about a subject or phenomenon—an end in itself. Evidence-based practice is based on the scholarship of research and evidence gathering and synthesis. It is a means for improving care for patients or effecting a change in a system that results in better care for patients, providers, and communities. It is a transformation of knowledge to new levels of understanding and integration. Changing to a model of evidence-based practice does not just happen; it requires the integration of a number of skills, including the use of good research and the synthesis of best information and other "evidences," including patient choice and professional expertise at its core. The DNP, with the advantage of expertise in practice built on a strong base of education and knowledge, is—and will continue to be—in the forefront of this movement to transform care.

References

Adib-Hajbaghery, M. (2007). Factors facilitating and inhibiting evidence-based practice in Iran. *Journal of Advanced Nursing, 58*(6), 566–575.

Agency for Healthcare Quality and Research. (2002). *Systems to rate the strength of scientific evidence, summary* (Technical Report No. 47). Retrieved from http://www.ahrq.gov/clinic/epcsums/strengthsum.htm

Agency for Healthcare Quality and Research. (2009). *Evidence-based practice centers.* Retrieved from http://www.AHRQ.gov/clinic/epc

AGREE Collaboration. (2001). *AGREE instrument.* Retrieved from www.agreecollaboration.org/instrument

American Association of Colleges of Nursing. (1999). *Position statement on defining scholarship for the discipline of nursing.* Retrieved from http://www.aacn.nche.edu/Publications/positions/scholar.htm

American Association of Colleges of Nursing. (2006). *The essentials of doctoral education for advanced nursing practice.* Retrieved from http://www.aacn.nche.edu/DNP/pdf/Essentials.pdf

American Nurses Credentialing Center. (2005). *Magnet recognition program overview.* Retrieved from http://www.medscape.com/partners/ancc/public/ancc

Andrews, T. (2008). Under pressure for a diagnosis: A case study review of pheochromocytoma genetics. *Clinical Scholars Review: The Journal of Doctoral Nursing Practice, 1*(2), 96–100.

Armson, H., Kinzie, S., Hawes, D., Roder, S., Wakefield, J., & Elmslie, T. (2007). Translating learning into practice. *Canadian Family Physician, 53*(9), 1477–1485.

Arthur, R., Marfell, J., & Ulrich, S. (2009). Outcomes measurement in nurse-midwifery practice. In R. M. Kleinpell (Ed.), *Outcome assessment in advanced practice nursing* (2nd ed.). New York: Springer.

Asch, S. M., Baker, D. W., Keesey, J., Broder, M., Schonlau, M., Rosen, M., et al. (2005). Does the collaborative model improve care for chronic heart failure? *Medical Care, 43*(7), 667–675.

Averis, A., & Pearson, A. (2003). Filling the gaps: Identifying nursing research priorities through the analysis of completed systematic reviews. *JBI Reports, 1*(3), 49–126.

Baker, C. M., Reising, D. L., Johnson, D. R., Stewart, R. L., & Baker, S. D. (1997). Organizational effectiveness: Toward an integrated model for schools of nursing. *Journal of Professional Nursing, 13*(4), 246–255.

Batalden, P. B., Nelson, E. C., & Roberts, J. S. (1994). Linking outcome measurements to continual improvement: The serial "V" way of thinking about improving clinical care. *Journal of Quality Improvement, 20*(4), 167–180.

Batalden, P. B., & Stoltz, P. K. (1993). A framework for the continual improvement of healthcare: Building and applying professional and improvement knowledge to test changes in daily work. *Joint Commission Journal of Quality Improvement, 19*(10), 424–447.

Berg, J. A. (2005). Creating a professional poster presentation: Focus on nurse practitioners. *Journal of the American Academy of Nurse Practitioners, 17*(7), 245–248.

Bernarde, S. F., Keogh, E., & Lima, M. L. (2007). Bridging the gap between pain and gender research: A selective literature review. *European Journal of Pain, 12*(4), 427–440. doi:10.1016.j.ejpain.2007.08.007

Bond, A. E., Draeger, C. R., Mandleco, B., & Donnelly, M. (2003). Needs of family members of patients with severe traumatic brain injury. *Critical Care Nurse, 23*(4), 63–71.

Boyer, E. L. (1990). *Scholarship reconsidered: Priorities of the professoriate*. The Carnegie Foundation for the Advancement of Teaching. San Francisco: Jossey-Bass.

Boyer, E. L. (1997). *Scholarship reconsidered: Priorities of the professoriate* (rev. ed.). The Carnegie Foundation for the Advancement of Teaching. San Francisco: Jossey-Bass.

Brown, S. J. (2005). Direct clinical practice. In A. B. Hamric, J. A. Spross, & C. M. Hanson (Eds.), *Advanced practice nursing: An integrative approach* (3rd ed., pp. 143–185). Philadelphia: W. B. Saunders.

Burns, N., & Grove, S. K. (2005). *The practice of nursing research: Conduct, critique, and utilization* (5th ed.). St. Louis, MO: Elsevier Saunders.

Burns, N., & Grove, S. K. (2009). *The practice of nursing research, appraisal, synthesis, and generation of evidence* (6th ed.). St. Louis, MO: Saunders.

Burns, S. (2009). Selecting advanced practice nurse outcome measures. In R. M. Kleinpell (Ed.), *Outcomes assessment in advanced practice nursing* (2nd ed.). New York: Springer.

Burns, S. M., & Earven, S. (2002). Improving outcomes for mechanically ventilated medical intensive care unit patients using advanced practice nurses: A 6-year experience. *Critical Nursing Clinics of North America, 14*(3), 231–242.

Bushnell, C. D., Hurn, P., Colton, C., Miller, V. M., del Zoppo, G., Elkind, M. S, et al. (2007). Advancing the study of stroke in women: Summary and recommendations for future research from an NINDS-Sponsored Multidisciplinary Working Group. *Stroke, 38*(5), e10.

Carey, M., Buchan, H., & Sanson-Fisher, R. (2009). The cycle of change: Implementing the best-evidence clinical practice. *International Journal for Quality in Health Care, 21*(1), 37–43. Retrieved from http:www//medscape.com/viewarticle/587379

Carnegie Foundation for the Advancement of Teaching. (1996). *Ernest L. Boyer* (Ninety-first Annual Report of the Carnegie Foundation for the Advancement of Teaching). Princeton, NJ: Author.

Cochrane Collaboration. (2004). *Cochrane reviewers' handbook*. London: The Cochrane Group.

Coe, R. (2002, September). *It's the effect size, stupid: What effect size is and why it is so important.* Paper presented at the Annual Conference of the British Educational Research Association, University of Exeter, England. Retrieved from http://www.leeds.ac.uk./educol/documents/0002182.htm

Collins, P. M., Golembeski, S. M., Selgas, M., Sparger, K., Burke, N., & Vaughn, B. B. (2008, January 25). Clinical excellence through evidence-based practice: A model to guide practice changes. *Topics in Advanced Practice E-Journal*. Retrieved from http://www.medscape.com/viewarticle/567682

Cooke, L., Smith-Idell, C., Dean, G., Gemmill, R., Steingass, S., Sun, V., et al. (2004). "Research to practice": A practical program to enhance the use of evidence-based practice at the unit level. *Oncology Nursing Forum, 31*(4), 825–832.

Craft-Rosenburg, M., Krajicek, M. J., & Shin, D. (2002). Report of the American Academy of Nursing Child-Family Expert Panel: Identification of quality and outcome indicators for maternal child nursing. *Nursing Outlook, 50*(2), 57–60.

Crotty, M. (1996). *Phenomenology and nursing research.* Melbourne, Australia: Churchill Livingstone.

D'Amour, D., Ferrada-Videla, M., San Martin-Rodriquez, L., & Beaulieu, M. D. (2005). The conceptual basis for interprofessional collaboration: Core concepts and theoretical frameworks. *Journal of Interprofessional Care, 19*(suppl 1), 116–131.

Decker, S., & Iphofen, R. (2005). Developing the profession of radiography: Making uses of oral history. *Radiography, 11*(4), 262–271.

Deming, E. W. (1986). *Out of crisis.* Cambridge, MA: MIT Press.

De Palma, J. A., & McGuire, D. B. (2005). Research. In A. B. Hamric, J. A. Spross, & C. Mittenson (Eds.), *Advanced nursing practice: An integrative approach* (3rd ed.). Philadelphia: Elsevier Saunders.

DiCenso, A., Cullum, N., & Ciliska, D. (1998). Implementing evidence-based nursing: Some misconceptions. *Evidence-Based Nursing, 1*(2), 38–39.

Diekelmann, N. L., Allen, D., & Tanner, C. A. (1989). *NLN criteria for appraisal of baccalaureate programs: A critical hermeneutic analysis.* New York: National League for Nursing.

Dohrn, J. (2008). Scaling up HIV treatment for pregnant women: Components of a midwifery model of care as identified by midwives in Eastern Cape, South Africa. *Clinical Scholars Review: The Journal of Doctoral Nursing Practice, 1*(1), 50–54.

Doran, D. M., & Sidani, S. (2007). Outcomes-focused knowledge translation: A framework for knowledge translation and patient outcomes improvement. *Worldviews on Evidence-Based Nursing, 4*(1), 3–13.

Dorn, K. (2004). Caring-healing inquiry for holistic nursing practice: Model for research and evidence based practice. *Topics in Advanced Practice Nursing E-Journal, 4*(4). Retrieved from http://www.medscape.com/viewarticle/496363

Doster, J. A., Purdum, M. D., Martin, L. A., Goven, A. J., & Moorefield, R. (2009). Gender differences, anger expression, and cardiovascular risk. *Journal of Nervous and Mental Diseases, 197*(7), 552–554.

Doumitt, G., Gattelliari, M., Grimshaw, J., & O'Brien, M. A. (2007). Local opinion leaders: Effects on professional practice and healthcare outcomes. *Cochrane Database Systematic Review,* Issue 4, Art. No. CD000125. doi:10.1002/14651858.CD000125.pub3

Doyle-Lindrud, S. (2008). Gestational breast cancer. *Clinical Scholars Review: The Journal of Doctoral Nursing Practice, 1*(1), 23–31.

Dreher, M. (1999). Clinical scholarship: Nursing practice as an intellectual endeavor. In Sigma Theta Tau International Clinical Scholarship Task Force, *Clinical scholarship resource paper* (pp. 26–33). Retrieved from http://www.nursingsociety.org/aboutus/PositionPapers /Documents/clinical_scholarship_paper.pdf

Duignan, P. (2006). *Outcomes model standards for systematic outcome analysis.* Retrieved from http://www.parkerduignan.com/oiiwa/toolkit/standards1.html

Durieux, P., Nizard, R., Ravaud, P., et al. (2000). A clinical decision support system for prevention of venous thromboembolism: Effect on physician behavior. *Journal of the American Medical Association, 283*(21), 2816–2821.

Edwards, S. D. (2001). *Philosophy of nursing: An introduction.* New York: Palgrave.

Fain, J. A. (2009). *Reading, understanding and applying nursing research* (3rd ed.). Philadelphia: F. A. Davis.

Fairman, J. (2008). Context and contingency in the history of post World War II scholarship in the United States. *Journal of Nursing Scholarship, 40*(1), 4–11.

Fawcett, J., & Garrity, J. (2009). *Evaluating research for evidence-based nursing practice.* Philadelphia: F. A. Davis.

Fawcett, J., Watson, J., Neuman, B., Hinton Walker, P., & Fitzpatrick, J. (2001). On nursing theories and evidence. *Journal of Nursing Scholarship, 33*(2), 115–119.

Fishbein, I., & Ajzen, M. (1980). *Understanding attitudes and predicting social behavior.* Englewood Cliffs, NJ: Prentice Hall.

Fitzpatrick, M. L., & Munhall, P. L. (2001). Historical research: The method. In P. L. Munhall (Ed.), *Nursing research: A qualitative perspective* (3rd ed.). Sudbury, MA: Jones and Bartlett.

French, P. (1999). The development of evidence-based nursing. *Journal of Advanced Nursing, 29*(1), 72–78.

Freshman, B., Rubino, L., & Chassiakos, Y. R. (2010). *Collaboration across the disciplines in health care.* Sudbury, MA: Jones and Bartlett.

Funk & Wagnalls New International Dictionary of the English Language (comprehensive millennium ed.). (2003). Chicago: Ferguson.

Gagan, M., & Hewitt-Taylor, J. (2004). The issues involved in implementing evidence based practice. *British Journal of Nursing, 13*(20), 1216–1220.

Gallagher, R. M. (2009). Participation of the advanced practice nurse in managed care and quality initiatives. In L. A. Joel (Ed.), *Advanced practice nursing: Essentials of role development* (2nd ed.). Philadelphia: F. A. Davis.

Giddens, A. (1982). *Profiles and critiques in social theory.* London: Macmillan.

Gifford, W., Davies, B., Edwards, N., Griffin, P., & Lybanon, V. (2007). Managerial leadership for nurses' use of research evidence: An integrative review of the literature. *World Views on Evidence Based Practice, 4*(3), 126–145.

Giorgi, A. (2000). Concerning the application of phenomenology to caring research. *Scandinavian Journal of Caring Science, 14*(1), 11–15.

Glanville, I., Schirm, V., & Wineman, N. M. (2000). Using evidence-based practice for managing clinical outcomes in advanced practice nursing. *Journal of Nursing Care Quality, 15*(1), 1–11.

Glasser, B. G., & Strauss, A. (1967). *The discovery of grounded theory.* Chicago: Aldine.

Goolsby, M. J., Klardie, K. A., Johnson, J., McNaughton, M. A., & Meyers, W. (2004). Integrating the principles of evidence-based practice into clinical practice. *Journal of the American Academy of Nurse Practitioners, 16*(3), 98–105.

Goolsby, M. J., Meyers, W. C., Johnson, J. A., Klardie, K., & McNaughton, M. A. (2004). Integrating the principles of evidence-based practice: Prognosis and the metabolic syndrome. *Journal of the American Academy of Nurse Practitioners, 16*(5), 178–186.

Griffin-Sobel, J. P. (2003). Evaluating an instrument for research. *Gastroenterology Nursing, 26*(3), 135–136.

Grol, R., Dalhuijsen, J., Thomas, S., Veld, C., Rutten, G., & Mokkink, H. (1998). Attributes of clinical guidelines that influence use of guidelines in general practice: Observational study. *British Medical Journal, 317*(7162), 858–861.

Gumei, M. K., Tiedje, L. B., & Oweis, A. (2007). Vaginal or cesarean birth: Toward evidence based practice. *American Journal of Maternal Child Nursing, 32*(6), 388.

Hallett, C. (1995). Understanding the phenomenological approach to research. *Nurse Researcher, 3*(2), 55–56.

Halligan, P. (2005). Poster perfect. *World of Irish Nursing and Midwifery, 13*(8), 49.

Handley, M., MacGregor, K., Schillinger, D., Sharifi, C., Wong, S., & Bodenheimer, T. (2006). Using action plans to help primary care patients adopt healthy behaviors: A descriptive study. *Journal of the American Board of Family Medicine, 19*(3), 224–231.

Hardicre, J., Devitt, P., & Coad, J. (2007). Ten steps to successful poster presentation. *British Journal of Nursing, 16*(7), 398–401.

Harvey, S. (1993). The genesis of the phenomenological approach to advanced nursing practice. *Journal of Advanced Nursing, 18*(4), 526–530.

Hawkins, R. C., & Clement, P. F (1984). Binge eating: Measurement problems and a conceptual model. In R. E. Hawkins, W. J. Fremouw, & P. F. Clement (Eds.), *The binge-purge syndrome: Diagnosis, treatment, and research* (pp. 229–251). New York: Springer.

Hebda, T., & Czar, P. (2009). *Handbook of informatics for nurses and healthcare professionals* (4th ed.). Upper Saddle River, NJ: Pearson/Prentice Hall.

Hodge, M. B., Asch, S. M., Olson, V. A., Kravitz, R. L., & Sauve, M. J. (2002). Developing indicators of nursing quality to evaluate nurse staffing ratios. *Journal of Nursing Administration, 32*(6), 338–345.

Holleman, G., Eliens, A., van Vliet, M., & van Acterburg, T. (2006). Promotion of evidence based practice by professional nursing associations: Literature review. *Journal of Advanced Nursing, 53*(6), 702–709.

Horsely, J. A., Crane, J., & Bingle, J. D. (1978). Research utilization as an organizational process. *Journal of Nursing Administration, 8*(7), 4–6.

Imberg, W. C. (2008). *The meaning of U.S. childbirth for Mexican immigrant women* (Doctoral dissertation). Available from ProQuest Dissertations and Theses database. (UMI No. 3318193)

Ingersoll, G. (2005). Generating evidence through outcomes management. In B. M. Melnyk & E. Fineout-Overholt (Eds.), *Evidence-based practice in nursing and healthcare: A guide to best practice*. Philadelphia: Lippincott Williams & Wilkins.

Ingersoll, G. L., McIntosh, E., & Williams, M. (2000). Nurse sensitive outcomes of advanced practice. *Journal of Advanced Nursing, 32*(5), 1272–1281.

Institute of Medicine. (2001). *Crossing the quality chasm: A new health system for the 21st century*. Washington, DC: National Academies Press.

Institute of Medicine. (2003). *Health professions education: A bridge to quality*. Washington, DC: National Academies Press.

International Development Research Center. (2009). *Confounding*. Retrieved from http://www.idrc.ca/en/ev-1-201-1-DO_TOPIC.html

Ironside, P. M. (2006). Reforming doctoral curricula in nursing: Creating multiparadigmatic, multipedagalogical researchers. *Journal of Nursing Education, 45*(2), 51–52.

Jackson, K. I., & Sheldon, J. M. (1998). Poster presentation: How to tell a story. *Pediatric Nurse, 10*(9), 36–37.

Jamtvedt, G., Young, J. M., Kristofferson, D. T., O'Brien, M. A., & Oxman, A. D. (2006). Audit and feedback: Effects on professional practice and healthcare outcomes. *Cochrane Database of Systematic Reviews, 2*, CD000259.

Johnston, L. (2005). Critically appraising quantitative evidence. In B. M. Melnyk & E. Fineout-Overholt (Eds.), *Evidence-based practice in nursing and healthcare: A guide to best practice.* Philadelphia: Lippincott Williams & Wilkins.

Kelly, D. R., Cunningham, D. E., McCalister, P., Cassidy, J., & MacVicar, R. (2007). Applying evidence in practice through small group learning: A qualitative exploration of success. *Quality in Primary Care, 15*(2), 93–99.

Kirchoff, K., & Beck, S. (1995). Using the journal club as a component of the research utilization process. *Heart and Lung: The Journal of Acute and Critical Care, 24*(3), 246–250.

Kitson, A., Harvey, G., & McCormack, B. (1998). Enabling the implementation of evidence-based practice: A conceptual framework. *Quality in Healthcare, 7*(3), 149–158.

Kleinpell, R. M. (2007, May). APNs invisible champions? *Nursing Management, 38*(5), 18–22.

Kleinpell, R. M. (2009). Measuring outcomes in advanced nursing practice. In R. M. Kleinpell (Ed.), *Outcome assessment in advanced nursing practice* (2nd ed.). New York: Springer.

Kohn, L. T., Corrigan, J. M., & Donaldson, M. S. (2000). *To err is human: Building a safer health system.* A report of the Committee on Quality of Health Care in America, Institute of Medicine. Washington, DC: National Academies Press.

Kovarsky, D. (2008). Representing voices from the life-world in evidence-based practice. *International Journal of Language and Communication Disorders, 43*(S1), 47–57.

Lambert, M. J., & Burlingame, G. M. (2009). Measuring outcomes in the state of Utah: Practice based evidence. *Behavioral Healthcare, 27*, 16–20. Retrieved from http://www.behavioral.net

Lanthier, E. (2002). *Correlation.* Retrieved from http://www.nvcc.edu/home/elanthier/methods/correlations-samples.htm

Leedy, P. D., & Ormrod, J. E. (2010). *Practical research: Planning and design.* Boston: Pearson.

Library of Congress. (n.d.). *American memory collection.* Retrieved from http://memory.loc.gov/ammem/index.html

Lopez-Bushnell, K. (2002). Get research-ready. *Nursing Management, 33*(11), 41–44.

Lowell, J. R. (1819–1891). *Scholarship.* Retrieved from http://quotationsbook.com/quote/22196

Luttik, M. L., Jaarsma, T., Lesman, I., Sanderman, R., & Hagedoorn, M. (2009). Quality of life in partners of people with congestive heart failure: Gender and involvement in care. *Journal of Advanced Nursing, 65*(7), 1442–1451. Epub April 30, 2009.

Lyder, C., & Fain, J. A. (2009). Interpreting and reporting research findings. In J. A. Fain (Ed.), *Reading, understanding, and applying research* (3rd ed., pp. 233–250). Philadelphia: F. A. Davis.

Maggs-Rapport, F. (2001). 'Best research practice': In pursuit of methodological rigour. *Journal of Advanced Nursing, 35*(3), 373–383.

Mak, Y. (2003). Use of hermeneutic research in understanding the meaning of desire for euthanasia. *Palliative Medicine, 17*(5), 395–402.

Marineau, M. L. (2005). *Exploring the lived experience of individuals with acute infections transitioning in the home with support by an advanced practice nurse using telehealth* (Doctoral dissertation). University of Hawaii at Manoa. (UMI Order No. AA13198369)

Marinopoulos, S. S., Dorman, T., Ratanawongsa, N., Wilson, L. M., Ashar, B. H., Magaziner, J. L., et al. (2007). Effectiveness of continuing medical education. *Evidence Reports in Technology Assessment, 14*, 1–69.

Masharani, V., Goldfine, I. D., & Youngren, J. F. (2009). Influence of gender on the relationship between insulin sensitivity, adiposity, and plasma lipids, in lean nondiabetic patients. *Metabolism.* Advance online publication. Retrieved from http://www.ncbi.nlm.nih.gov/pubmed/19604524

McCaughan, D., Thompson, C., Cullum, N., Sheldon, T. A., & Thompson, D. R. (2002). Acute care nurses' perceptions of barriers to using research information in clinical decision-making. *Journal of Advanced Nursing, 39*(1), 46–60.

McCloskey, D. J. (2008). Nurses' perceptions of research utilization in a corporate health care system. *Journal of Nursing Scholarship, 40*(1), 39–45.

McCollum, M., Hanson, L. S., Lu, L., & Sullivan, P. W. (2005). Gender differences in diabetes mellitus and effects on self-care activity. *Gender Medicine, 2*(4), 246–254.

McEwen, M., & Wills, E. M. (2007). *Theoretical basis for nursing* (2nd ed.). Philadelphia: Lippincott Williams & Wilkins.

McQueen, J., Miller, C., Nivison, C., & Husband, V. (2006). An investigation into the use of a journal club for evidence-based practice. *International Journal of Therapy and Rehabilitation, 13*(7), 311–316.

McSherry, R. (2002). *Evidence informed nursing: A guide for clinical nurses.* London: Routledge.

MedPage Today. (n.d.). *Guide to Biostatistics.* Retrieved from http://www.medpagetoday.com/Medpage-Guide-to-Biostatistics.pdf

Melnyk, B., & Cole, R. (2005). Generating evidence through quantitative research. In B. Melnyk & E. Fineout-Overholt (Eds.), *Evidence-based practice in nursing and healthcare* (pp. 239–281). Philadelphia: Lippincott Williams & Wilkins.

Melnyk, B., & Fineout-Overholt, E. (2002). Putting research into practice. Rochester ARCC. *Reflections on Nursing Leadership, 28*(2), 22–25.

Melnyk, B., & Fineout-Overholt, E. (2005). *Evidence-based practice in nursing and healthcare.* Philadelphia: Lippincott Williams & Wilkins.

Minnick, A. (2009). General design and implementation challenges in outcomes assessment. In R. M. Kleinpell (Ed.), *Outcomes assessment in advanced practice nursing* (2nd ed.). New York: Springer.

Miracle, V. (2008). Effective poster presentations. *Dimensions of Critical Care Nursing, 27*(3), 122–124.

Mitchell, P. H., Ferketich, S., & Jennings, B. M. (1998). Quality health outcomes model. *Image: Journal of Nursing Scholarship, 30*(1), 43–36.

Moccia, P. (1987). *Nursing theory: A circle of knowledge* [Videorecording]. New York: National League for Nursing.

Monico, E. P., Moore, C. L., & Calise, A. (2005). The impact of evidence based medicine and evolving technology on the standard of care in emergency medicine. *The Internet Journal of Law, Healthcare and Ethics, 3*(2).

Munhall, P. (1994). *In women's experience.* New York: National League for Nursing.

Munhall, P. (2007) A phenomenological method. In P. L. Munhall (Ed.), *Nursing research: A qualitative perspective* (4th ed.). Sudbury, MA: Jones and Bartlett.

National Organization of Nurse Practitioner Faculties. (2005). *Nurse practitioner faculty practice: An expectation of professionalism.* Retrieved from www.nonpf.org/FPStatement2005final.pdf

Naylor, M. D., Brooten, D., Campbell, R., Jacobsen, B. S., Mezey, M. D., Pauley, M. V., et al. (1999). Comprehensive discharge planning and home follow-up of hospitalized elders: A randomized clinical trial. *Journal of the American Medical Association, 281*(7), 613–620.

Newhouse, R. P., Dearholt, S. L., Poe, S. S., Pugh, L. C., & White, K. M. (2008). *Johns Hopkins nursing evidence-based practice model and guidelines: Instructor's guide.* Indianapolis, IN: Sigma Theta Tau International.

Nolan, M. (2005). Reconciling tensions between research, evidence-based practice and user participation: Time for nursing to take the lead. *International Journal of Nursing Studies, 42*(5), 503–505.

O'Grady, E. T. (2008). Advanced practice registered nurses: The impact on patient safety and quality. In *Patient safety and quality: An evidence-based handbook for nurses.* Retrieved from http://www.ahrg.gov/qual/nurses/bk/docs/O'Grady.E-Aprn.pdf

Oman, K. S., Duran, C., & Fink, R. (2008). Evidence-based policy and procedures: An algorithm for success. *Journal of Nursing Administration, 38*(1), 47–51.

Padilla, G. V., Ferrell, B., Grant, M. M., & Rhiner, M. (1990). Defining the content domain of quality of life for cancer patients with pain. *Cancer Nursing, 13*(2), 108–115.

Patton, M. Q. (1990). *Qualitative evaluation and research methods* (2nd ed.). Newbury Park, CA: Sage Publications.

Pesut, B., & Johnson, J. (2007). Reinstating the 'Queen': Understanding philosophical inquiry in nursing. *Journal of Advanced Nursing, 61*(1), 115–121.

Peterson, L. A., Woodward, L. D., Urech, T., Daw, C., & Sookanan, S. (2006). Does pay-for-performance improve the quality of health care? *Annals of Internal Medicine, 145*(4), 265–272.

Polit, D. F., & Hungler, B. P. (1997). *Essentials of nursing research: Methods, appraisal, and utilization* (4th ed.). Philadelphia: Lippincott-Raven.

Porter, S. (1996). Qualitative research. In D. F. S. Cormack (Ed.), *The research process in nursing* (3rd ed., pp. 113–122). Oxford: Blackwell Science.

Pravikoff, D. S., Tanner, A. B., & Pierce, S. T. (2005). Readiness of U.S. nurses for evidence-based practice. *American Journal of Nursing, 105*(9), 40–51.

Prochaska, J. O., & DiClemente, C. C. (1986). Toward a comprehensive model of change. In W. R. Miller and N. Heather (Eds.), *Treating addictive behaviors: Processes of change.* New York: Plenum Press.

Prosser, H., Almond, S., & Walley, T. (2003). Influences on GP's decision to prescribe new drugs: The importance of who says what. *Family Practice, 20*(1), 61-68.

Rasgon, N., Shelton, S., & Halbreich, U. (2005). Perimenopausal mental disorders: Epidemiology and phenomenology. *CNS Spectrums: The International Journal of Neuropsychiatric Sciences, 10*(6), 471–478.

Reavy, K., & Tavernier, S. (2008). Nurses reclaiming ownership of their practice: Implementation of an evidence-based model and process. *Journal of Continuing Education in Nursing, 39*(4), 166–172.

Reed, P., & Shear, N. C. (2004). *Perspectives on nursing theory* (4th ed.). Philadelphia: Lippincott Williams & Wilkins.

Reeves, M. J., Fonarow, G. G., Zhao, X., Smith, E. E., Schwamm, L. H., & Get with the Guidelines Stroke-Steering Committee and Investigators. (2009). Quality of care in women with ischemic stroke in the GWTG program. *Stroke, 40*(4), 1127–1133. doi:10:1161./ Stroke AHA.108.543/57

Rosenstock, I. M. (1966). Why people use health services. *Milbank Fund Quarterly, 44*, 94–127.

Rosswurm, M. A., & Larrabee, J. (1999). A model for change to evidence based practice. *Image: Journal of Nursing Scholarship, 31*(4), 317–322.

Russell, C., & Gregory, D. (2003). Evaluation of qualitative research studies. *Evidence-Based Nursing, 6*(2), 36–40.

Rutledge, D. N., & Bookbinder, M. (2002). Processes and outcomes of evidence-based practice. *Seminars in Oncology Nursing, 18*(1), 3–10.

Rycroft-Malone, J., Kitson, A., Harvey, G., McCormack, B., Seers, K., Titchen, A., et al., (2002). Ingredients for change: Revisiting a conceptual framework. *Quality and Safety in Health Care, 11*(2), 174–180.

Rycroft-Malone, J., Seers, K., Titchen, A., Harvey, G., Kitson, A., & McCormack, B. (2004). What counts as evidence in evidence-based practice? *Journal of Advanced Nursing, 47*(1), 81–90.

Sackett, D. L., Richardson, W. S., Rosenberg, W. T., & Haynes, R. B. (1997). *Evidence-based medicine: How to practice and teach evidence-based medicine.* New York: Churchill Livingstone.

Samson, L. (2006). *Building capacity for health disparities research.* Grant 1P20MD001816-01 from the National Center on Minority Health and Health Disparities, National Institutes of Health, Bethesda, MD.

Scarbrough, M. L., & Landis, S. E. (1997). A pilot study for the development of a hospital based immunization program. *Clinical Nurse Specialist, 11*(2), 70–75.

Schmidt, N., & Brown, J. M. (2009). *Evidence-based practice for nurses: Appraisal and application of research.* Sudbury, MA: Jones and Bartlett.

Schulman, L. S. (1993). Teaching as community property: Putting an end to pedagogical solitude. *Change, 25*(6), 6–7.

Scott-Findley, S., & Pollack, C. (2004). Evidence, research and knowledge: A call for conceptual clarity. *Worldviews on Evidence Based Nursing, 1*(2), 92–97.

Sheratt, C. (2005). The journal club: A method for occupational therapists to bridge the theory-practice gap. *British Journal of Occupational Therapy, 68*(7), 301–306.

Sigma Theta Tau International Clinical Scholarship Task Force. (1999). *Clinical resource paper.* Retrieved from www.nursingsociety.org/aboutus/PositionPapers/Documents/clinical_scholarship_paper.pdf

Simmons-Mackie, N. N., & Damico, J. S. (2001). Intervention outcomes: Clinical applications of qualitative methods. *Topics in Language Disorders, 21*(4), 21–36.

Singleton, J., & Levin, R. (2008). Strategies for learning evidence-based practice: Critically appraising clinical practice guidelines. *Journal of Nursing Education, 47*(8), 380–383.

Soumarai, S. B., McLauglin, T. J., Gurwitz, J. H., Guadagnoli, E., Hauptman, P. J., Borbas, C., et al. (1998). Effect of local medicine opinion leaders on quality of care for acute myocardial infarction. *Journal of the American Medical Association, 279*(17), 1358–1363.

Spitzer, R. L., Devlin, M., Walsh, B. T., Hasin, D., Wing, R., Marcus, M., et al. (1992). Binge eating disorder: A multi-site field trial of the diagnostic criteria. *International Journal of Eating Disorders, 11*(3), 191–203.

Stetler, C. B. (1994). Refinement of the Stetler/Marram model for application of research findings to practice. *Nursing Outlook, 42*(1), 15–25.

Stetler, C. B., & Marram, G. (1976). Evaluating research findings for applicability in practice. *Nursing Outlook, 24*(9), 559–563.

Strauss, A., & Corbin, J. (1994). *Basics of qualitative research: Grounded theory procedures and techniques.* Newbury Park, NJ: Sage Publications.

Strauss, A., & Corbin, J. (1998). *Basics of qualitative research: Techniques and procedures for developing grounded theory.* Thousand Oaks, CA: Sage Publications.

Stroud, S. D., Erkel, E. A., & Smith, C. A. (2005). The use of personal digital assistants by nurse practitioner students and faculty. *Journal of the American Academy of Nurse Practitioners, 17*(2), 67–75.

Stull, A., & Lanz, C. (2005). An innovative model for nursing scholarship. *Journal of Nursing Education, 44*(11), 493–497.

Taft, L. B., Stolder, M. E., Knutson, A. B., Tamke, K., Platt, J., & Bowles, T. (2004). Oral history: Validating contributions of elders. *Geriatric Nursing, 25*(1), 38–43.

Timmerman, G. M. (1999). Using a women's health perspective to guide decisions made in quantitative research. *Journal of Advanced Nursing, 30*(3), 640–645.

Titler, M. G. (2002). Use of research in practice. In G. LoBiondo & J. Haber (Eds.), *Nursing research methods: Critical appraisal and utilization* (5th ed.). St. Louis, MO: Mosby.

Titler, M. G., Klieber, C., Steelman, V., Goode, C., Rakel, B., Barry-Walker, J., et al. (1994). Infusing research into practice to promote quality care. *Nursing Research, 43*(5), 307–313.

Trim, S. (2008). Journal club offers new opportunities. *Kai Tiaki Nursing New Zealand, 14*(11), 23.

Tropello, P. G. D. (2000). *Origins of the nurse practitioner movement, an oral history* (Doctoral dissertation). Rutgers, State University of New Jersey–New Brunswick, and University of Medicine and Dentistry of New Jersey. (UMI Order No. AAI9970979)

Tymkow, C., Shen, J. J., & MacMullen, N. (2006). Project 2: Emergency room usage among uninsured patients with access to a primary care provider. In L. Samson (Ed.), *Building capacity for health disparities research.* Grant 1P20MD001816-01 from the National Center on Minority Health and Health Disparities, National Institutes of Health, Bethesda, MD.

van Manen, M. (1990). *Researching lived experiences: Human science for an action sensitive pedagogy.* Albany, NY: State University of New York Press.

Watkins, C., Harvey, I., Langley, C., Gray, S., & Faulkner, A. (1999). General practitioners' use of guidelines in the consultation and their attitudes to them. *British Journal of General Practice, 49*(438), 11–15.

Webber, P. B. (2008). The Doctor of Nursing Practice degree and research: Are we making an epistemological mistake? *Journal of Nursing Education, 47*(10), 466–472.

Yegdich, T. (1999). In the name of Husserl: Nursing in pursuit of the things-in-themselves. *Nursing Inquiry, 7*(1), 29–40.

Zuzelo, P. R. (2007). Evidence-based nursing and qualitative research: A partnership imperative for real-world practice. In P. L. Munhall (Ed.), *Nursing research: A qualitative perspective* (4th ed.). Sudbury, MA: Jones and Bartlett.

CHAPTER 4

Information Systems/Technology and Patient Care Technology for the Improvement and Transformation of Health Care

Susan F. Burkart-Jayez

The "soul of informatics" demands proactive engagement of all health care profes-
sionals to address our fundamental educational needs for this new paradigm—a par-
adigm where values and technologies are virtually inseparable. How do we prepare
practitioners, educators, and researchers? . . . How are we preparing our profes-
sionals and future academic, practice, and research leaders for a whole new world?
—CONNIE WHITE DELANEY

The American Association of Colleges of Nursing's (AACN) *Essentials of Doc-*
toral Education for Advanced Nursing Practice (2006, p. 12) identifies "foundational outcome competencies deemed essential for all graduates of a
Doctorate of Nursing Practice (DNP) program regardless of specialty or
functional focus." This chapter addresses Essential IV in preparing DNP
graduates to "utilize information systems to evaluate programs of care, outcomes of care, and care systems" and to "provide leadership within healthcare systems and/or academic settings related to the use of information
systems." For the full recommendation, see Figure 4-1.

According to Kingsley and Kingsley (2009), "there is a substantial generation gap between college professors and their students . . . [S]tudents are
more comfortable in a technology rich environment, but that doesn't equate
to knowledge [and/or] critical thinking skills needed to locate, filter, and
evaluate information found on line. A core competency for operating in an
electronic environment is information literacy . . . [the ability] to apply new
knowledge, manage individual and aggregate level information, and assess
the efficacy of patient care technology."

■ **Figure 4-1 Essential IV: Information Systems/Technology and Patient Care Technology for the Improvement and Transformation of Health Care**

DNP graduates are distinguished by their abilities to use information systems/technology to support and improve patient care and healthcare systems, and provide leadership within healthcare systems and/or academic settings. Knowledge and skills related to information systems/technology and patient care technology prepare the DNP graduate to apply new knowledge, manage individual and aggregate level information, and assess the efficacy of patient care technology appropriate to a specialized area of practice. DNP graduates also design, select, and use information systems/technology to evaluate programs of care, outcomes of care, and care systems. Information systems/technology provide a mechanism to apply budget and productivity tools, practice information systems and decision supports, and web-based learning or intervention tools to support and improve patient care.

DNP graduates must also be proficient in the use of information systems/technology resources to implement quality improvement initiatives and support practice and administrative decision-making. Graduates must demonstrate knowledge of standards and principles for selecting and evaluating information systems and patient care technology, and related ethical, regulatory, and legal issues.

The DNP program prepares the graduate to:

1. Design, select, use, and evaluate programs that evaluate and monitor outcomes of care, care systems, and quality improvement including consumer use of health care information systems.

2. Analyze and communicate critical elements necessary to the selection, use, and evaluation of health care information systems and patient care technology.

3. Demonstrate the conceptual ability and technical skills to develop and execute an evaluation plan involving data extraction from practice information systems and databases.

4. Provide leadership in the evaluation and resolution of ethical and legal issues within healthcare systems relating to the use of information, information technology, communication networks, and patient care technology.

5. Evaluate consumer health information sources for accuracy, timeliness, and appropriateness.

Source: American Association of Colleges of Nursing. (2006). *The essentials of doctoral education for advanced nursing practice.* Retrieved from http://www.aacn.nche.edu/DNP/Essentials.pdf. Reprinted with permission.

The nature of this topic is such that the most efficient use of the material presented is as a guide to building the knowledge, skills, abilities, and toolkits needed to achieve the outcomes recommended by the AACN. Topic background is presented to underscore the saliency of the author's suggestions, but the benefit of this chapter is best realized by performing the tasks as they are presented.

Information Systems/Technology

Computer Literacy and Competency

When faced with novel subspecialty information, it is important to learn the language of the domain. A brief glossary can be found in Appendix 4-2 at the end of the chapter, and terms used that are contained in the glossary are italicized in the text. Because *informatics* is an evolving field, concepts related to it change rapidly; therefore, the terminology continues to expand and evolve as national efforts at consensus continue. The most exciting aspect of the information to follow is that it brings the reader to the plan developed for *healthcare information technology (HIT)*. The target date for national implementation of competence in *computer literacy, information technology (IT)*, and *healthcare informatics* is 2014 (Kobalusk McGee, 2009). This guide is "just in time" training.

Over the years, multiple studies have looked at nursing students' and staff nurses' computer competency. Koivunen (2008, p. 302) "identified different ways of learning computer use and barriers to use; evaluating computer skills; performing a literature search; reflecting findings against the literature search on the most effective teaching and learning computer skills." Although the psychiatric nursing population was the domain of interest, the findings are generalizable to all nursing practice sites. The work identified learning methods and barriers to learning computer skills and evaluated the individual nurses' level of skill. This information was then used as the basis for developing more effective methods for achieving computer facility. Nurses' computer skills were evaluated using the European Computer Driving License/International Computer Driving License test (ECDL/ICDL) (ECDL, 2009).

Many institutions of higher education for nursing now have basic requirements for nursing students regarding information technology. One example is

Marshall University (2009). The first-year course, as described on the university's website, covers a basic understanding of computer *hardware* and *software* and how a computer works, *word processing*, the use of spreadsheets, and an ability to use software programs. Additionally, every course in the nursing program has a computer component in which students use hospital information systems to access patient data, conduct library searches through discipline-specific searches, and use spreadsheets as a management tool.

Building Internet Resources

Table 4-1 contains a non-exhaustive list of information *websites* used in preparing this section and useful in DNP-level practice. At this juncture, with text in hand, log on to the *Internet*, open your *browser*, and type each site's *URL* from the table into the browser's address field, one at a time. After typing each URL, select "Favorites" from the toolbar, and "add to" from the drop-down menu. At task completion, the reader will have a beginning collection of places in which to explore in depth the topics discussed in this chapter. Additionally, the list will present the latest in acquiring computer literacy or competency and accessing quality clinical care standards.

Authors such as Eley et al. (2008, pp. 19–20) have explored nurses' computer competence. The results of the participants' self-assessed computer expertise were as follows: 50% felt that they required more computer or information technology training, and 25% felt that their current skill level was a barrier. Those who received on-the-job computer training believed the training was adequate and timely. These nurses felt that training, although available, was not emphasized as an option, and that training interfered with the nurse's workload. The group in this study favored a national standard for nursing computer competency.

Computer and Internet skills are necessary for the successful implementation of new IT applications in patient care (Koivunen, 2008, pp. 302–314; TIGER Initiative, n.d., 2007, 2009). *Computer literacy* is the ability to use computers to perform a variety of tasks. *Computer competency* is the ability to demonstrate proficiency in use of software applications such as Microsoft Word, Excel, and PowerPoint, and knowledge in computer terminology, hardware selection, and simple maintenance functions. Literacy is an attribute; competency is the reproducible evaluation of the skills and knowledge related to an attribute. According to Wojner (2001, pp. 202–203), "technology is only as good as the skills and knowledge of the clinicians using it

■ Table 4-1   Information Technology–Related Websites

Nursing Informatics Working Group (NIWG)	http://www.amia.org/niwg
Alliance for Nursing Informatics	ANI and the TIGER initiative: http://www.allianceni.org/tiger.asp
Nelson: Patient Care Technology and Safety	http://www.ahrq.gov/qual/nurseshdbk/docs/ PowellG_PCTS.pdf
American Library Association	http://www.ala.org/ala/mgrps/divs/aasl/guidelinesandstandards/ guidelinesandstandards.cfm
Centers for Disease Control and Prevention	http://www.cdc.gov
National Guidelines Clearinghouse	Clinical guidelines: http://www.ngc.gov
Nursing Informatics	Competency lists: http://www.nursing-informatics.com/niassess/index.html
Project SAILS	https://www.projectsails.org/abouttest/skillsets.php? page=aboutTest#id1#id1
European Computer Driving License	http://www.ecdl.co.uk
Agency for Healthcare Research and Quality	http://www.ahrq.gov
Health Information Technology	http://healthit.hhs.gov
Health Information Technology Scholars Program	http://www.hits-colab.org
American Library Association	Information literacy: http://www.ala.org/ala/acrl/acrlissues/ acrlinfolit/infolitoverview/introtoinfolit/introinfolit.htm
National Academies Press	Institute of Medicine's collection of work on healthcare quality improvement issues: http://www.nap.edu
The Joint Commission	http://www.jointcommission.org/sentinelevents
Marshall University	Marshall University nursing competency requirements: http://www.marshall.edu/academic-affairs/MU_Info/mpcomp.htm
National League of Nursing	http://www.nln.org/aboutnln/PositionStatements/ informatics_052808.pdf
Agency for Healthcare Research and Quality	Patient safety work by AHRQ: http://www.psnet.ahrq.gov
Presidential message	Presidential call for electronic health records by 2014: Executive order 13,410 at http://www.whitehouse.gov

(continues)

■ Table 4-1   **Information Technology–Related Websites** (CONTINUED)

The Leapfrog Group	Private agency for quality: http://www.leapfroggroup.org
Quality Forum	Private agency for quality: http://www.qualityforum.org
Institute for Healthcare Improvement	Private agency for quality: http://www.ihi.org
Healthcare Quality	Quality and safety issues in nursing: http://www.qsen.org/about/overview
Robert Wood Johnson Foundation	Healthcare technology projects: http://www.rwjf.org
Safe Practices for Better Healthcare: 2006 Update	http://www.ihi.org/Topics/PatientSafety/SafetyGeneral/ Literature/SafePracticesforBetterHealthcare2006Table1.htm
TIGER	TIGER summit site: http://www.tigersummit.com
Informatics Competencies	University of Utah: http://www.nurs.utah.edu/informatics/ competencies.htm
Tech Terms Dictionary	http://www.oasismanagement.com/TECHNOLOGY/GLOSSARY/

. . . [T]he effect of technology varies . . . as a result of the different methods used to prepare and teach the clinicians to use it."

The Technology Informatics Guiding Education Reform (TIGER) initiative (TIGER, 2009), involving over 1,100 nursing content experts, completed three years of work in developing a ten-year plan for nursing's path toward computer/information/informatics literacy for patient care as one domain requiring curriculum development (Figure 4-2). The TIGER initiative is a large-scale example of outcomes management: methodically unraveling the issue, significance, and outcomes of patient care. One of the focus areas of the TIGER initiative is defining the basic technology competency curriculum for nurses. Standardized proficiency in healthcare technology will ensure that variance in efficacy of technology use by individuals will be dampened. The collaborative was funded by federal grants from the National Library of Medicine, National Institutes of Health, and the Department of Health and Human Services, and by grants from the Robert Wood Johnson Foundation and the Agency for Healthcare Research and Quality (AHRQ), among others. The initiative's sponsorship (Table 4-2) is worth mentioning and is indirect evidence of the importance of incorporating computer and technology into nursing's educational base. Each of these entities has its own website. For

The TIGER Informatics Competencies Team have organized and harmonized the informatics competencies into four primary categories:

1. Basic Computer Competencies
2. Information Literacy Competencies
3. Information Management and Informatics Competencies
4. Clinical Information Management Competencies

Component of the TIGER Nursing Informatics Competencies Model	Standard	Standard-Setting Body
Basic Computer Competencies	European Computer Driving Licence	European Computer Driving Licence Foundation
Information Literacy	Information Literacy Competency Standards	American Library Association
Information Management	Electronic Health Record Functional Model–Clinical Care Components	Health Level Seven (HL7)
	European Computer Driving Licence–Health	European Computer Driving Licence Foundation

Basic Computer Competencies

European Computer Driving Licence (ECDL) Foundation
http://ecdl.com

- The ECDL syllabus is maintained and periodically updated by the not-for-profit ECDL Foundation. The ECDL Foundation makes arrangements with entities in various countries to localize the ECDL syllabus. Outside of Europe, ECDL is known as International Computer Driving Licence. ICDL is available in the United States through CSPlacement.

CSPlacement
www.csplacement.com

- Offers CSP Basic, an e-learning course and a certification exam that is substantially equivalent to the TICC recommendation of a first and significant step towards basic computer competency.
- Offers CSP, an e-learning course and a certification exam that is substantially equivalent to the entire ECDL syllabus.

■ Figure 4-2   Recommendations of the TIGER Informatics Competencies Team

Source: The above work is entirely excerpted from the TIGER website and is the sole creation and property of same.

Healthcare Information Management System Society (HIMSS)
www.himss.org
- Has a new certificate called Health Informatics Training System (HITS). The HITS program of e-learning, testing, and certification contains content that is substantially equivalent to the TICC recommendation of a first and significant step towards basic computer competency, as well as other content.

Information Literacy

Information literacy builds on computer literacy. Information literacy is the ability to

- identify information needed for a specific purpose
- locate pertinent information
- evaluate the information
- apply it correctly

By January 2011, all practicing nurses and graduating nursing students will have the ability to:

1. Determine the nature and extent of the information needed
2. Access needed information effectively and efficiently
3. Evaluate information and its sources critically and incorporate selected information into his or her knowledge base and value system
4. Individually or as a member of a group, use information effectively to accomplish a specific purpose
5. Evaluate outcomes of the use of information

Resources

American Library Association
http://www.ala.org/ala/mgrps/divs/acrl/standards/informationliteracy
competency.cfm
- The ALA's report "Information Literacy Competency Standards for Higher Education" identifies the competencies recommended above as standards. The report also lists performance indicators and outcomes for each standard. A faculty member or instructor can effectively use this report to

■ Figure 4-2   Recommendations of the TIGER Informatics Competencies Team
(CONTINUED)

create a more detailed syllabus and/or lesson plan(s) to implement the TICC information literacy competencies.

The Information Literacy in Technology
http://www.ilitassessment.com
- The iLIT test assesses a student's ability to access, evaluate, incorporate, and use information. It is a commercially available test and may be of use in demonstrating proficiency in information literacy.

Information Management

Information management is the underlying principle upon which TICC Clinical Information Management Competencies are built. Information management is a process consisting of 1) collecting data, 2) processing the data, and 3) presenting and communicating the processed data as information or knowledge.

Recommendation	Timeline for Adoption
Schools of nursing and healthcare delivery organizations will implement the information competencies	By January 2012
Schools of nursing and healthcare delivery organizations will implement the transformed ECDL-Health syllabus items listed above.	By January 2012

Resources

HL7 EHR System Functional Model
http://www.hl7.org/EHR/
- This ANSI standard can be used by nursing instructors in schools of nursing and healthcare delivery organizations to develop curriculum to impart the recommended information management competencies to all practicing nurses and graduating nursing students.

ICDL-Health Syllabus
http://www.ecdl.com Click products, then ECDL Health

■ Figure 4-2   Recommendations of the TIGER Informatics Competencies Team
(CONTINUED)

- A significant portion of the HL7 EHR System Functional Model is covered by the ECDL-Health Syllabus. The ECDL-Health Syllabus was developed by the ECDL Foundation to extend the foundation of basic computer competency skills that are not industry specific into the healthcare industry.

Digital Patient Record Certification (DPRC)
http://dprcertification.com
- The ECDL Foundation partners with an organization in each country that wishes to use ICDL-Health to localize the syllabus for use in that country. In the United States, the Digital Patient Record Certification localizes the ICDL-Health syllabus.

Health Information System Management Society
www.himss.org
- The HITS program, sponsored in the United States by the Health Information System Management Society, uses a more international version of the ICDL-Health syllabus.

Clinical Information Management Competencies

TICC has transformed the Direct Care components of the HL7 EHR System Functional Model into these recommended Clinical Information Management Competencies for nurses (of the 70+ listed, a sample follows):

Using an EHRS, the nurse can:

Identify and Maintain a Patient Record
Manage Patient Demographics
Present Ad Hoc Views of the Health Record
Manage Medication Lists
Manage Problem Lists
Manage Patient-Specific Care and Treatment Plans
Manage Medication Administration
Manage Clinical Documents and Notes
Interact with Clinical Workflow Tasking
Interact with Clinical Task Assignment and Routing
Facilitate Patient, Family and Care Giver Education
Facilitate Communication with Medical Devices

For complete information log on to: http://www.tigersummit.com/

■ Figure 4-2 Recommendations of the TIGER Informatics Competencies Team
(CONTINUED)

■ Table 4-2   Sponsors of the TIGER Initiative

Alliance for Nursing Informatics
American Health Information Management Association
American Medical Informatics Association
American Nurses Association
American Nursing Informatics Association
Apptis
Audience Response Systems
Capital Area Roundtable on Informatics in Nursing
Cerner Corporation
Clinical Information Technology Program Office
CliniComp International
CPM Resource Center
Eclipsys
Elsevier
GE Healthcare Systems
Healthcare Information and Management Systems Society
IBM
Independence Foundation
Marion J. Ball
McKesson
MITRE Corporation
Siemens
Sigma Theta Tau International
Tenet Healthcare
Thomson Healthcare
University of Maryland, Baltimore County

further background, readers are invited to go to their browser, type each organization's name into the search box, and *browse* areas of interest.

A second task is to visit and interact with the TIGER summit website (which should now be in your Favorites list). View each of the tabs across the top of the site for a complete map of nursing's competency needs for the immediate and long-term future. This site presents the proposed curriculum content changes that will be introduced into all levels of nursing education over the next ten years. Patricia Hinton-Walker, one of the foundational leaders of the TIGER initiative, offered the following in a personal communication (4/21/09):

The T.I.G.E.R. initiative is now moving into phase III. The focus of T.I.G.E.R III is integration throughout the nursing profession and with interdisciplinary colleagues. The work of one of the T.I.G.E.R Collaborative groups was to develop a Virtual Demonstration Center. This center will be the vehicle for much of the dissemination and learning that needs to take place connected with other collaboratives such as: education, leadership, staff development, integrating the informatics competencies that the informatics collaborative developed. The T.I.G.E.R Phase III team is just coming together to explore funding and new partnerships that will allow the T.I.G.E.R initiative to move forward with integration through dissemination and development of learning platforms in order to facilitate the integration. Additionally, a major focus of T.I.G.E.R III will be to explore funding and partnerships needed to develop the Virtual Demonstration Center for national and future International access.

The third task is to learn about the ECDL/ICDL by accessing the ECDL/ICDL site (ECDL, 2009). Table 4-3 provides an overview of the ECDL concept. After reviewing the content of this table, the reader should log on to the Internet and click on the Favorites *icon*; the drop-down list should include www.ecdl.co.uk. It is recommended the reader thoroughly explore the site to get a sense of the future changes that need to occur in the nursing curriculum to embrace computer competency. How is it that the EDCL/ICDL is identified as core to computer/information literacy/competency? In addition to the recommendations of the TIGER summit (2009), other nursing scholars have testified to the utility of this toolkit. According to Jones (2005), the ECDL is currently used in teaching basic IT skills to staff in all industries, not just health care. In a survey conducted in the United Kingdom, nurses who had ECDL certification responded that they were saving up to 30 minutes of time a day, which was then available for direct patient care. This study produced information on computer competency's impact on how nurses spend their time after the implementation of healthcare information technology.

Kossman (2008, p. 70) notes that the recommendations of the Institute of Medicine (IOM) to improve patient safety include the use of information technology to automate medication delivery systems, collect patient clinical data, and provide clinical decision support. Time burden studies (Kossman, 2008; Lee, 2007; Breslin, 2004) looking at the impact of *electronic health record (EHR)* use on nurses' time, using a variety of methodologies that included time–motion studies, work sampling, and self-report, had varied results, show increased, decreased, and neutral time burdens with EHRs.

■ Table 4-3   The ECDL

The core certification in the ECDL Foundation's product range is the ECDL/ICDL, the world's leading end-user computer skills certification program. The ECDL/ICDL is designed to cover the key concepts of computing, their practical applications, and their use in the workplace and society. The certification test that this series prepares students to take is a part of earning the European Computer Driving Licence (ECDL) 4.0 certification.

Module 1: Concepts of Information Technology (IT)

Requires the candidate to have an understanding of some of the main concepts of IT at a general level.

Module 2: Using the Computer and Managing Files

Requires the candidate to demonstrate knowledge and competence in using the common functions of a personal computer and its operating system.

Module 3: Word Processing

Requires the candidate to demonstrate the ability to use a word processing application on a computer.

Module 4: Spreadsheets

Requires the candidate to understand the concept of spreadsheets and to demonstrate the ability to use a spreadsheet application on a computer.

Module 5: Database

Requires the candidate to understand some of the main concepts of databases and demonstrate the ability to use a database on a computer.

Module 6: Presentation

Requires the candidate to demonstrate competence in using presentation tools on a computer.

Module 7: Information and Communication

Module 7 is divided into two sections. The first section, Information, requires the candidate to understand some of the concepts and terms associated with using the Internet and to appreciate some of the security situations. In the second section, Communication, the candidate is required to understand some of the concepts of electronic mail (e-mail) together with having an appreciation of some of the security considerations associated with using e-mail.

Source: ECDL Foundation. http://www.ecdl.com. Reprinted with permission.

Doctorally prepared advance practice nurses (APNs) must be competent in computers, information technology, and informatics to be able to transform *data* into information used in executive decision making. Standardized competency is the first step. Because the experts in various nursing and healthcare information organizations proposing computer competency curricula recommend the EDCL/ICDL as foundational, the reader is encouraged to achieve EDCL/IDCL certification, regardless of level of educational preparation (Jones, 2005, pp. 70–71; TIGER, 2007).

In the literature, many subscribe to the core requirement of computer literacy for nurses. "Curriculum Strategies to Improve Baccalaureate Nursing Information Technology Outcomes" (Fetter, 2009, p. 4), for example, identifies "enhancing information technology (IT) competence as one of nursing's most significant and urgent priorities," which has vast potential to reduce health errors and improve care quality, access, and cost-effectiveness. In 2004 the Department of Health and Human Services called for "IT to be completely integrated into patient care" and noted that "the Veterans Administration (VA) is currently close to realizing this goal" (Fetter, 2009). The strategy outlined in Fetter's article includes policy-based incentives for the networking of nursing programs, clinical agencies, vendors, and accrediting bodies in order to introduce standard IT and information literacy and competency into nursing education and practice.

Information Literacy

According to the Nursing Informatics Working Group's (NIWG) history page,

> Information literacy builds on computer literacy, taking the ability to find the information and adding the ability to evaluate and apply it. With respect to nursing practice, information literacy is the ability to identify information needed for a specific purpose, locate pertinent information, evaluate the information and apply it correctly. (Englebardt & Nelson, 2002)

The steps and skills needed for providing the best patient care in a technology-rich environment presented on the NIWG website include the ability to determine what information is needed by using critical thinking and assessment skills. The nurse should find the information based on all available resources, including colleagues, policies, and literature in various formats; evaluate the information using critical thinking and evaluation of the validity of the source; put the information into practice; and evaluate whether use of the information resulted in improved patient care.

According to the American Library Association (ALA), *information literacy* is defined as the set of skills needed to find, retrieve, analyze, and use information. The next task for the reader is to access the ALA site for the latest in information literacy. The American Association of School Librarians (AASL), a division of the ALA, describes the information-literate student as one who

- Accesses information efficiently and effectively
- Evaluates information critically and competently
- Uses information accurately and creatively
- Pursues information related to personal interests
- Appreciates literature and other creative expressions of information
- Strives for excellence in information seeking and knowledge generation
- Recognizes the importance of information to a democratic society
- Practices ethical behavior in regard to information and information technology
- Participates effectively in groups to pursue and generate information (ALA, 1998)

Kent State University in Ohio has developed and maintains a Standardized Assessment of Information Literacy Skills (SAILS) (see Table 4-4 for details). The SAILS website defines the skills required to find, retrieve, critically evaluate, and implement information. The tools supplied are sufficient for the student to achieve information literacy through self-study, or as a basis for curriculum design (Radcliff et al., 2007). Doctoral-level nurses need to be experts in critically evaluating the available information using multiple sources.

Berwick et al. (1991, p. 153) noted that more time spent on training in the use of basic tools translates into more rapid gains. He gives examples of information literacy found in everyday practice: Pareto diagrams (representing largest to smallest frequency), line graphs/run charts (identifying trends over time), pie charts (showing relative parts of a whole), bar graphs (comparing categorical data), histograms (showing frequency distribution of continuous data such as time, weight, size, or temperature), and control charts (determining whether a process can be considered stable, and thus predictable, or unstable, and thus unpredictable). Such information presentation is common, yet not all viewers are fully knowledgeable as to the concepts behind these graphics, much less when to use which type. As one becomes information literate, one gains the ability to generate data and to transform these data into information

■ Table 4-4 Project SAILS

Developing a Research Strategy

- Describes a general process for searching for information.
- Identifies keywords that describe an information source (e.g., book, journal article, magazine article, website).
- Identifies the appropriate service point or resource for the particular information need.
- Uses the website of an institution, library, organization, or community to locate information about specific services.
- Uses various technologies to manage the information selected and organized.
- Determines whether information satisfies the research or other information need.

Selecting Finding Tools

- Distinguishes among indexes, online databases, and collections of online databases, as well as gateways to different databases and collections.
- Selects appropriate tools (e.g., indexes, online databases) for research on a particular topic.
- Identifies the differences between freely available Internet search tools and subscription or fee-based databases.
- Determines when some topics may be too recent to be covered by some standard tools (e.g., a periodicals index) and when information on the topic retrieved by less authoritative tools (e.g., a Web search engine) may not be reliable.

Searching

- Demonstrates an understanding of the concept of Boolean logic and constructs a search statement using Boolean operators.
- Demonstrates an understanding of the concept of proximity searching and constructs a search statement using proximity operators.
- Demonstrates an understanding of the concept of nesting and constructs a search using nested words or phrases.
- Demonstrates an understanding of the concept of keyword searching and uses it appropriately and effectively.
- Demonstrates an understanding of the concept of truncation and uses it appropriately and effectively.
- Narrows or broadens questions and search terms to retrieve the appropriate quantity of information, using search techniques such as Boolean logic, limiting, and field searching.

■ Table 4-4   Project SAILS (CONTINUED)

- Demonstrates how searches may be limited or expanded by modifying search terminology or logic.

Using Finding Tool Features

- Describes the structure and components of the system or tool being used, regardless of format (e.g., index, thesaurus, type of information retrieved by the system).

- Identifies the source of help within a given information retrieval system and uses it effectively.

- Identifies what types of information are contained in a particular system (e.g., all branch libraries are included in the catalog; not all databases are full text; catalogs, periodical databases, and websites may be included in a gateway).

- Determines appropriate means for recording or saving the desired information (e.g., printing, saving to disc, photocopying, taking notes).

- Uses help screens and other user aids to understand the particular search structures and commands of an information retrieval system.

- Demonstrates an awareness of the fact that there may be separate interfaces for basic and advanced searching in retrieval systems.

- Describes search functionality common to most databases regardless of differences in the search interface (e.g., Boolean logic capability, field structure, keyword searching, relevancy ranking).

- Selects among various technologies the most appropriate one for the task of extracting the needed information (e.g., copy/paste software functions, photocopier, scanner, audio/visual equipment, or exploratory instruments)

Retrieving Sources

- Demonstrates an understanding of the fact that items may be grouped together by subject in order to facilitate browsing.

- Describes some materials that are not available online or in digitized formats and must be accessed in print or other formats (e.g., microform, video, audio).

- Retrieves a document in print or electronic form.

- Describes various retrieval methods for information not available locally.

Evaluating Sources

- Demonstrates an understanding that some information and information sources may present a one-sided view and may express opinions rather than facts.

(continues)

■ **Table 4-4   Project SAILS** (CONTINUED)

- Demonstrates an understanding that some information and sources may be designed to trigger emotions, conjure stereotypes, or promote support for a particular viewpoint or group.

- Searches for independent verification or corroboration of the accuracy and completeness of the data or representation of facts presented in an information source.

Documenting Sources

- Identifies different types of information sources cited in a research tool.

- Identifies citation elements for information sources in different formats (e.g., book, article, television program, Web page, and interview).

- Locates information about documentation styles either in print or electronically (e.g., through the library's website).

Understanding Economic, Legal, and Social Issues

- Identifies and discusses issues related to privacy and security in both the print and electronic environments.

- Demonstrates an understanding that not all information on the Web is free (i.e., some Web-based databases require users to pay a fee or to subscribe in order to retrieve full text or other content).

- Participates in electronic discussions following accepted practices (e.g., "Netiquette").

- Legally obtains, stores, and disseminates text, data, images, or sounds.

Source: Radcliff, C. J., Salem, J. A., Jr., O'Connor, L. G., & Gedeon, J. A. (2007). *Project SAILS skill sets for the 2008–2009 academic year*. Retrieved from https://www.projectsails.org/abouttest/skillsets.php. Modified with permission.

for executive decision making. McNeil et al. (2003, p. 345), who surveyed nurses at the exit from their education program regarding their IT skills, found that "e-mail use, bibliographic retrieval via library-based resources or the Internet, use of the Internet and World Wide Web, and use of presentation graphics software were most frequently cited as computer competency skills acquired. Information technology tools such as remote monitoring devices, online consumer health tools, and hand-held computers were examples given by the group studied as examples of information literacy skills." This indicated a need for nursing curricula to include information management (literacy) as found in daily nursing practice. The American Association of School Librarians maintains a list of the "25 best teaching and learning sites" for information management, literacy, and technology-based tools (ALA, 2000).

Informatics

Thede (2003, p. 6) writes that Scholes and Barber first used the term "informatics" in 1980 in an address to MEDINFO, and that *nursing informatics* is "the use of computer technology in all endeavors: services, education and research." Thede further states that "informatics offers many benefits for health care: the ability to create and use aggregated data, to prevent errors, and to provide better medical records." According to Thede, the National Center for Nursing Research proposed seven areas for nursing informatics: "using data, information, and knowledge for patient care; defining data in nursing care; acquiring and delivering knowledge about patient care; creating new tools for patient care from new technologies; integrating systems; and evaluating the effects of nursing systems." Fifteen years later, nursing education still struggles with the core curriculum to ensure students and graduates are able to achieve competency in these areas.

Ornes (2007, p. 75) emphasizes that "Nursing [p]rograms must integrate informatics content into their curricula to prepare nurses to use information technology" and cites the observation of Staggers (2002, p. 384) that nurses need "fundamental information management and computer technology skills" so they can "use existing information systems and available information to manage their practice."

The National League for Nursing's (NLN) position statement on preparing the next generation of nurses for practice (2008) addresses incorporating informatics competencies into nursing education, noting that informatics is one of the Institute of Medicine's five quality and safety competencies. The other quality and safety competencies are patient-centered care, teamwork and collaboration, evidence-based practice, and quality improvement and safety. The NLN further recommends forming partnerships between clinicians and informatics people at the agency level to "help faculty and students develop competence in informatics, and to ensure that all faculty members have competence in computer literacy, information literacy, and informatics" (NLN, 2008) (Table 4-5).

One often-cited master list of competencies was developed by Staggers et al. (2002, pp. 384–385) and is available through the University of Utah website listed in Table 4-1. This study, reported by Page (2004), had as its focus

■ Table 4-5   Recommendations of the National League of Nursing

The National League for Nursing recommends the following for faculty, administrators, and its own leaders and members:

For Nurse Faculty

- Participate in faculty development programs to achieve competency in informatics.
- Designate an informatics champion in every school of nursing to:
  (a) help faculty distinguish between using instructional technologies to teach vs. using informatics to guide, document, analyze, and inform nursing practice, and
  (b) translate state-of-the-art practices in technology and informatics that need to be integrated into the curriculum.
- Incorporate informatics into the curriculum.
- Incorporate ANA-recognized standard nursing language and terminology into content.
- Identify clinical informatics exemplars, those drawn from clinical agencies and the community or from other nursing education programs, to serve as examples for the integration of informatics into the curriculum.
- Achieve competency through participation in faculty development programs.
- Partner with clinicians and informatics people at clinical agencies to help faculty and students develop competence in informatics.
- Collaborate with clinical agencies to ensure that students have hands-on experience with informatics tools.
- Collaborate with clinical agencies to demonstrate transformations in clinical practice produced by informatics.
- Establish criteria to evaluate informatics goals for faculty.

For Deans/Directors/Chairs

- Provide leadership in planning for necessary IT infrastructure that will ensure education that prepares graduates for 21st-century practice roles and responsibilities.
- Allocate sufficient resources to support IT initiatives.
- Ensure that all faculty members have competence in computer literacy, information literacy, and informatics.
- Provide opportunities for faculty development in informatics.
- Urge clinical agencies to provide hands-on informatics experiences for students.
- Encourage nurse-managed clinics to incorporate clinical informatics exemplars that have transformed nursing practice to provide safe quality care.

■ **Table 4-5 Recommendations of the National League of Nursing**
(CONTINUED)

- Advocate that all students graduate with up-to-date knowledge and skills in each of the three critical areas: computer literacy, information literacy, and informatics.
- Establish criteria to evaluate outcomes related to achieving informatics goals.

For the National League for Nursing

- Disseminate this position statement widely.
- Seek external funding and allocate internal resources to convene a think tank to reach consensus on definitions of informatics, competencies for faculty and students, and program outcomes that include informatics.
- Participate actively in organizations that focus on education in nursing informatics to ensure that recommendations from those organizations are congruent with the NLN's positions on curriculum.
- Use ETIMAC and its task groups to:
  (a) develop programs for faculty, showcase exemplar programs, and
  (b) disseminate outcomes from the think tank.
- Encourage and facilitate accrediting bodies, regulatory agencies, and certifying bodies to reach consensus on definitions related to informatics and minimal informatics competencies for practice in the 21st century.

Source: National League for Nursing. (2008, May 9). *Preparing the next generation of nurses to practice in a technology-rich environment: An informatics agenda*. Retrieved from http://www.nln.org/aboutnln /PositionStatements/informatics_052808.pdf. Reprinted with permission.

the production of a research-based master list of informatics competencies, differentiated by level of nursing practice. Informatics knowledge is the theory; informatics skills are the methods, tools, and techniques; and computer literacy is learning how to manipulate computer technology.

Lin et al. (2007, p. 54) defined informatics competency as the knowledge and skills necessary to use computers and information technology in nursing practice. One of their suggested competencies was in basic programming skills using software such as Microsoft Excel. In their report, Lin et al. state that the conceptual framework for nursing informatics competency includes "hardware, software and network concepts; computer application principles; computer use skills; programming design; computer limitations; personal and social issues; and attitudes toward computers." Charles (2008, p. 22) presents informatics in the context of *evidence-based medicine (EBM)* as using tested, objectively measurable care guidelines and following best practices to reduce variability in care outcomes. The Evidence-Based Practice page (www.ahrq.gov/clinic/epcix.htm) on AHRQ's website provides information on EBM and the informatics available for incorporating guidelines into practice for the DNP.

Kirkley (2004, p. 94) explains how the use of clinical IT in bedside nursing mirrors magnet-level qualities. She describes a *computer information system (CIS)* introduced within a healthcare agency in 1998 that had an online decision support system (DSS), clinical documentation, care planning, and *computerized physician order entry (CPOE)*. The core nursing functions included results reporting, clinical documentation, medication charting, patient assessments, and performance reports, thus giving nurses the knowledge they need to make informed decisions at the point of care. At the facility studied, all educational materials, policies, and procedures were consolidated online for open access to all staff, and nurses completed competency training by computer. This supported the magnet aspect that nurses are accountable for their own practice as well as the coordination of care.

Patient Care Technology

Technology is not a panacea: although designed to serve as a safety defense to prevent or minimize the effects of adverse events, when used inappropriately or poorly implemented, technology can contribute to errors and adverse events. Technology has the potential to reduce adverse events in four ways: eliminate errors, reduce error occurrence, detect errors early, and mitigate the effects of errors after they occur.
—NELSON (2004)

What is patient care technology (PCT)? According to Audrey Nelson in *Patient Safety and Quality: An Evidence-Based Handbook for Nurses*, (2004, p. 652) "Patient care technologies can be classified in many ways ... : direct nursing care delivery technology, indirect nursing care delivery technology, communication technology, patient and nurse protective devices, nurse protective devices, patient assessment, monitoring and surveillance, patient assistive devices, remote monitoring, continued learning, and pattern identification. Well-designed technology allows nurses to focus on care-giving functions and promoting the health of patients." Table 4-6 presents some of the daily tools requiring competent use by nurses. The reader's fourth task is to access the patient safety information at http://www.ahrq.gov/qual/nurseshdbk/docs/PowellG_PCTS.pdf. Current APN practice includes the "hospitalist" role, that is, providing oversight of the care provided to the inpatient population in various settings. Doctorally prepared

■ Table 4-6   Technology Commonly Used by Nurses

Direct Nursing Care Delivery Technology

Barcode medication administration
IV pumps
Feeding pumps

Indirect Nursing Care Delivery

Robotics
Radio frequency identification
Electronic inventory systems
Computerized staffing systems

Communication with People Distanced by Place and Time

Electronic medical records
Electronic ordering systems
Communication devices (cell phones, PDAs, Voicera paging systems)

Patient Assessment, Monitoring, and Surveillance

Telemetry
Bedside monitoring
Ventilators
Video surveillance
Stethoscope
Sphygmomanometer
Thermometer
Otoscope
Ophthalmoscope
Pulse oximetry

Remote Patient Monitoring

Telemedicine and Telehealth

Pattern Identification (to learn from errors and systems influences on adverse events)

Electronic medical records
Workload and staffing data systems

Continuous Learning

Distance learning
Video conferencing
Online training

Patient Protective Devices

Wandering alarms
Fall alarms

(continues)

■ Table 4-6 Technology Commonly Used by Nurses (CONTINUED)

Nurse Protective Devices

Mechanical lifts
Hand sanitizer dispensers

Source: Powell-Cope, G., Nelson, A. L. & Patterson, E. S. (2008). Patient care technology and safety. In R. G. Hughes (Ed.), Patient safety and quality: *An evidence-based handbook for nurses* (AHRQ Publication No. 08-0043). http://www.ahrq.gov/qual/nurseshdbk/docs/PowellG_PCTS.pdf. Modified with permission.

APNs need to be familiar, if not facile, with each of the patient care technology types, because they both oversee and provide direct patient care.

The Joint Commission (The Joint Commission, 2008) reported that adverse events related to health care/information technology arise from several sources, including lack of inclusion of frontline staff in developing and implementing new technologies, poor human–machine interfaces, absence of use of best-practices information, and poor resourcing for maintaining technologies once implemented. Recommendations to avoid unintended or adverse outcomes include involving end users in examining care processes for potential risks prior to implementing technological changes. Also recommended are training programs for all levels of clinicians and staff involved in the use of technology.

The disconnect between available technology and clinical utility is addressed by Wojner (2001, p. 205), who views technology as "only as good as the skills and knowledge of the clinicians using it" and notes that "the effect of technology varies between hospitals as a result of the different methods used to prepare and teach the clinicians to use it . . . particularly patient monitoring technologies." Wojner describes a common disconnect between the specific use of technology and the availability of devices, using pulse oximetry as an example. In collecting data on critically ill patients, one measure commonly collected is the pulse oximetry reading, without considering the utility of the information rendered. Patients treated for gastrointestinal bleeds or myocardial infarction in the emergency room are as likely to have pulse oximetry monitoring as the patient with chronic obstructive pulmonary disease, pneumonia, or pulmonary embolism. However, the information obtained is crucial to the latter group, and less so for the former. An analogy is monitoring body temperature in the suspected septic patient versus the patient with an acute orthopedic injury: A task is performed because the technology is available, and data are obtained and recorded, but the data are not necessarily essential in evaluating the presumed condition. The utility of the pulse oximetry measurement is for supplemental oxygen and other pulmonary-related interventions, yet the information is collected regardless of diagnosis as part of a routine task. Thus, Wojner cautions us that "the use of technology in healthcare must be tempered by education, training, and appropriate application in order to be of optimal benefit to patient outcomes."

Breslin et al. (2004, p. 275) evaluated one type of patient care technology, listed in Table 4-6 as "Communication with People Distanced by Place and Time," specifically, the use of Voicera wireless systems. The wireless Voicera system consists of a communication device worn by the user for all types of communications processes on inpatient units. Data collected for the study focused on the most prevalent communications processes, which included inbound communications from physicians, patients, patients' families, pharmacies, and laboratories, and outbound communications to physicians, intravenous therapy services, and ancillary departments. Using wireless technology on one nursing unit netted a time savings of more than 3,400 hours per year, or the equivalent of 1.7 full-time employees. This approximates an additional 3 hours per 8-hour shift available for direct patient care without increasing staffing levels, decreasing the probability of *nursing-sensitive adverse events*.

Conversely, Nelson (2004) notes, "given that 5,000 types of medical devices are used by millions of health care providers around the world, device related problems are inevitable." Common pitfalls include poor design, poor design interface with the intended application (patient-centered care), poor planning for technology-driven practice changes, and poor technology maintenance after implementation. This has led to the concept of "yet-to-be errors"—adverse events caused by unforeseen outcomes of using new technology. According to Simpson (2009, p. 203), the best way to eliminate human-induced errors is to improve human behavior. For nurses, better behavior results in better care. Standard competency assessment in the use of technology is one facet of improving behavior. Performance management, or monitoring patient care indicators, can also improve nursing behaviors by helping nurses map outcomes to practice through objective feedback on the individual's efficacy in providing care. Nurses have incredible knowledge and influence on healthcare outcomes, yet there is often variation in the quality of nursing care and in nurse-sensitive outcomes. The gap between knowledge and practice needs to be closed (Murphy, 2008). According to Delaney (personal communication 10/1/09) "all technology will change practice as will practice influence technology."

In work completed by Lee (2007, p. 109), patients' perceptions of nurses' behavior in the use of information in health care was found to fall into three categories: increased work efficiency (providing everyday care information; more time on patient care and less on documentation), privacy and confidentiality issues (because of easy data access), and satisfaction of relationships (didn't care about PDA use as long as they got the care they needed or didn't see difference in care). The use of technology-based tools by nurses was found to be of no concern to patients as long as the tools did not interfere with direct patient care.

Transformation of Health Care

Quality

> *Between the health care we have and the care we could have lies not just a gap, but a chasm. Failing to use available science is costly and harmful: it leads to overuse of unhelpful care, underuse of effective care and errors in execution. Simple innovations spread faster than complicated ones.*
>
> —BERWICK (2003, P. 1969)

Although the need for curriculum changes to integrate technology into nursing education has been discussed in the literature for nearly 30 years, the complexities of the innovations are a barrier. Until now, there has been little in policy and funding at the national level to encourage the changes required. However, the $21 billion allocated for health IT programs in the American Recovery and Reinvestment Act of 2009 will create career opportunities and fuel educational programs for professionals to acquire a mix of technology and clinical expertise with information technology (Kobalusk McGee, 2009). In the first year of incentives, hospitals can receive up to $1.5 million for effectively using electronic medical record (EMR) systems, while doctor practices can eventually earn around $40,000. It is estimated that only 20% of hospitals currently have fully functional HIT/EMR systems. With hospitals and other clinical practice sites making the leap to computerized patient records, the nursing education system will need to respond rapidly with appropriate classroom and practical training.

Technology affects safety (e.g., order entry decreases prescribing errors) and effectiveness (e.g., via clinical reminders) and enhances patient-centered care (e.g., by increasing clinical knowledge through Web resources), timeliness (e.g., e-health), and efficiency, all domains of interest for DNP clinical care and professional education. According to a report by Clancy (2009), better-quality health care using IT means making patient information available at the point of care at any time and to all team members in order to provide the right treatment, without delay, using best-practice guidelines, while preventing medical errors. An EMR coordinates patient care by "giving multiple providers access to the same, accurate and current information, extending medical resources to underserved populations through Telehealth, measuring performance for comparing providers by linking front end processes (DSS to assist in providing treatment) and back end feed-back systems to show outcomes."

Goldstein (2008, pp. 709–710) concurs that health information technology "facilitates the transparency and sharing of information that already exists— essential for improving the quality of care, reducing costs and reducing health care disparities." The IOM is an advocate of HIT/EMR, viewing it as fundamental to patient safety. Goldstein describes four essential components: a fully functional EMR with the ability to collect and store patient data electronically; an EMR capable of making information available to providers on request; computerized clinician order entry (often referred to as CPOE); and the ability to access computerized decision support. A minimally functional EMR has limited CPOE and limited DSS. Table 4-7 presents recommendations made by the National Quality Forum (NQF) regarding CPOEs.

Outcomes Management

Wojner's (2001) book *Outcomes Management: Applications to Clinical Practice* includes a self-instruction module introducing *outcomes management* (OM) and the use of technology in health care. If outcomes management is not part of the student's current course of study, this text will serve to help the reader understand its concepts and how computer competency is core to building outcomes management plans.

One of this chapter author's recent research projects in outcomes management was to measure the impact of technology on bedside acute care and intensive care nurses' time in rendering patient care. The project,

■ Table 4-7 National Quality Forum's Safe Practices, Care Settings, and Specifications for Computerized Prescriber Order Entry Systems

Practice and Care Settings	Additional Specifications
12. Implement a computerized prescriber order entry (CPOE) system built upon the requisite foundation of reengineered evidence-based care, an assurance of healthcare organization staff and independent practitioner readiness, and an integrated information technology infrastructure. *Applicable Clinical Care Settings:* Acute care hospitals, although incremental implementation may be necessary in rural areas (as defined by the U.S. Census Bureau) and/or small community hospitals.	Providers enter orders using an integrated, electronic information management system that is based on a documented implementation plan that includes or provides for the following: ■ Risks and hazards assessment to identify the performance gaps to be closed, including a lack of standardization of care; high-risk points in medication management systems such as at the point of order entry and at the point that the medication is administered; and the introduction of disruptive innovations. ■ Prospective re-engineering of care processes and workflow. ■ Readiness of integrated clinical information systems that include, at a minimum, the following information and management systems: Admit Discharge and Transfer (ADT); laboratory with electronic microbiology output; pharmacy; orders; electronic medication administration record (including patient, staff, and medication identification) (eMAR); clinical data repository with clinical decision support capability; scheduling; radiology; and clinical documentation. ■ Readiness of hospital governance, staff, and independent practitioners, including Board governance, senior administrative management, frontline caregivers, and independent practitioners. The following CPOE specifications: ■ facilitates the medication reconciliation process; ■ is part of an electronic health record information system or an existing clinical information system that is bidirectionally and tightly interfaced with, at a minimum, the pharmacy, the clinical documentation department (including medication administration records), and laboratory systems to facilitate the review of all orders from all providers; ■ is linked to prescribing error prevention software with effective clinical decision support capability; ■ requires prescribers to document the reasons for any override of an error prevention notice; ■ enables and facilitates the timely display and review of all new orders by a pharmacist before the administration of the first dose of medication, except in cases in which a delay would cause harm to a patient; ■ facilitates the review and/or display of all pertinent clinical information about the patient, including allergies, height

■ Table 4-7   National Quality Forum's Safe Practices, Care Settings, and Specifications for Computerized Prescriber Order Entry Systems (CONTINUED)

Practice and Care Settings	Additional Specifications
	and weight, medications, imaging, laboratory results, and a problem list—all in one place; ■ categorizes medications into therapeutic classes or categories (e.g., penicillin and its derivatives) to facilitate the checking of medications within classes and retains this information over time; and ■ can check the medication ordered as part of providing effective clinical decision support for dose range, dosing, frequency, route of administration, allergies, drug-drug interactions, dose adjustment based on laboratory results, excessive cumulative dosing, and therapeutic duplication.

Source: National Quality Forum. (2006). Safe practices for better healthcare: 2006 update. Table 1. Retrieved from http://www.qualityforum.org/About_NQF/CSAC/Safe_Practices_Table.aspx. Reprinted with permission.

Research Collaborative: Examining the Connection Between Patient Care, Nursing Sensitive Adverse Events, and Environment of Care Intensity (Burkart-Jayez & Spath, 2008; see Appendix 4-1), funded by a seed grant from the American Organization of Nurse Executives (AONE), was a small-scale outcomes management evaluation built on computer literacy, technology literacy, information literacy, and informatics competency. The method used was nurses' self-report. The two objectives of the research/quality improvement study were (1) to measure the distribution of nursing time constraints for direct, indirect, unit-support, and stand-by activities (with a subset of computer usage tasks for medication administration and all documentation) on a nursing care unit basis; and (2) to analyze known adverse events, in the context of the derived intensity factor (IF), in order to evaluate for the existence of a relationship not yet described in nursing literature. Competencies required by the researcher, acquired over the course of completing the study, included all of the basics recommended as core computer competencies for all nurses and others in health care. Weak competencies in technology selection, software selection, and advanced information literacy were barriers in the course of conducting the study, and illustrate the need for the curricula of doctorally prepared APNs to include standard competencies as proposed by the TIGER II initiative.

Buerhaus et al. (1997) argued that nurses must know what needs to be done or not done (clinical competency), whether that which requires clinical expertise is occurring (outcomes managed), and why they are doing what they are doing (information competency). The study by Burkart-Jayez and Spath (2008) was a means of quantifying the time burdens unintentionally introduced by healthcare technology and of identifying activities performed by nurses that did or did not require clinical expertise. Data for nursing time obligations were collected for direct care, indirect care, unit support, and "other" computerized patient record systems (all computer time except *bar coded medication administration [BCMA]*) This information was then analyzed for significance.

Overall, with the exception of BCMA time, nurses' reported times are similar, with near identical graphs, as evidenced in the unit comparison line graph in Attachment I of Appendix 4-1. Direct patient care time recorded ranged from 26.6% to 30.6%. Literature cites 27% as the point at which nursing-sensitive adverse events are more likely than not to occur. Nurses' time with their patients often approached the near-minimum level for uneventful care. The predicted "down time" (breaks, lunch periods, in-services) was 10.4%; however, nurses reported only 7.9% down time. Nurses invested more time than resourced in order to care for their patients and still could not exceed 30% direct patient care time. Time spent on technology-based tasks approached 39.9%. This is significant because staffing models are based on patient acuity and volume and do not take into account the time dedicated to technological adaptations for standard nursing tasks (medication administration and documentation within an EMR). Thus, nurse-to-patient staffing ratios for direct care are underestimated by up to 39.9%.

Unit support time (activities requiring no nursing education/licensure) averaged 10.1% of nurses' time. Delegation of such activities would thus return 10.1% of nursing time to patient-centered activities. The study demonstrated a "hidden" time commitment—the technology used for documentation and administration of medications accounted for up to 41% of nurses' time. In up to 11% of their workday, nurses continue to provide services that do not require a nurse's education/licensure. Results indicate that with formal training in healthcare technology, using the above-described time demands on bedside nurses on technology-related activities, a 30-minute addition of time available for direct care translates into approximately 17% more time.

Houston (1996, p. 147) defines outcomes management in health care as the use of aggregate variance data to change a system of healthcare practices, where variance is any event that alters patient progress toward the expected outcome. Sources of variance include practitioner behavior (competency), the severity of illness (as with high-risk patients), and practice patterns that either expedite care or inhibit delivery of care. Although technology has the potential for vast improvements in the provision of health care, without competency in the end user, adequate training, and resources for continued maintenance of equipment and user performance, technology can be the source of "yet-to-be" errors. It is incumbent on nurse educators and nurse clinicians to be fully aware of the purpose of each technological innovation, and on nurse scientists, both at the bedside and the podium, to have the requisite knowledge skills and abilities to function in the coming conversion to an electronic environment.

Conclusion

What is the emerging image of nurse clinicians? They will be certified competent in computer, information, and informatics technology. Their day will begin with an electronic overview of each patient's treatment plan. In a technology-rich environment, nurses will have wireless communication devices for instant contact with other members of the healthcare team. For bedside nurses, portable computer stations will be within steps of their patients, supplemented by laptop computers on rolling stands, and will be used for documentation, data collection on patient outcomes, and dispensing of medications using bar-coding technology. Supplies for the patient's care (dressings/linen, etc.) will be stored in closets that open to the room and the corridor; assistive personnel will stock these "nurse-servers" and inventory use with handheld bar-coding. Each day will bring the capacity for face-to-face follow-up with patients in their home using *telehealth* networks, as well as live and Web-based educational opportunities.

Moving patients safely will include such devices as inflatable transfer mats placed under patients as they travel from their unit to other departments for procedures, which will forgo the multiple-staff manual lift. For example, after hip surgery, patients will begin near-immediate rehabilitation using ceiling-based lifts with walking slings, eliminating the fear of falling and the pain that initial weight bearing brings.

The work area will be less noisy as phones and call bell systems give way to wireless devices. In addition, wireless tools will transmit vital signs and other monitoring modalities directly into the computer-based medical record, eliminating the need for transcription of data and the potential errors associated with redundant or manual documentation. Throughout their shift, nurses' workload and staffing data will be monitored for the purpose of adjusting staffing levels. Throughout the day, with careful resourcing and maintenance of the tools used, and the ongoing education of the end users, nurses will have garnered more time for direct patient care, thus decreasing the opportunities for the occurrence of nursing-sensitive adverse events.

For APNs, many of the same tools will augment their provision of services. Faced with challenging patient care issues, the DNP APN can access a DSS for clinical pathways and best practices and collect outcomes data for improving patient care. All of this is available now, with the goal of widespread adaptation by 2014. APNs must be familiar with all forms of patient care technology, because they both oversee and provide direct patient care.

How, then, to prepare for this impending future? Achieve basic computer literacy with such tools as the ECDL/ICDL, basic information competency using websites such as that of the ALA, and basic informatics competency through any distance learning website, and begin exploring the use of outcomes management in daily processes. All of these competencies can be obtained by self-study while awaiting the redesign of the nursing curriculum. Early training and adaption to technology, although not without risk, will improve each patient's receipt of safe, efficient, and effective care.

For the DNP-prepared ANP, information, computer, and technologic literacy and competency are already essential in daily practice. The quality and quantity of information available to the healthcare consumer and provider continues to expand. Knowing how to provide the right care the right way, with the right outcome, is no longer sufficient. Patients are no longer apt to be passive recipients of healthcare services. The DNP must be able to communicate with these patients using technology and information-based platforms, including telehealth, e-mail, Web-based health education, and EBM. As hospitalists, the DNP APN must understand the time burdens associated with patient care technology when implementing plans of care, and balance innovation with insight into the nursing process.

References

American Association of Colleges of Nursing. (2006, October). *The essentials of doctoral education for advanced nursing practice.* Washington, DC: Author. Retrieved from http://www .aacn.nche.edu/DNP/pdf/Essentials.pdf

American Library Association. (2000). *Information literacy standards for student learning* [Brochure]. Retrieved from http://www.ala.org/ala/mgrps/divs/aasl/aaslpubsandjournals/information powerbook/ip_brochure.pdf

Berwick, D. (2003). Disseminating innovations in health care. *JAMA, 289*(15), 1969–1975.

Berwick, D., Roessner, J., & Godfrey, A. B. (1991). *Curing health care: New strategies for quality improvement.* San Francisco: Jossey-Bass.

Breslin, S., Greskovich, W., & Turisco, F. (2004, September). Wireless technology improves nursing workflow and communications. *CIN: Computers, Informatics, Nursing, 22*(5), 275–281.

Buerhaus, P. I., Clifford, J., Erickson, J. I., Fay, M. S., Miller, J. R., Sporing, E. M., et al. (1997). Executive nurse leadership. Summary of the Harvard Nursing Research Institute's Follow-up conference. *JONA, 27*(4), 12–20.

Burkart-Jayez, S., & Spath, D. (2008). *Research protocol: Research collaborative: Examining the connection between patient care, nursing sensitive adverse events, and environment of care intensity.* AONE seed grant.

Burke, L., & Weill, B. (2005). *Information technology for the health professions* (2nd ed.). Upper Saddle River, NJ: Pearson/Prentice Hall.

Charles, R. (2008, December). Making the most of EBM: Evidence-based medicine moves forward with clinical decision support (Decision Support/EBM). *Health Management Technology, 29*(12), 22–23.

Clancy, C. M. (2005, September 9). Health information technology and the "quality movement." *Second Health IT Summit.* Washington, DC: Agency for Healthcare Research and Quality. Retrieved from www.ahrq.gov/news/sp090905.htm

Eley, R., Fallon, T., Soar, J., Buikstra, E., & Hegney, D. (2008, October). The status of training and education in information and computer technology of Australian nurses: A national survey. *Journal of Clinical Nursing, 2758*(10), 17–20.

Englebardt, S. P., & Nelson, R. (2002). *Health care informatics: An interdisciplinary approach.* St. Louis, MO: Mosby.

Fetter, M. S. (2009). Curriculum strategies to improve baccalaureate nursing information technology outcomes. *Journal of Nursing Education, 48*(2), 78–85.

Goldstein, M. M., & Blumenthal, D. (2008). Building an information technology infrastructure. *Journal of Law, Medicine & Ethics, 36*(4), 709–715.

Houston, S. (1996). Getting started in outcomes research. *AACN, 7*(1), 146–152.

Institute of Medicine. (2001). *Crossing the quality chasm: A new health system for the 21st century.* Washington, DC: National Academies Press.

The Joint Commission. (2008, December 11). *Safely implementing health information and converging technologies* (Issue Brief No. 42, p. 1). Available: http://www.jointcommission.org /SentinelEvents/SentinelEventAlert/sea_42.htm

Jones, J. R. (2005, November 16). Driving the information highway: The NHS IT strategy is an opportunity for nurses to get ahead of the game. *Nursing Standard, 70*(2).

Kingsley, K. V., & Kingsley, K. (2009). A case study for teaching inforamtion literacy skills. *BMC Medical Education, 9,* 7.

Kirkley, D. (2004, June). Clinical IT: Powering up data analysis for the nurse executive [Data analysis to inform executive decision making: EMRs and other CIS functionality provide the hard data needed to guide these types of high-level decisions]. *Nursing Economics, 22*(3), 147–156. From *The use of data-mining in a large acute care hospital.* 2003, Poster session presented at American Association of Nurse Executives.

Koivunen, M., Valimaki, M., Jakobsson, T., & Pitkanen, A. (2008, September). Developing an evidence-based curriculum designed to help psychiatric nurses learn to use computers and the internet. *Journal of Professional Nursing, 24*(5), 302–314.

Kolbasuk McGee, M. (2009, February 11). Stimulus bill will stimulate health IT adoption, jobs. *Information Week,* 1. Retrieved from http://www.informationweek.com/news/healthcare /showArticle.jhtml?articleID=213900067

Kossman, S. P., & Scheidenhelm, S. L. (2008, March/April). Nurses' perceptions of the impact of electronic health records on work and patietn outcomes. *CIN: Computers, Informatics, Nursing, 26*(2), 69–77.

Lee, T-T. (2007, March/April). Patients' perceptions of nurses' bedside use of PDAs. *CIN: Computers, Informatics, Nursing, 25*(2), 106–111.

Lin, J-S., Lin, K-C., Jiang, W-W., & Lee, T-T. (2007). An exploration of nursing informatics competency and satisfaction related to network education. *Journal of Nursing Research, 15*(1), 54–65.

McNeil, B. J., Elfrink, V. L., Bickford, C. J., Pierce, S. T., Beyea, S. C., Averill, C., et al. (2003, August). Nursing information technology knowledge, skills, and preparation of student nurses, nursing faculty, and clinicians: A U.S. survey. *Journal of Nursing Education, 42*(8), 341–349.

Murphy, J. (2008, November 11). Decision support for nurses: Moving to an evidence-based approach (My Two Cents). *Health Data Management, 16*(11).

National League for Nursing. (2008, May 9). *Preparing the next generation of nurses to practice in a technology-rich environment: An informatics agenda* (Position Statement). Retrieved from http://www.nln.org/aboutnln/PositionStatements/informatics_052808.pdf

National Quality Forum. (2006). *Safe practices for better healthcare: 2006 update. Table 1.* Retrieved from http://www.qualityforum.org/About_NQF/CSAC/Safe_Practices_Table.aspx

Nelson, A., Powell-Cope, G., Gavin-Dreschnack, D., Quigley, P., Bulat, T., Baptiste, A. S., et al. (2004, September). Technology to promote safe mobility in the elderly. *Nursing Clinics of North America, 39*(3), 649–671.

Ornes, L. L., & Gassert, C. (2007, February). Computer competencies in an BSN program. *Journal of Nursing Education, 46*(2), 75–78.

Page, A (Ed.). (2004). *Keeping patients safe. Transforming the work environment of nurses.* Washington, DC: National Academies Press.

Powell-Cope, G., Nelson, A. L., & Patterson, E. S. (2008, March). Patient care technology and safety. In R. G. Hughes (Ed.), *Patient safety and quality: An evidence-based handbook for nurses* (Prepared with support from the Robert Wood Johnson Foundation). AHRQ Publication No. 08-0043. Rockville, MD: Agency for Healthcare Research and Quality.

Radcliff, C. J., Salem, J. A., Jr., O'Connor, L. G., & Gedeon, J. A. (2007). *Project SAILS skill sets for the 2008–2009 academic year.* Retrieved from http://www.projectsails.org/abouttest /skillsets.php

Scholes, M, & Barber, B. (1980). Towards nursing informatics. In D. A. D. Lindberg, and S. Kaihara (Eds.), *Medinfo 1980* (pp. 70–73). Amsterdam, The Netherlands: North-Holland.

Simpson, R. L. (2009, March). The softer side of technology: How IT helps nursing care. *Nursing Administration Quarterly, 28*(4), 302–305.

Staggers, N., Gassert, C. A., & Curran, C. (2002, November/December). A Delphi study to determine informatics competencies for nurses at four levels of practice. *Nursing Research, 51*(6), 383–390.

The TIGER Initiative. (2007). *Technology Informatics Guiding Education Reform.* Retrieved from http://www.tigersummit.com.

Thede, L. Q., Allen, M., & Pierce, S. T. (2003). *Informatics and nursing: Opportunities and challenges* (2nd ed.). Philadelphia: Lippincott Williams & Wilkins.

Wojner, A. W. (2001). Outcomes management: Applications to clinical practice. St. Louis, MO: Mosby.

Research Protocol: Research Collaborative: Examining the Connection Between Patient Care, Nursing Sensitive Adverse Events, and Environment of Care Intensity*

Susan F. Burkart-Jayez, ND, RN, ANP-C
Deborah Spath, MSN, RN

The facility in which the project occurred experienced the nursing sensitive adverse events (NSAE) common to all healthcare facilities: medication errors, falls, decubitus, and unanticipated deaths.

An intensity factor (IF) of the nursing units' workload was calibrated for each unit, based on historical workload data, as a measure of activity within a patient care unit as a whole (Attachment A, Table 1). Initially developed by others as a tool for calculating gaps in staffing strength, an earlier project by the PI used this factor: Findings from the project held promise for being used to forecast and avert work environment conditions conducive to nursing sensitive adverse events.

The project objectives:

1. To measure the distribution of nursing time constraints for direct, indirect, unit-support, and stand-by activities (with a subset of computer usage tasks for medication administration and all documentation), on a nursing care unit basis, and

---

*The material presented does not represent the Department of Veterans Affairs, Veterans Health Administration, or the Samuel S. Stratton VAMC. The project was funded by the American Organization of Nurse Executives (AONE) through the support of the Albany Research Institute.

2. To analyze known adverse events, in the context of the derived IF in order to evaluate for the existence of a relationship not yet described in nursing literature.

Significance of Project

Health care quality research supports that a minimum of 27% nursing time spent in direct care is the lower limit necessary to positively impact nursing sensitive adverse events.

In linking processes and outcomes, such as workflow and nursing sensitive adverse events (NSAE), we can identify what needs to change and how, and what happens because of factor modification. This protocol is an example of outcomes management: Data pertaining to workload, nurse's time obligations in the direct care setting, and NSAE were analyzed for opportunities in improving patient outcomes, using both qualitative and quantitative data. Currently, the institution uses the Root Cause Analysis (RCA) methodology to look at events with serious patient care impact. The teams are clinically based, can range from three to eight members, and take a cumulative 49 to over 100 hours. The average salary at the institution for nursing was $37.00/hour at the time of calculation (the first three-quarters of fiscal year 2003). Given the diverse composition of the teams, this figure is a fair estimate of hourly costs. All figures are estimates, based on existent data, and represent the least possible scenario cost (Burkart-Jayez, 2004). The sample cost of current activities for monitoring/managing NSAE is shown in Attachment B, Table 2b, and represents a potential for cost avoidance should an early warning be developed for adverse patient outcomes. Simply put, the figures calculated for the monitoring events without outcomes management can be viewed as "the cost of doing nothing," because monitoring never ends. One intended outcome of this project is the derivation of a mathematical portent of adverse events for evaluation against other, more complex structure issues (such as staff mix, staff education level, and staff expertise), that can be readily analyzed in subsequent studies.

Background

As Buerhaus et al. (1997) propose, nurses must know that which needs to be done or not done, that what requires clinical expertise is occurring, and that we know why we are doing what we are doing. Thus, by defining time utilization at the bedside, using categories of direct care, indirect care, unit support, and "other" activities, the first step toward understanding the facility specific work environment was taken. This process engaged the bedside nurses in the research process from its inception and fostered ever essential participation in the activities and results that follow.

Perkins et al. (2000) describe outcomes management as relying on clinical resource management, quantitative and qualitative analyses, and indicators that are patient, provider, or organizationally focused. In linking processes and outcomes, such as workflow and NSAE, we can identify what needs to change and how, and what happens because of factor modification. This pilot is an example of outcomes management: Inspection of data pertaining to workload, nurses' time obligations in the direct care setting, and NSAE will be analyzed for opportunities in improving patient outcomes, using both qualitative and quantitative data.

Aiken (1997), Laschinger et al. (2003), and Perkins et al. (2000), among others, articulate the linkage between processes and outcomes, organizational attributes and outcomes, and working conditions and outcomes. Aiken suggests that unraveling this linkage between factors and outcomes will create a new understanding of ways to improve quality of patient care and patient centered outcomes.

Common indicators of NSAE identified in nursing literature include medication errors, intravenous device associated infections, and transfusion error rates per thousand bed days of care (BDOC). The National Quality Forum also identifies skin breakdown, hospital-acquired urinary tract infections, pneumonia and upper gastrointestinal bleeds, cardiac arrest, falls, length of stay, adverse drug events, patient and family complaints, and surgical wound infections as issues responsive or sensitive to nursing care (www.qualityforum.org, 2004). Factors initially proposed to be analyzed in this project included falls, medication errors, nosocomial infections, decubitus, and mortality. Nosocomial infections are analyzed as a facility annual rate, and are compared to annual average IF, BDOC, Nursing Task, and NSAE rates per thousand BDOC. The additional indicator calculated for this project as a potential risk adjustment is an IF—the "busy"-ness of the nurses' work environment. BDOC captures one patient's journey through the system. An IF shows intensity of the work environment based on each patient's journey; that is, each patient has one BDOC, but may have been treated on several nursing care units within one 24-hour interval. For example, a patient with heart disease may be admitted to the Emergency Room, transferred to the ICU for stabilization/observation, transferred to the Operating/Recovery Room for stent placement, and transferred back to the ICU. Once stable, the patient could then be transferred to an Acute Care Nursing ward. In theory, up to five different nursing teams would have provided care to this patient, but the patient would only be counted once in the average daily census (ADC), which is based on the patient's location at midnight. By demonstrating the actual number of patients served in a 24-hour period as a percentage of the ADC upon which staffing methods are based, nurse leaders will have an additional tool for illustrating nurse staffing requirements. (See Attachment A, Table 1.)

Goals of Outcomes Management (OM) include increasing quality of care and decreasing adverse events. Quality is the degree to which patient care services increase the probability of positive outcomes and reduce the probability of negative outcomes. Care process components of technical, interpersonal, and professional skills contribute to variation in outcome and recognize the provider skill in delivery of care (Houston, 1996).

As noted by Woods (2002), as healthcare professionals, we will be called on more and more to communicate what we are doing to ensure patient safety. This project set out to reduce adverse events in a population of patients through the strengthening of workload assessment processes and by enumerating core responsibilities for the nursing staff. Inherent to this project was the need to collect, analyze, and interpret data for communication of safety issues to leadership and frontline staff.

Flood (1994) identifies that evidence from organizational theory on evaluation suggests that voluntary, internal monitoring is most effective in change management because people respond to information about their performance; thus, a self-reporting methodology was used. These processes are related to better quality of care. The nursing leaders at the project's facility want the culture to be one of nursing excellence. They agree with Aiken et al.'s (1997) position that unraveling the linkage between organization attributes/culture and outcomes can provide significant understanding of ways to improve quality of care and patient outcomes. These leaders supported the proposed project as a tool in linking processes and outcomes: The co-PI is the facility Associate Director for Patient and Nursing Services (Nurse Executive).

Outcome indicators for patient care efficacy align with organizational features such as nursing surveillance, nurse-clinician communication/collaboration, and the quality of the work environment. Adverse events may be an even more sensitive marker of organizational quality than other types of performance measures such as cost, length of stay, and patient satisfaction. For example, mortality rates are associated with organizational processes such as communication. The greater the degree of reciprocal interdependence (exchange of time, expertise, and resources), the greater the effect on outcomes (Mitchell, 1997). Some of the factors Mitchell cites include technology, RN to patient ratio (nurse staffing intensity), professional expertise (competency, skill mix), professional influences (autonomy), and collaboration and coordination of care, all facets of nursing's domain (Mitchell, 1997).

A subset of mortality data, failure to rescue (FTR), described on http://www.qualityindicators.ahrq.gov (2003) "as preventable death related to complications of hospitalization" and "the key indicator of quality of professional care," was collected through review by the PI of charts of those patients who died during the interval studied. FTR has limitations as an indicator of quality. One limitation is the variation in definition of FTR. Dr. Lucian Leape, of the Harvard School of Public Health, proposes conservatively that 1 in 25 patients (4%) are harmed by errors, and an overall increase in deaths comes almost entirely from adding "failure to rescue" (FTR) (AHRQ, 2004). Dr. Leape describes FTR as a delay in recognizing and intervening on behalf of a patient who becomes suddenly ill. Examination of all of the to-date identified NSAE, as well as mortality data, coupled with analysis of workload, as part of the second objective may produce tools for continued event avoidance.

Project

Upon expedited review and approval of the proposal by the facility's Institutional Review Board (IRB), the PI met with nursing staff on each unit to explain the project. (See Attachment E, Figure 2.) Common activities specific to a unit's provision of nursing care and services were identified and determined to be one of four categories, based on nursing literature: direct care, indirect care, unit support, and stand-by time. The nursing staff self-assessed/recorded their activities for aggregation using a paper workload collection tool. (See Attachment C, Figure 2.) In the cases in which a staff nurse was more comfortable with being assessed by an observer logging his or her activities, the staff nurse was then observed by the PI. As the project continued, nurses initially committed to data collection found that participation was an additional time constraint. This necessitated the PI capturing data to complete the baseline. Data was collected three times for each shift for all acute care units—two medical-surgical units and the Intensive Care Unit (ICU). This approach has been validated as an accurate workload measurement method (Carson, 2001). The data was anonymously aggregated into direct care, indirect care, unit support, and "other" categories, and a subset of computer-based tasks, producing a profile of the patient care environment in real time. Concurrently, data collected from multiple databases of workload proxies included:

1. Average Daily Census (ADC): measured as the number of patients present within a facility at midnight, by unit.
2. Mortality data were retrieved from the Automated Medical Information System (AMIS) and converted to a rate per thousand BDOC.
3. Nosocomial events (infections, decubitus formation) were to be extracted from secondary diagnoses at discharge as a function of date and location only; the only readily accessible information was for skin ulcer and infection rates, due to coder-staffing limitations.

Data for the latter were examined for fiscal year (FY) 2005 through FY 2006 (October 1, 2004 through September 30, 2006) as a baseline. All of the data were received as an anonymous aggregate from primary sources. Neither individual patients nor individual employees were identifiable from the data sets used, because the sole purpose was to identify trends. The Admission-Discharge-Transfer (ADT) factor was used to calculate an IF, and was also transformed into a nominal/quantitative set of low-average-high and critical levels. This manipulation has been used in the prior work of the principal investigator and yields information reflecting the intensity of the environment in which nurses work. (See Attachment A.)

The invasion of privacy of individual patients and employees was assessed as of minimal risk: Data received by the PI had no patient identifiers, rather only anonymous aggregate numbers by category of occurrence, date, and patient care location. Only the PI and co-PI had access to data collected for the study prior to analysis. The physical security of all information was safeguarded. Computer access codes were not shared, and the workstation for data storage was locked when not in use and located in a locked office. Data was backed up on floppy discs and stored in a locking file cabinet within the PI's locked office.

The project took place at a tertiary care facility with 53 acute care (10 intensive unit), 50 long-term care, and 10 acute behavioral care beds. The scope of the project initially included all in-patient units, but was reduced to examining the acute care units in order to facilitate project progress/completion.

Data Collection Activities

1. Pearson Correlations were conducted for the following:
   a. Falls
   b. Med errors
   c. Ulcers
   d. Operator-related medication errors
   e. Deaths/FTR

Manipulations included comparison of indicators to each other, to BDOC and to the calculated IF. (See Attachment G, Table 5.)

2. Nursing time obligations were collected for:
   a. Direct care
   b. Indirect care
   c. Unit support
   d. Other
      i. CPRS/all computer time except BCMA use, and
      ii. BCMA use

These are demonstrated in Attachment H.

Findings

Summary of Time Analysis

1. Overall, with the exception of BCMA time, nursing reported times are similar, with near identical graphs as evidenced in the Unit Comparison line graph. (See Attachment H, Table 6, and Attachment I, Graphs 9–12.)
2. Direct patient care time recorded ranged from 26.6% to 30.6%; literature cites 27% as the point at which nursing sensitive adverse events are more likely than not to occur. Nurses' time with their patients is at the near minimum level for uneventful care.

3. The predicted "down time" (other) is 10.4% (based on contract-defined rest breaks), yet nurses report only 7.9% other (breaks, lunch periods, in-services). Nurses invested more time each shift, and still could not exceed 30% direct patient care time.

4. Time spent on technology-based tasks approached 39.9%. This is significant in that staffing models are based on patient acuity and volume and do not take into account the time dedicated to technological adaptations for standard nursing tasks (medication administration and documentation within an electronic medical record). Thus, nurse-to-patient staffing ratios are underestimated by up to 39.9%.

5. Unit support time (activities requiring no nursing education/licensure) averaged 10.1%. Delegation of such activities would thus return 10.1% of nursing time back to patient-centered activities.

Evaluation of Time Analysis

1. A more precise method of analyzing nursing time spent on technology-based activities would support the reported time. One method would involve running file reports for both BCMA and CPRS use time. The total staffing available for each shift reported could then be used to calculate the exact amount of available nursing time spent on these tasks.

2. Identification of recurring, non-nursing tasks would lend itself to shifting such workload to alternate staff resources.

3. Although initially proposed as a time study, it will be useful to analyze the time totals in comparison to adverse events rates at the unit/shift level.

Summary of the Connection between NSAE and IF

These findings suggest that calculation of a unit's IF based on "real-time" unit activity could contribute to quality patient care through informing nursing leadership as to current patient activity and nursing unit workload in development of an overarching nurse staffing model. For example, end-of-shift census and acuity of care as a basis for the number of nursing staff required for the next shift captures one moment in the eight-hour work shift (the total number of patients and their needs "category" at the end of the tour). The acuity of care level is based upon 20-plus-year-old measures, in a time of open-ended lengths of stay. (See Attachment J, Figure 3.) Twenty years later, patients who we would categorize as "1" and perhaps "2" on a 5-point scale would not necessarily meet current admission and length of stay criteria. The IF, on the other hand, calculates the actual number of patients served in the same time period, taking into account the patients who have been admitted into, transferred into and out of, and discharged from a particular unit, and patients who have met a much more complex standard for hospitalization.

The calculation of an IF may serve as an "early warning system": that is, as the IF reaches the high to critical range, patients may be at a higher risk for skin ulcer formation and adverse events contributing to unanticipated death. Quality assurance and/or nursing research would further illuminate these findings.

For now, for one facility's acute care and intensive care units, information on time demands on direct care, and the impact of patient flow on patient care have been identified. This information may be useful in staffing level/bed availability determinations. Future work on the identified trends by nursing researchers can clarify the connection between patient care, NSAE, and the intensity of the environment of care.

Conclusion

The distribution of nursing time constraints for direct, indirect, unit-support, and stand-by activities were calculated for two acute medical-surgical nursing units and one intensive care unit. A "hidden" time commitment, the technology used for documentation and administration of medications, accounted for up to 41% of nurses' time. Nurses continue to provide services that do not require a nurse's education/licensure for up to 11% of their workday. The latter provides an opportunity to shift workload to appropriate ancillary staff, resulting in a relative "professional nurse staffing increase" of 11%. An in-depth analysis of nursing-computer time, using time reports from each computer application, would yield more precise data that are illustrative of the impact of technology on nursing resources allocated for direct care.

As examined in previous work (Burkart-Jayez, 2004), nursing outcomes management requires attention to and intervention focused on the indicators identified in literature as reflective of quality nursing care: medication errors, infections, transfusion errors, skin breakdown, hospital acquired urinary tract infections, pneumonia and upper gastrointestinal bleeds, cardiac arrest, falls, length of stay, adverse drug events, patient and family complaints, and surgical wound infections rates per thousand bed days of care. The addition of an "outcomes manager"—a nursing clinician dedicated to monitoring all NSAE—would be valuable in examining occurrence of and contributing factors to such events, followed by an intervention/prevention plan. Such a clinician would be in the position of providing evidence-based guidance to nursing staff. This guidance would enhance the patient care environment and improve access to quality care.

References

Aiken, L. H., Sochalski, J., & Lake, E. T. (1997). Studying outcomes of organizational change in health services. *Medical Care, 35*(11), NS6–NS18.

Agency for Healthcare Research and Quality. (2003). *National healthcare quality report.* Rockville, MD: U.S. Department of Health and Human Services. Retrieved from http://www.ahrq. gov/qual/nhqr03/fullreport/index.htm

Bradley, C. (2001, January). *Staffing strategies, beyond the numbers and ratios.* Paper presented at the meeting of The Forum on Healthcare Leadership, Philadelphia, PA.

Buerhaus, P. I., Clifford, J., Erickson, J. I., Fay, M. S., Miller, J. R., Sporing, E. M., et al. (1997). Effective nursing leadership: Summary of the Harvard Nursing Research Institute's follow-up conference. *JONA, 27*(4), 12–20.

Burkart-Jayez, S. (2004). Nursing Doctorate Project: Nursing competency assessment and outcomes management.

Cochrell, P. (2001, January). *Patient classification systems for a new era of care delivery.* Paper presented at the meeting of The Forum on Healthcare Leadership, Philadelphia, PA.

Couvaras, C. (2001, January). *The impact of admissions, transfers, and discharge on budgeting and scheduling.* Paper presented at the meeting of The Forum on Healthcare Leadership, Philadelphia, PA.

Curtin, L. (2001, January). *Keynote.* Paper presented at the meeting of The Forum on Healthcare Leadership, Philadelphia, PA.

DeGroat, H. (2001, January). *Improving staffing precision policies and practice.* Paper presented at the meeting of The Forum on Healthcare Leadership, Philadelphia, PA.

Drenkard, K. N. (2001). Creating a future worth experiencing. *JONA, 31*(7–8), 364–376.

Flood, A. B. (1994). The impact of organizational and managerial factors on the quality of care in health care organizations. *Medical Care Review, 51*(4), 381–428.

Houston, S. (1996). Getting started in outcomes research. *AACN, 7*(1), 146–153.

Kleinpell, R., Gawlinski, A., McCloy, K., & Jesurum, J. (1998). Measuring outcomes in cardiovascular APN practice. In R. Kleinpell (Ed.), *Outcomes Assessment in Advance Practice Nursing* (pp. 131–188). New York: Springer.

Kleinpell, R. (1997). Whose outcomes. Patients, providers, or payers? *Nursing Clinics of North America, 32*(3), 513–520.

Laschinger, H. K., Almost, J., & Tuer-Hoedes, D. (2003). Workplace empowerment and magnet hospital characteristics. *JONA, 33*(7–8), 410–422.

Mitchell, P. H., & Shortell, S. M. (1997). Adverse outcomes and variations in organization of care delivery. *Medical Care, 35*(Suppl. 11), NS19–NS32.

Perkins, S. B., Connerney, I., & Hastings, C. E. (2000). Outcomes management: From concepts to application. *AACN, 11*(3), 339–350.

Pischke-Winn, K., & Minnick, A. (1996). Project management: Lessons learned from introducing a multitask environmental workers program. *JONA, 26*(6), 31–38.

Raphael, S. (2001, January). *Nursing quality indicators: Tools for safe staffing.* Paper presented at the meeting of The Forum on Healthcare Leadership, Philadelphia, PA.

Rundall, T. G., Starkweather, D. B., & Norrish, B. R. (1998). *After restructuring: Empowerment strategies at work in America's hospitals.* San Francisco: Jossey-Bass.

Wojner, A. W. (1997). Outcomes management: From theory to practice. *Critical Care Nursing Quarterly, 19*(4), 1–15.

Woods, D. K. (2002). Realizing your market influence, Part 1. Meeting patient needs through collaboration. *JONA, 32*(4), 189–195.

List of Abbreviations

ADC	Average Daily Census
ADT	Admissions/Discharges/Transfers
BCMA	Bar Coding Medication Administration
BDOC	Bed Days of Care
CA	Competency Assessment
CNS	Clinical Nurse Specialist
FTR	Failure to Rescue
ICU	Intensive Care Unit
IF	Intensity Factor
JC	The Joint Commission
LOS	Length of Stay
NCPC	Nursing Clinical Practice Council
ND	Nursing Doctorate
NE	Nurse Executive
NPR	Nursing Peer Review
NSAE	Nursing Sensitive Adverse Events
OM	Outcomes Manager
PM	Performance Management
RCA	Root Cause Analysis
RM	Risk Manager

Definitions

Complication or adverse event: "An injury caused by medical management rather than by the underlying disease or condition of the patient." In general, adverse events prolong the hospitalization, produce a disability at the time of discharge, or both. Used in this report, complication does not refer to the sequelae of diseases, such as neuropathy as a "complication" of diabetes. Throughout the report, "sequelae" is used to refer to these conditions (www.qualityforum.org).

Patient safety indicators: Specific quality indicators that also reflect the quality of care inside hospitals, but focus on aspects of patient safety. Specifically, PSIs screen for problems that patients experience as a result of exposure to the healthcare system, and that are likely amenable to prevention by changes at the system or provider level.

Preventable adverse event: An adverse event attributable to error is a "preventable adverse event." A condition for which reasonable steps may reduce (but not necessarily eliminate) the risk of that complication occurring.

Quality: "Quality of care is the degree to which health services for individuals and populations increase the likelihood of desired health outcomes and are consistent with current professional knowledge." In this definition, "the term *health services* refers to a wide array of services that affect health...(and) applies to many types of health care practitioners (physicians, nurses, and various other health professionals) and to all settings of care. . . ."

Quality indicators: Screening tools for the purpose of identifying potential areas of concern regarding the quality of clinical care. For the purpose of this report, we focus on indicators that reflect the quality of care inside hospitals. Quality indicators may assess any of the four system components of health care quality, including patient safety (see below), effectiveness (i.e., "providing services based on scientific knowledge to all who could benefit, and refraining from providing services to those not likely to benefit), patient centeredness, and timeliness (i.e., "minimizing unnecessary delays").

Rate based indicators: Indicators for which the primary purpose is to identify the rate of a complication rather than to identify specific cases.

Attachment A

Table 1. Calculation of Unit- and Facility-Specific Intensity Factors

Unit	Bench-Mark Range of ADT/month*	Range of ADT for 24 months by nursing unit	Average ADT for 24 months by nursing unit	Low 1	Average 2	High 3	Critical 4	Average Intensity Factor (IF) For Project Interval	Average nominal value for project interval
Intensive Care	85-98	81-143	112	23-71	72-119	120-167	>168	1.59	3
Acute Care- 7B	50-55	206-238	238	14-42	43-71	72-101	>101	1.45	4
Acute Care- 8B	50-55	158-259	104	14-42	43-71	72-101	>101	1.38	4

ADC=Average Daily Census

ADT (per 24 hour period)=Admissions+Discharges+Transfers

IF=Intensity Factor=ADT + ADC/ADC

Low-Average-High-Critical: unit values using industry standard as pivot point for quartile averages

*After Covaras, 2001

Developed in collaboration with Kate Toms, PhD

For inclusion in Burkart-Jayez, S. (2004). "Competency Assessment and Outcomes Management", for Rush College of Nursing, Chicago, December 2004, Nursing Doctorate (unpublished).

Attachment C

Figure 1. Workload Collection Tool

Date_____ Hour_____ AM/PM   WARD: ICU/7B/8B   RN LPN NA

	0			5			5			5			5			5			5
D																						
BC																						
I																						
CP																						
U																						
O																						

NB: Actual tool has 12 5-minute marks across face, and is double sided=2 hours of time

D= Direct: Admission, assessment, VS, crisis, IV care, transfusions, ADL care, discharge, skills requiring scope of practice/competency assessment, teaching (family/patient), procedures
BC= BCMA
I=Indirect: Report, MD rounds, documentation, patient classification, care plan, narcotic counts
CP=CPRS/any computer use
U=Unit-Support: Transport, supplies, audits, empty/stock linen, wait, food trays, "down time," errands off of unit
O=Other: Committee/staff meetings, personal time, breaks, personal phone calls

Table 3.b Approximate Cost of Risk Management of Nursing Sensitive Adverse Events, FY 2003

Activity	
RCA	$35,834.50
ADE	$88,882.20
Case reviews	$9,800.00
Total estimated review costs	$134,096.70

RCA=Root Cause Analysis: Team-based adverse event reviews, calculated from number of staff hours/salary rates in participating on each RCA for FY 2003.
ADE=Number of medication errors x % of errors likely to cause harm x recovery cost of harm, FY 2003
Case Reviews=Number of patient care charts reviewed by an RN x 2 hours average review time x average facility salary for RN, FY 2003.

From Burkart-Jayez, S. (2004). "Competency Assessment and Outcomes Management," Nursing Doctorate Project, Rush College of Nursing, Chicago, December 2004.

Attachment G. Pearson Correlation of Indicators Evaluated and Graphs Demonstrating Individual Correlations

Table 5. Correlations

			₿	₿		₿		
₫	₿	1	₿	*	₿	0	5	
	₿		₿	0	₿	9	0	
	N	2	2	2	2	2	2	
₿ ₿	₿	₿	1		₿	₿		
	₿	₿		₿	₿	₿	₿	
	N	2	2	2	2	2	2	
₿ ₿	₿	*		1		₿	*	
	₿	0	₿		₿	₿	₿	
	N	2	2	2	2	2	2	
₿ ₿	₿	₿	₿		1	₿	5	
	₿	₿	₿	₿		₿	8	
	N	2	2	2	2	2	2	
Þ	₿	0	₿	₿	₿	1	₿	
	₿	9	₿	₿	₿		₿	
	N	2	2	2	2	2	2	
₿ ₿	₿	5		*	5	₿	1	
	₿	0	₿	₿	8	₿		
	N	2	2	2	2	2	2	

Attachment H.

Table 6. Comparison of Nursing Time-Task Categories in Minutes

Unit	BCMA	Direct	Indirect	Computer	Unit Support	Other	Total	Total
8B	561	1545	811	1160	456	518	5051	
	11.11%	30.59%	16.06%	22.97%	9.03%	10.26%		
7B	1293	1602	453	947	787	347	5429	
	23.82%	29.51%	8.34%	17.44%	14.50%	6.39%		
ICU	1068	1274	749	1060	292	339	4782	
	22.33%	26.64%	15.66%	22.17%	6.11%	7.09%		

Attachment I.

Graph 9

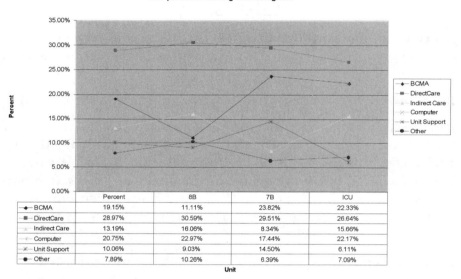

Comparison of Nursing Time Categories

	Percent	8B	7B	ICU
BCMA	19.15%	11.11%	23.82%	22.33%
DirectCare	28.97%	30.59%	29.51%	26.64%
Indirect Care	13.19%	16.06%	8.34%	15.66%
Computer	20.75%	22.97%	17.44%	22.17%
Unit Support	10.06%	9.03%	14.50%	6.11%
Other	7.89%	10.26%	6.39%	7.09%

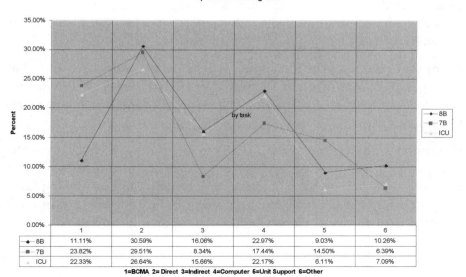

Unit comparisons-Nursing Time

	1	2	3	4	5	6
8B	11.11%	30.59%	16.06%	22.97%	9.03%	10.26%
7B	23.82%	29.51%	8.34%	17.44%	14.50%	6.39%
ICU	22.33%	26.64%	15.66%	22.17%	6.11%	7.09%

1=BCMA 2= Direct 3=Indirect 4=Computer 5=Unit Support 6=Other

Glossary

Bar coded medication administration (BCMA): Use of a scanner to identify medication to be administered to a patient and ordered in an electronic medical record.

Boot: To load the operating system into memory (Burke & Weill, 2005).

Browse: (1) In database systems, to browse means to view data. Many database systems support a special browse mode, in which you can flip through fields and records quickly. Usually, you cannot modify data while you are in browse mode. (2) In object-oriented programming languages, to browse means to examine data structures. (3) To view formatted documents. For example, you look at Web pages with a Web browser. "Browse" is often used to mean the same as "surf."

Browser: Short for *Web browser*, a software application used to locate and display Web pages. The two most popular browsers are Microsoft Internet Explorer and Mozilla Firefox. Both of these are graphical browsers, which means that they can display graphics as well as text. In addition, most modern browsers can present multimedia information, including sound and video, although they require plug-ins for some formats.

Computer competency: The ability to demonstrate proficiency in use of software applications such as Microsoft Word, Excel, and PowerPoint, and knowledge in computer terminology, hardware selection, and simple maintenance functions.

Computer information system (CIS): A computer system that usually includes an online decision support system, clinical documentation, care planning, and computerized physician order entry. The core nursing functions of such systems include results reporting, clinical documentation, medication charting, patient assessments, and performance reports.

Computer literacy: The level of expertise and familiarity someone has with computers. Computer literacy generally refers to the ability to use applications rather than to program. Individuals who are very computer literate are sometimes called power users.

Computerized physician/provider order entry (CPOE): Use of a software application for the ordering of medications, laboratory/radiology testing, consultation, and referral requests. The CPOE is the electronic replacement for paper prescriptions, and written/verbal orders in both the in-patient and outpatient setting, and is cited as an important tool to avoidance of medical errors and provision of patient safety.

Data: (1) Distinct pieces of information, usually formatted in a special way. All software is divided into two general categories: data and programs. Programs are collections of instructions for manipulating data. (2) The term *data* is often used to distinguish binary machine-readable information from textual human-readable information. For example, some applications make a distinction between data files (files that contain binary data) and text files (files that contain ASCII data).

Database: An organized collection of information that is easy to maintain, sort, and search (Burke & Weill, 2005).

Database management system (DBMS): Application software that allows the user to enter organized lists of data and easily edit, sort, and search them (Burke & Weill, 2005).

Electronic health record (EHR): An EMR is a type of healthcare information technology, which is the digital version of the patient's medical file. A fully functional EHR allows recording of patient information and demographics, results viewing and management, order entry management (including e-prescribing), and clinical decision support. A minimally functional EHR lacks full order entry capabilities and clinical decision support. Also known as an electronic medical record (EMR).

Electronic medical record (EMR): See *electronic health record (EHR)*.

Evidence-based medicine (see also evidence-based practice): Integration of the best available evidence from the scientific literature with clinical judgement and expertise in making healthcare decisions for the individual patient.

Graphical user interface (GUI): An operating environment or interface that allows users to interact with the computer by clicking on icons with a mouse (Burke & Weill, 2005).

Hardware: An object or objects that you can actually touch, such as disks, disk drives, display screens, keyboards, printers, boards, and chips. In contrast, software is untouchable. Software exists as ideas, concepts, and symbols, but it has no substance. Books provide a useful analogy. The pages and the ink are the hardware, whereas the words, sentences, paragraphs, and the overall meaning are the software. A computer without software is like a book full of blank pages—you need software to make the computer useful, just as you need words to make a book meaningful.

Healthcare information technology (HIT): Use of computer hardware and software for the processing, storage, and retrieval of healthcare-related information, including all clinical components of care and administrative data. An example of HIT is the electronic health record (EHR).

Healthcare informatics: The integration of computer science, information science, and healthcare. Examples of tools in healthcare informatics include clinical guidelines, electronic heath records, patient care technology devices, and databases of healthcare outcomes.

Icon: A small picture that represents an object or program. Icons are very useful in applications that use windows, because with the click of a mouse button you can shrink an entire window into a small icon. (This is sometimes called minimizing.) To redisplay the window, you merely move the pointer to the icon and click (or double click) a mouse button. (This is sometimes called restoring or maximizing.) Icons are a principal feature of a *graphical user interface (GUI)*.

Informatics: The integration of information and information management with electronic processing and communication technology.

Information literacy: Set of abilities allowing individuals to recognize when information is needed and to locate, evaluate, and use information appropriately (Association of Colleges and Research Libraries, 2000). Information literacy is the ability to identify information needed for a specific purpose, locate pertinent information, evaluate the information, and apply it correctly (Englebardt & Nelson, 2002).

Information technology (IT): The broad subject concerned with all aspects of managing and processing information, especially within a large organization or company. Because computers are central to information management, computer departments within companies and universities are often called IT departments. Some companies refer to this department as IS (information services) or MIS (management information services).

Internet: A global network connecting millions of computers. More than 100 countries are linked into exchanges of data, news, and opinions. Unlike online services, which are centrally controlled, the Internet is decentralized by design. Each Internet computer, called a host, is independent. Its operators can choose which Internet services to use and which local services to make available to the global Internet community. Remarkably, this anarchy by design works exceedingly well.

Medical informatics: The use of technology to organize information on health care (Burke & Weill, 2005).

Nursing informatics: The use of computer technology in all nursing endeavors: services, education, and research (Scholes & Barber, 1980, in Thede, 2003). The use of computer technologies in carrying out nursing functions (Hannah et al., 1994, in Thede, 2003). A combination of computer science, information science, and nursing science designed to assist in the management and processing of nursing data, information, and knowledge to support the practice of nursing and the delivery of nursing care (Graves & Corcoran, 1989, cited in Thede, 2003).

Nursing-sensitive adverse events (NSAE): Failure to rescue, nosocomial infections, pressure ulcers, falls, medication errors, transfusion errors.

Operating system: The most important program that runs on a computer. Every general-purpose computer must have an operating system to run other programs. Operating systems perform basic tasks such as recognizing input from the keyboard, sending output to the display screen, keeping track of files and directories on the disk, and controlling peripheral devices such as disk drives and printers.

Outcomes management: The use of aggregate variance data to change a system of healthcare practices, where variance is any event that alters patient progress toward the expected outcome. Sources of variance include practitioner behavior (competency), the severity of illness (as with high-risk patients), and practice patterns that either expedite care or inhibit delivery of care (Houston, 1996).

Software: Anything that can be stored electronically. Software is often divided into two categories: systems software, which includes the *operating system* and all the utilities that enable the computer to function; and applications software, which includes programs that do real work for users, such as word processors, spreadsheets, and *database management systems*.

Technology: (1) (a) The application of science, especially to industrial or commercial objectives. (b) The scientific method and material used to achieve a commercial or industrial objective. (2) Electronic or digital products and systems considered as a group. (3) Anthropology. The body of knowledge available to a society that is of use in fashioning implements, practicing manual arts and skills, and extracting or collecting materials.

Telehealth: Telemedicine and other health-related activities using telecommunication lines and computers, including education, research, public health, and administration of health services (Burke & Weill, 2005).

URL: Abbreviation of *uniform resource locator;* the global address of documents and other resources on the *World Wide Web*. The first part of the address is called a protocol identifier and indicates what protocol to use; the second part is called a resource name and specifies the IP address or the domain name where the resource is located. The protocol identifier and the resource name are separated by a colon and two forward slashes.

Web browser: See *Browser*.

Websites: Files in which information on the Web are stored (Burke & Weill, 2005).

Word processing: Using a computer to create, edit, and print documents. Of all computer applications, word processing is the most common. To perform word processing, you need a computer, a special program called a word processor, and a printer. A word processor enables you to create a document, store it electronically on a disk, display it on a screen, modify it by entering commands and characters from the keyboard, and print it on a printer.

World Wide Web (Web or WWW): The part of the Internet that is most accessible and easiest to navigate, organized as sites with hyperlinks to one another (Burke & Weill, 2005).

For a more detailed lexicon, see http://www.oasismanagement.com/ TECHNOLOGY/GLOSSARY.

CHAPTER 5

Healthcare Policy for Advocacy in Health Care

Angela Mund

There are three critical ingredients to democratic renewal and progressive change in America: good public policy, grassroots organizing and electoral politics.
—PAUL WELLSTONE

Introduction

In 2001, the Institute of Medicine (IOM) challenged all healthcare professionals to improve the quality of patient care with an emphasis on increasing its safety, effectiveness, efficiency, equitability, timeliness, and patient centeredness (IOM, 2001). To create widespread change in the delivery of health care and in the structure of America's health systems, policies supporting quality improvement must be researched, developed, funded, and implemented. The complexity of today's healthcare environment and the increase in volume of scientific knowledge demand the involvement of nurses educated in the legislative process and prepared to influence policy on the local, state, and national levels.

Advanced practice registered nurses (APRNs) have the advantage of an appreciation of the patient care experience and the challenges of working within complex healthcare systems. However, those unique experiences must be combined with an education in the intricacies of policy and politics in order to create true and effective change. Policy activism translates into patient advocacy. In 1992, Ham described five basic elements critical to understanding the inherent complexity of policy. These elements are just as relevant today and include the following concepts:

1. Reviewing policies includes studying formal decisions and actions.
2. A policy may include a network of interacting decisions rather than a single decision.
3. Policies change over time.
4. Policies that were *not* acted on should also be included when reviewing policy making.
5. It is important to identify the policies that were created out of clear decision-making and to use that information to develop an effective process of policy making. (Hewison, 1999, p. 1378)

During the creation of the American Association of Colleges of Nursing's (AACN) *Essentials of Doctoral Education for Advanced Nursing Practice*, the AACN recognized and supported the integral relationship between policy and practice. Therefore, the AACN included the curricular requirement of instruction in "health care policy for advocacy in health care" in the *Essentials* (AACN, 2006). According to the AACN, doctorally educated nurses will have the tools to engage in and serve as leaders in the development and implementation of healthcare policy that affects financing, regulation, quality improvement, and equitable access to health care.

The ability to effectively engage in influencing policy can be created by obtaining an understanding of the foundations of nursing policy, the elements of the political process, and the relationship between leadership and policy making. APRNs can be at the forefront of changing the system of healthcare delivery in the United States by shaping local and legislative decision-making processes. In 2000, Rains and Carroll asserted that there has never been a greater need for nurses to be involved in the political process in order to ensure the best use of shrinking resources, provide affordable health care for all, and advocate for changes in healthcare policy.

History of the Relationship Between Nursing and Policy Making

The integration of nursing and policy is not a new concept. During the Crimean War, Florence Nightingale recognized the connection between policies made by Parliament and the British soldiers' poor living conditions (Ennen, 2001). Nurses' policy involvement has waxed and waned since the 19th century, when Nightingale exerted influence on the public policies of sanitation and infection control practices. There was a lack of political interest and influence in the early 20th century (Milstead, 2008, p. 2). After a few decades of silence, individual nurse leaders such as Lillian Wald and

Lavina Dock spoke up and publically supported suffrage, women's rights, nursing licensure, and the right to health care (Rubotzky, 2000). Nursing as a collective field, however, did not speak out on the issues. In 1985, Huston described several factors explaining nurses' lack of political involvement, including the "socialization to view power and politics negatively and the invisibility of nurses in the media" (Rains & Carroll, 2000, p. 37). From the 1970s through the 1990s, nurses were gaining in the areas of nursing science and education, use of technological knowledge and clinical skills, and in the creation of a new paradigm of advanced practice nursing. Advanced practice nurses were now confronted with understanding the political and practice implications of state and national legislation and with creating policies that supported the continued advancement of the profession.

During the 1970s, the Department of Health, Education, and Welfare created the Committee to Study Extended Roles for Nurses. This committee recommended further studies on cost-benefit analysis and attitudes toward the use of APRNs and recommended increased federal funding for nurse practitioners (Hamric, Spross, & Hanson, 2000). The 1970s also brought battles over prescriptive authority, the right for APNs to use the word *diagnose*, and the right to directly bill Medicare for nurse anesthesia services (Hamric et al., 2000). The 1980s brought the concepts of cost containment and diagnosis-related groups and the associated legislation that would have an impact on APRN practice. Nurse practitioners and nurse anesthetists encouraged lawmakers and the Health Care Financing Administration, currently the Centers for Medicare and Medicaid Services, to create policies and pass legislation concerning reimbursement procedures that would support the profession of advanced practice nursing. In 1989, nurse anesthetists became the first APRN group allowed to obtain direct reimbursement from Medicare, for anesthesia services. The passage of this legislation is considered to be "one of the greatest lobbying achievements not only of the American Association of Nurse Anesthetists (AANA) but of the whole of nursing" (Bankart, 1993, p. 167).

Throughout the 20th century, nursing organizations were created and led by nurses who acknowledged the need for involvement in the policy arena, the necessity of professional leadership, and the importance of strong grassroots efforts by their nurse members. The 1990s were a decade of growth in the numbers of APNs and of both nurse practitioner and nurse anesthetist programs. Comprehending the increased complexity of patients and of healthcare systems, APRN educational programs transitioned to requiring a master's-level education for entry to practice. APRN organizations continued to develop a voice, while the American Nurses Association (ANA), realizing the need for access to legislators, moved its headquarters to Washington, D.C. (Hamric et al., 2000; Milstead, 2008).

As we begin the 21st century, conflicts over physician supervision, prescriptive authority, scope of practice, equal access to healthcare providers, and the quality, safety, and cost-effectiveness of health care are still being waged at the state and federal levels. The recent incorporation of policy into the APN role and the Doctor of Nursing Practice degree requirements is leading to a resurgence of interest in the responsibility of influencing healthcare reform, the promotion of global health, and the protection of the profession.

Influencing the Health Policy Agenda

Public policy is created by governmental legislation and involves laws and regulations. It has been defined as "the purposeful, general plan of action developed to respond to a problem that includes authoritative guidelines" (Sudduth, 2008, p. 171). According to Mason, Leavitt, and Chafee (2002), "public policy often reflects the value, beliefs and attitudes of those designing the policy" (p. 8). Public policy can be further divided into social policy, which concerns communities, and then into health policy, which focuses on the health of the individual (Mason et al., 2002). The word *politics* has both positive and negative connotations. On one hand, it brings to mind images of corruption, misbehavior, and "politics as usual." However, politics should also have positive undertones as the decision-making process whereby APRNs can influence the development of legislation and the allocation of resources. Doctor of Nursing Practice (DNP) graduates are well positioned to influence the content and quality of healthcare legislation. Along with their extensive clinical background and a well-developed comprehension of the issues, APRNs must have a working knowledge of the language of legislation and regulation.

The Process of Legislation

The legislative process is rarely the very linear, rational process described in textbooks. Instead, it is a process whereby competing interests attempt to influence policy making by making bargains, trading votes, and using

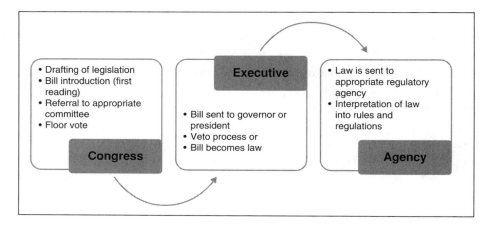

■ Figure 5-1   Movement of a bill.

rhetoric to convince legislators that their policy agenda is the best. APRNs have the opportunity and responsibility to educate lawmakers as legislation moves through the legislative bodies and government agencies. Figure 5-1 notes the basic steps of moving a bill through the state or federal process. In the federal policy arena, proposed legislation is called a bill until it is passed by both houses of Congress and signed into law by the president. At the state level, a bill moves via a similar process and is passed by the state legislature and signed into law by the governor.

Although APRNs can draft legislation, it is more common to partner with an interested and supportive legislator in either the state or federal House of Representatives or the Senate. The drafting process may include only a small number of persons or may involve a significant number of interested parties. It will be beneficial at this stage to allow any stakeholder nursing groups to review the language of the proposed legislation. Why is this important? Not all language is viewed the same by all groups, and what may be good for one APRN group may be detrimental to another. The time to find this discrepancy is not during the hearing phase, when the ability to influence legislation may be limited by time constraints and lack of coalition support.

The greater the political power of the sponsoring legislator, the greater the probability of successfully passing a piece of legislation. The likelihood of successful passing of legislation will also improve if supportive legislators introduce the bill to both chambers of Congress at the same time. Bipartisan support from both Republican and Democratic sponsors further increases the likelihood of successful movement of legislation through Congress. Following the drafting of the legislation, the senator or representative will introduce the proposed legislation to the chamber; the legislation will then be referred to the proper committee, typically based on the recommendation of the sponsoring legislator. The bill is given a number corresponding to the chamber in which it was introduced (e.g., S.252). The details of each bill can be found at www.thomas.gov. The selection of the "proper" committee is based primarily on the appropriateness of the committee but can also be a political decision based on whether members of the committee support or oppose the proposed legislation. In theory, members usually author bills that will be referred to the committees where they have jurisdiction. While the legislation is in committee, interested parties and stakeholders may be invited to submit written or oral testimony either supporting or refuting the legislation. The legislation then undergoes a process called markup in which the committee debates the legislation, discusses the flaws, and amends the legislation as necessary.

During this process, APRNs should be prepared to serve as content experts while advocating for the profession of nursing and shaping the healthcare agenda. It is imperative at this point to know the "enemies" of your legislation and be able to generate a strategy for managing controversy. Well-prepared testimony includes a description of who is doing the testifying (e.g., a family nurse practitioner in a rural practice), the background of the issue, and why the legislation is supportive or detrimental in resolving the issue. Effective testimony must also include what the APRN testifying would like the committee to do. Submitting oral testimony may be a stressful situation, but the key to presenting a logical, persuasive report is to prepare in advance. When preparing testimony, it is very important to be able to discuss the issue in great detail, know the influential legislators on the committee, and include the potential impact on patient care.

Once the committee agrees on the content and language of the bill, it is then moved to the Senate or House floor and voted upon by the members. The submitting committee must create a report to accompany the bill. The report includes such information as the intent of the legislation, the potential financial implications, dissenting opinions, and amendments to the initial bill. The bill may be referred back to committee, approved, or voted down.

Meanwhile, "companion legislation" is introduced in the other chamber of Congress, typically with similar wording; however, rarely is the wording exactly the same. The passage of the original legislation in one chamber encourages the forward movement of the companion legislation in the other chamber. Following the passage of both companion bills, one in the Senate and one in the House, the bill may be moved to a conference committee to work out any differences. The conference committee is composed of both senators and representatives. Both chambers must concur and approve their respective bills prior to the bill passing out of Congress and moving to the executive branch. If the bill does not come out of committee prior to the end of the legislative session, the bill is dead and must be reintroduced during the following session.

An important role for APRNs during this phase is to contact their representatives or senators and to build coalitions with other professional associations. The importance of creating these relationships prior to the introduction of any legislation will become evident as the bill moves through Congress. Nurses must not wait until the proposed legislation is being voted on—this is too late! Instead, nurses must be involved during the very early stages. Although the emphasis of influencing legislation often lies within the Congress, at the federal level the executive branch has the power to either veto the legislation or to sign the legislation. Again, a similar process occurs at the state level. Another import factor to consider is the power of the office of governor or president in supporting or blocking the legislative effort.

The Process of Regulation

An equally important but maybe more complex segment of policy is regulation. Regulation is the implementation process of legislation and occurs at both the state and federal levels. After a bill is passed through Congress and signed into law by the president, it is sent to a regulatory agency within the government, which then interprets the law and creates the rules and regulations that shape the way the new law is executed. Congress rarely includes explicit directions for implementation within the legislation and, in fact, may be purposefully vague. Again, stakeholders are invited to comment on the proposed draft of the rules and regulations. It is important not to overlook this phase since a hard-fought battle to produce legislation favorable for nursing may become something completely different during the regulatory process. Conversely, if policy cannot be changed in the legislative arena,

APRNs may be able to persuade the regulatory agency to publish rules that are favorable to nursing. This may be a dangerous game to play, because regulations must be consistent with the enabling statute. In the event that the regulation is inconsistent with the law, the law supersedes the regulation.

Federal agencies of interest to APRNs include the Department of Health and Human Services, the Centers for Medicare and Medicaid Services (CMS), the Department of Veterans Affairs, the Indian Health Service, and the Armed Forces. CMS is the primary agency regulating reimbursement for APRN services, including supervision requirements. Prior to a regulation being put into effect, two steps must occur. First, the proposed rule is published in the *Federal Register* and information is included on how the public can participate in the process by providing comment and attending the meetings (Loversidge, 2008). The second step involves the agency considering all the information and deciding on a course of action. The final regulation is then published in the *Federal Register* and becomes effective after 30 days. The *Federal Register* is a daily journal of the government of the United States containing the public notices of all the government agencies, executive orders, and presidential proclamations. All of the information from the *Federal Register* is in the public domain and can be accessed by any APRN at www.gpoaccess.gov/fr/index/html. Many professional organizations have paid staff to monitor the *Federal Register* for regulations that may have an impact on APRNs.

Boards of nursing, medicine, and pharmacy are examples of state regulatory agencies that may create rules and regulations affecting nurses and the delivery of health care within states. These agencies have the power to control entry into the profession, monitor and discipline licensees, and ensure continued competency of licensees (Loversidge, 2008). State agencies obtain their rulemaking authority through enabling laws. An enabling law is "one in which the state legislature delegates to an administrative agency the authority to adopt regulations to implement the law's purposes" (Tobin, 2001, p. 113). In essence, enabling laws give regulatory agencies the power to create rules and regulations. APRNs should assist in maintaining a collegial relationship between their state professional organizations and the board of nursing. Most appointments to state boards are made by the governor and necessitate the support of legislators and professional organizations. APRNs must be represented on boards of nursing to monitor the actions of the board and offer recommendations related to advanced nursing practice.

Boards of medicine may attempt to regulate nursing practice through language concerning supervision and collaboration. Therefore, it is advisable for APRNs to be aware of the regulatory agenda of all state boards that may have an interest in limiting APRNs' scope of practice and patient access. This involvement may include having an APRN presence at the board meetings of nursing and non-nursing state boards. When reviewing proposed regulations, it is important to understand the intent of the regulation and evaluate the language of the regulation for possible limits to APRN scope of practice and reimbursement. Other possible avenues to influence the regulatory process include seeking appointment to CMS panels, providing testimony at regulatory hearings, obtaining a position on advisory panels to the National Council of State Boards of Nursing (NCSBN), or agreeing to serve as an APRN expert during drafting of regulatory policy.

The NCSBN is a coalition of state boards of nursing that provides an avenue for state boards to examine regulatory issues and "counsel together on matters of common interest and concern affecting public health safety and welfare," including performing policy analysis, licensure, and research (NCSBN, n.d.). In 2008, the NCSBN partnered with the APRN Consensus Work Group and created the Consensus Model for APRN Regulation. The Consensus Model grew out of a concern that because each state determines the legal scope of practice and the criteria for entry to practice and competence through certification examinations, the ability of APRNs to move between states is limited and access to health care for patients may decrease. The Consensus Model promotes a uniform regulatory process based on nationally accepted standards for certification, licensure, and practice. All APRN stakeholder professional associations were invited to comment on the proposed Consensus Model. The APRN Model Act on Rules and Regulations was approved by the NCSBN in August 2008. It was essential throughout this process that all APRN groups had a place at the table and were able to discuss concerns with the regulatory language, create a coalition of a wide variety of nursing groups, and generate a model that all of the nursing stakeholders could support. However, as language from the Consensus Model begins to appear in proposed state legislation, it is imperative that APRNs monitor the legislative language to ensure that the intent of the model is correctly displayed in the legislation.

Therefore, in policy making, it is important to consider all phases and potential areas for influence throughout the entire process. Although similarities exist between states, APRNs should also understand the peculiarities of their state of licensure and the differences between federal and state legislation and regulation. APRNs can influence policy by providing proactive solutions to the problems facing health care rather than lamenting the problems. The solutions should contain information on practicality, feasibility, financial implications, and the benefits for the profession of nursing and for overall health care. Armed with an understanding of the background of policy making, the APRN will be able to build coalitions, foster grassroots lobbying efforts, and cultivate effective lobbying skills.

Professional Organizations, Grassroots Lobbying, and Coalition Building

The powerful combination of a united political voice through professional organizations and the grassroots efforts of APRNs has the power to influence the healthcare agenda. Through membership dues and other revenue sources, professional organizations have the resources to create a network of federal government lobbyists, state government political affairs directors, and political action committees.

Strength in numbers and coalition building are an important part of creating political influence. Membership in a professional organization is the responsibility of all APRNs. Table 5-1 lists examples of APRN professional organizations. Professional organizations all have healthcare advocacy on their agenda, but their approach to influencing policy varies. The yearly legislative agenda for each professional organization is based on the current policy climate, the presence of pro-nursing members of Congress on important committees, and the current needs of the profession. Some organizations have offices based in Washington, D.C., with paid office staff, professional lobbyists, and political action committees. Others operate primarily on a grassroots-type scale, with members providing the majority of the legislative work. Regardless of the organizational makeup, all members should maintain a two-way channel of communication to facilitate the flow of policy information and generate a network of involved members for grassroots lobbying efforts.

It is important to remember that political decisions are not made in the Senate or House chamber on the day of the vote but in offices throughout the legislative session. Decisions may be based on external pressures from other legislators, constituents, friends, and professional groups. A poten-

■ Table 5-1   APRN Professional Organizations

American Academy of Nurse Practitioners (AANP)
American Association of Colleges of Nursing (AACN)
American Association of Nurse Anesthetists (AANA)
American College of Nurse Midwives (ACNM)
American Nursing Association (ANA)
American Organization of Nurse Executives (AONE)

tially powerful grassroots approach to influencing policy is to become involved in the election campaign of an official running for public office. Involvement may range from knocking on doors to discuss the campaigner's stance on the issue of access to health care to hosting a fundraising event. Visibility is critical. When elected, the legislator will remember the supporters who were involved in the early stages of his or her run for a position in the local, state, or federal government. An indication of effective involvement can be when a legislator introduces an APRN to another legislator with the words "the APRNs were with me from the beginning." This early involvement translates into an open-door policy with the legislator for members of the organization.

Lobbying is not a dirty word but an important part of the legislative process bound by ethical rules of conduct. Lobbyists are registered, educated professionals hired by both state and federal organizations to influence decisions made by legislators. One approach to influence legislation is to ensure that the legislators have all the pertinent information prior to making a decision on a certain piece of legislation. For example, in the recent healthcare bill, a legislator who has a reputation of being "CRNA friendly" proposed an amendment for reimbursement for pain management services. However, the wording covered only physician services. After a discussion with the AANA lobbyist, the amendment was changed.

Because healthcare professional organizations are composed of members with full-time careers in the clinical arena, lobbyists are an integral part of influencing the healthcare agenda. Lobbyists are able to be continuously available during the legislative process. The lobbyists have cultivated relationships with legislative staff and understand the inner workings of Congress. Professional lobbying activities performed on behalf of an organization can include monitoring ongoing and proposed legislation, developing an agenda of legislative goals, advising on distribution of political action committee funds, communicating with the membership, and educating members during grassroots lobbying efforts. Lobbyists often assist in creating a voice for the professional organization in developing oral and written testimony. Professional lobbyists do not create the message. APRNs have the message; the lobbyist just knows how to get the message to the right people and in the correct manner.

Legislators are more likely to listen to the concerns of their constituents and to support the efforts of a group of constituents. APRNs must take on the professional responsibility of advocating for nursing and healthcare reform by contacting their representatives and senators in Congress. APRNs have the ability to tell the story of their patients who cannot afford preventive health care, or the small-town hospital that is closing due to budget cuts, or the patient who does not have access to health care due to lack of providers. Personal stories told by a clinician in one of the most respected and trusted professions can be a powerful tool for influencing legislation. Also, storytelling can be the least intimidating entry into the world of grassroots lobbying. When APRN DNP students share their personal difficulties in obtaining funding for education and for research, it creates a more lasting impression than when a nonstudent discusses the challenges of financing education. Professional organizations play a significant role in preparing the membership and alleviating some of the fears of grassroots lobbying.

For example, the AANA's Federal Government Affairs Office creates "Action Alerts" to encourage members to contact their representatives or senators. A portion of the AANA website contains the information that members who are certified registered nurse anesthetists (CRNAs) can use to contact their legislators. At a yearly assembly held in Washington, D.C., the staff at the AANA's D.C. office educates CRNAs on the legislative process as a whole, on the current issues facing health care and healthcare reform, and on the issues specific to CRNAs. A portion of the assembly is spent practicing for lobbying, including the dos and don'ts of presenting the issues and very specific details on the agenda for lobbying visits to Capitol Hill. Attending these professional meetings can be a very empowering experience, creating an understanding of what one individual, as part of a larger organization, can do to advocate for the profession of nursing and for the health of the nation. Table 5-2 lists examples of effective lobbying techniques.

■ Table 5-2　Effective Lobbying

- Lobby in person or on paper.
  - □ Send letters to your member of Congress when necessary.
  - □ Obtain face time with legislators early on and throughout their term(s).
  - □ Make an appointment rather than just drop by (not just in Washington, but at home too).
  - □ Be professional in appearance and demeanor.
  - □ Be punctual.
- Understand how the policy-making process works.
  - □ Attend educational "boot camps."
  - □ Maintain two-way communication with your professional organization regarding the organization's legislative agenda.
- Use your professional organization's lobbyist.
- Cultivate relationships with key legislative staff.
  - □ Take the time and opportunity to educate staff on nursing issues.
- Research your issues.
  - □ Be knowledgeable, confident, and articulate.
  - □ Know the number and status of the bill you are supporting or opposing (www.thomas. gov).
- Research the legislator you will be lobbying.
  - □ Build legislative profiles.
  - □ Is there a healthcare provider in the legislator's family?
  - □ Is the legislator on a committee with jurisdiction over healthcare issues? Is he or she the chair of the committee or a ranking member?
- Drive the discussion.
  - □ Tell your story.
  - □ Provide credible, "at the bedside" information about the impact of policies on health care.
  - □ Discuss the impact of proposed legislation on the individual in his or her district—on constituents, the healthcare consumer, and the overall health of the United States.
  - □ Never bash or speak poorly of your adversaries' position on the legislation.
  - □ If applicable, ask the legislator to sign on to cosponsor a bill you are supporting.
- Stay in touch.
  - □ Send a handwritten thank you note as follow-up.
  - □ Include your business card and how to contact you for questions or assistance.
  - □ Flaunt your credentials!
- Exemplify professionalism.
  - □ Focus on advocacy, trust, knowledge, and competency.
  - □ Focus on the unique role, skills, and pivotal position of APRNs in the healthcare system.

Another essential aspect of lobbying is appreciating the roles and responsibilities of congressional staff. Each member of Congress has a chief of staff, also called an administrative assistant (AA), who is responsible for overseeing the overall management of the office, including managing the media and public relations and serving as a political advisor. Legislative directors are responsible for the "day-to-day legislative activities and may have more policy expertise" (Wakefield, 2008, p. 70). Legislative assistants (LAs), often post-college interns or fellows participating in a fellowship program, have the most contact with special interest groups such as nursing professional organizations. LAs can be very influential because they advise the member of Congress on health policy issues. They control what information is presented to the member of Congress and what groups get face time with the senator or representative. LAs are assigned to a specific issue, such as health or veteran's affairs; this does not mean that the LA is an expert in that area, however! When meeting with an LA for the first time, it is crucial to determine what he or she knows about advanced practice nursing and nursing's stance on healthcare issues. It is important to spend time educating the LA, in a non-defensive, noncondescending manner, regarding APRN practice and the professional organization's legislative agenda. Even if the exact goal of the lobbying visit was not met, the LA will have obtained a greater understanding of APRNs, including those with doctoral educations, which may increase the probability that a DNP may be sought out for advice on proposed legislation. An established relationship with the member of Congress's health LA will serve as a communication conduit for information regarding upcoming legislation and committee hearings.

Although the blend of money and politics may not always appear like a good combination, a strong political action committee (PAC) will increase access to and gain the attention of members of Congress. A PAC is a "group that is formed by an industry or an issue oriented organization to raise and contribute money to the campaign of political candidates who likely can advance their issue" (Twedell & Webb, 2007, p. 279). PACs have been involved in the campaign process over the last 60 years. Two types of PAC exist: separate segregated funds (SSFs) and nonconnected committees. SSFs are established and administered by organizations, whereas nonconnected committees are not sponsored by any organization (Federal Election Commission, 2009). Nursing PACs collect funds from their membership, pool the money, research the candidates, and distribute the money to legislators who are more likely to support the agenda of the nursing organization. PACs may contribute primarily to Democratic or Republican candidates, but often the PAC may be nonpartisan, supporting the candidate with similar priorities or the candidate who is influential on healthcare issues.

As Congress addresses campaign reform, PACs have come under increased scrutiny and have been required to increase transparency in regard to sources of funding, donation amounts to candidates, and relationships with Congress. The Federal Election Campaign Act of 1971 prohibited organizations from using their general funds and membership dues to fund campaign contributions, and the Bipartisan Campaign Reform Act of 2002 placed further limits on contributions (Twedell & Webb, 2007). Nurse anesthetists (NAs), nurse practitioners (NPs), clinical nurse specialists (CNSs), and certified nurse midwives (CNMs) have APRN-specific PACs. The American Nurses Association's PAC also contributes to candidates that support APRN issues.

Physician groups and pharmaceutical companies continue to have the top-spending PACs in health care, which often translates into greater political influence. During the 2008 election cycle, the only nursing PAC to break into the top ten PACs was that of the American Association of Nurse Anesthetists. Interestingly, the American Society of Anesthesiologists led PAC contributions from specialty physician groups (Center for Responsive Politics, 2009). According to the U.S. Department of Health and Human Services, in 2004 there were 240,460 APRNs (Health Resources and Services Administration, 2007). If each APRN donated $50 to his or her PAC, the resultant $12 million could move APRN PACs toward the top of the list of influential healthcare PACs. Information regarding individual PACs, including where the money comes from, how it is spent, and the overall worth of each PAC, can be found at www.opensecrets.org/index.php. With nursing's positive public image and a well-funded PAC, imagine the possibilities to influence legislation and advocate for improved quality and access to health care.

Coalition building is an effective approach to obtaining legislative and regulatory approval for an organization's policy agenda. Coalitions may last for the short term or long term, with the objective of combining resources to achieve a common goal. Nursing organizations can form coalitions either with other healthcare organizations or between APRN groups. For example, a coalition of over 30 nursing organizations created the Nursing Community Consensus Document (2008) requesting improved funding for doctoral education and calling for the removal of the rule that limits traineeship grants for doctoral education. Although the emphasis is on increasing nursing faculty, the importance of removing the cap on doctoral grants for entry-level doctoral students should not go unnoticed. According to Rice (2002, p. 122), the essential ingredients for strong coalitions include "leadership, membership, and serendipity." As in all organizations, it is important to have a leader who can organize the work of the coalition and a leader who can motivate the group to stay on target (Rice, 2002). This could be an important venue for a DNP. Membership is essential to increase the productivity and the visibility of the organization. Coalitions may be formed by unforeseen opportunities. For example, proposed state legislation to remove the collaboration requirement for prescriptive authority may bring together the state nursing association and the state APRN organizations.

Just as there are benefits for organizations in coming together, there are also potential pitfalls and challenges to effective functioning of the group. When forming a coalition, it is essential to have all the right people: members who will work hard and people with a stake in the common goal (Rice, 2002). One of the challenges of working in a group of differing organizations is the presence of differing perspectives. Although the group may have one common goal, each member organization may have contradictory perspectives on other goals. When this occurs, it is essential to have a leader, potentially one with a DNP degree, who will seek out diverse opinions, allow members to agree to disagree, and "work toward achieving decisions which members can live with" (Rice, 2002, p. 128). Also, although opposing organizations may not agree on all topics, it is important to handle conflict effectively in order to maintain a working relationship if the need for collaboration does occur.

Coalitions may be created for the purpose of countering a threat to the ability of member organizations to practice to the full scope of their professional licensure. The Coalition for Patients' Rights (CPR) is composed of 35 organizations representing a variety of licensed healthcare professionals. With strength in numbers and a diverse group of providers, the aim of CPR is to offset the efforts of the American Medical Association's Scope of Practice Partnership (SOPP) initiative, which is designed to limit patients' choice of healthcare providers and ultimately patient access to health care (CPR, n.d.) Some coalitions may be formed without the express purpose of policy making. However, the data obtained by these nursing groups can be used to give a statistical significance to a proposed legislative agenda item. The Interagency Collaborative on Nursing Statistics (ICONS) "promotes the generation and utilization of data, information, and research about nurses, nursing education, and the nursing workforce" (ICONS, 2006).

Coalitions of like-minded organizations may join forces to ensure a seat at the table while the details of the composition of healthcare reform legislation are debated. The Patients' Access to Responsible Care Alliance (PARCA) is a coalition of nonphysician organizations that "aims to provide federal policymakers with access to information from all areas of the healthcare community . . . and is committed to quality cost-effective care and ensuring patients have options in the delivery of such care" (PARCA, n.d.). The inclusion of nondiscriminatory language for reimbursement for services provided by a nonphysician is critical for the future of APRNs and for equitable access to health care for all. An example of PARCA-supported antidiscrimination language is as follows:

SEC.___PROHIBITION ON DISCRIMINATION AGAINST HEALTHCARE PROVIDERS

Notwithstanding any other provision of this Act (or an amendment made by this Act), a health insurance issuer to which this Act (or amendment) applies shall not discriminate with respect to participation, reimbursement, covered services or indemnification under a health plan or other health insurance coverage against any health care provider who is acting within the scope of that provider's license or certification under applicable State law.

PARCA is composed of nursing APRN organizations, the American Academy of Audiology, the American Chiropractic Association, the American Optometric Association, the National Association of Social Workers, and others. As evidenced by the composition of PARCA, an important aspect to consider when building effective coalitions is the significance of connecting diverse groups, including both depth and breadth of professions.

Healthcare Reform

Due to increasing healthcare costs, "the insecurity resulting from basing healthcare insurance on employment," and the significant number of uninsured, the American public grew increasingly dissatisfied with the state of health care in the United States throughout the 1990s (Schroeder, 1993, p. 945). In 1993, the Clinton administration attempted to reform health care in the United States. The proposed national Health Security Act (HSA) of

1993 included guaranteed comprehensive benefits, limitations on health insurance premiums, and increased emphasis on quality, and mandated employers to provide insurance coverage through regulated health maintenance organizations (National Health Security Plan, 1993). The proposed plan, spearheaded by then First Lady Hillary Clinton, had significant opposition from conservatives, small business owners, and the health insurance industry because of its cost and complexity, significant government oversight and control, and the potential to limit patient healthcare choices. In the end, legislation for healthcare reform was not passed.

Because of the difficulty in creating a coalition for support and the appearance of political shenanigans, the American public's interest in healthcare reform declined during the time that the HSA legislation was drafted. For the first time, nursing, the largest group of healthcare providers, had a significant presence during the debate over how to reform the U.S. healthcare system. This presence was due to the work of a small group of nurses who understood the importance of creating legislative relationships and of suggesting solutions to the problem, and who demonstrated a "willingness to compromise in the present to secure the greater gain in the future" (Milstead, 2008, p. 20).

In advance of the presidential and legislative impetus to restructure the healthcare system, the ANA created a task force in 1989 to begin work on an agenda to reform health care. Nursing's *Agenda for Healthcare Reform*, published in 1992, focused on the contribution that reforming health systems would have on improving access to care while controlling cost and improving outcomes. The agenda called for a "federal standard of uniform basic benefits package for all US citizens and residents financed through public-private partnerships using a variety of healthcare providers including provisions for community health and quality measurement" (Trotter Betts, 1996, p. 4). Despite the failure of the HSA, the activism during this period allowed nurses to obtain increased visibility in the policy arena and develop skills in policy making. Nursing and the ANA came out better informed, with greater access to legislators, and better armed for the next legislative challenge (Trotter Betts, 1996; Rubotzky, 2000).

Blendon and Benson, in a 2001 review regarding American opinions on health policy over the last 50 years, found that "Americans may have expressed dissatisfaction with private health insurance and managed care but most don't trust the federal government to take over as a single-payer provider or are satisfied enough with their current medical payment arrangements" (cited in Jamelske, Johs-Artisensi, Taft, & German, 2009, p. 17). However, given the 2008 downturn in the economy, Americans and Congress are again concerned with enacting some variety of healthcare reform. With the rising cost of healthcare premiums and the increase in the number of Americans who are uninsured or underinsured, Americans have begun to realize that the potential to lose coverage in the future does exist. So, healthcare reform once again is on the forefront of the federal legislative agenda. Policy lessons learned during the previous attempts at healthcare reform have set the stage for organized nursing to influence policy that will ensure improved health care for all Americans. It remains to be seen whether the changes in healthcare delivery will look like the failed sweeping reform attempted during the Clinton administration or a more incremental reform policy. An incremental healthcare reform policy would begin with small changes, allowing for the addressing of political dynamics at each stage. Influential policy makers exist on both sides of the plan for reform: creation of an immediate, all-encompassing change versus making small adjustments at regular intervals. Political influence developed by the ANA and nursing leaders in the 1980s and 1990s must be sustained throughout the upcoming legislative challenges during the anticipated long road to sustainable healthcare financing reform.

APRNs are skilled at applying the nursing process to the clinical care of the patient. The nursing process—assess, diagnose, plan, implement, and evaluate—can also be used to apply policy to practice by analyzing the current state of health care in the United States and constructing a possible solution. Begin with an assessment of the situation. A bipartisan report released by the U.S. Senate Finance Committee on May 18, 2009, noted that "46 million Americans lack health insurance coverage, employer-sponsored health care premiums have increased 117 percent between 1999–2008, and annual health care spending is expected to outpace annual growth in the overall economy by 2.1 percent in the next ten years. Also, in 2009, health spending will increase 5.5 percent while gross domestic product is expected to decrease 0.2 percent" (Senate Finance Committee, 2009).

The next step in the process is to identify or diagnose the problem. Armed with data from government sources including the Department of Health and Human Services, Centers for Disease Control and Prevention, and the Centers for Medicare and Medicaid Services, APRNs can recognize many of the problems in healthcare systems, including a healthcare delivery system that does not provide access to all Americans, the uncontrolled rise in health-care cost, and the lack of preventive health care.

Following a diagnosis of the problem, the biggest challenge then becomes how to plan for resolution of the crisis while anticipating potential obstacles. According to Malone (2005), obstacles to policy intervention include "lack of media attention, ideological opposition from those in decision-making positions, lack of money, advocacy leadership struggles and efforts from those actively opposed" (p. 141). The doctorally prepared advanced practice nurse will be prepared, informed, and empowered to challenge any Congress or presidential administration to support a healthcare policy that meets the six aims of the IOM: safe, effective, patient centered, timely, efficient, and equitable (IOM, 2001). The search for innovative solutions while using the resources at hand may prove to be more difficult than anticipated, as evidenced by the failure of the Clinton plan. How can the United States ensure equal access to high-quality care for all Americans while controlling cost? Is the U.S. nursing workforce substantial enough to handle the potential influx of patients into the healthcare system? APRNs may be asked to provide expert testimony, serve as content experts, and garner support from legislators during this stage of the process.

While the legislation is being implemented, APRNs must continue their political activism with vigilance and a skeptical eye regarding any drafts, testimony, or regulations that do not support the intent of the reform legislation. The last step of the process—which should actually occur throughout the progression of legislation—is to evaluate whether the legislation works. Formative evaluation of the policy process should occur from the beginning. Did APRNs become involved, and how effective were they? What were the obstacles to policy legislation and implementation? Were the obstacles recognized early in the process? Does the legislation meet the six aims of the IOM? Does the legislation provide for equal access to providers and for patients? How will outcomes be measured, and will they be measured equitably for all providers? Will this plan be sustainable?

In this author's opinion, true healthcare reform will require a paradigm shift, moving from simply increasing the national budget to reevaluating and revolutionizing the way health care is delivered in the United States. Outdated approaches to reimbursement should be replaced, provider discrimination should be prevented, research for evidence-based health care should be supported, and information technology should be employed to provide for seamless patient care and evaluation of outcomes.

Long-Standing Policy Goals

Prior to advocating for improvements in health care, it is crucial to understand the issues that have been at the forefront of nursing policy and politics for over four decades and that continue to warrant nursing's legislative and regulatory involvement. According to Malone (2005, p. 139), "it is important to understand the recent history of any policy issue to better understand the obstacles and resources in play."

Nursing Workforce Development

As the demand for health care rises and the demographics of our population change, the nursing profession continues to be challenged with an overall nursing workforce shortage. Although the primary factor behind the nursing workforce shortage changes over time, "consistent factors include unfavorable working conditions, relatively low income potential, more satisfying alternative job opportunities, and lack of nursing faculty" (McHugh, Aiken, Cooper, & Miller, 2008, p. 6). Doctorally prepared APRNs and nursing faculty are drawn from the relatively small pool of baccalaureate-prepared nurses; therefore, deficiencies in the number of registered nurses affects APRN vacancy rates and, ultimately, may limit patient access to care. Vacancy rates change over time relative to the changing economic times and healthcare market. Therefore, when advocating for legislative change concerning workforce development, it is necessary to have updated facts on past and current vacancy rates, the impact of past funding efforts on the shortage of nurses, and the impact of vacancy rates on healthcare delivery. For example, data from the U.S. Bureau of Labor Statistics (BLS) has been used to support the need for educational funding due to a projected need for a 23% increase in registered nurses by 2016 (BLS, 2007). Additional information in the BLS *Occupational Outlook Handbook* reports that all four APRN specialties (CNS, CRNA, CNM, and NP) will be in "high demand particularly in medically underserved areas" and "relative to physicians, these RNs increasingly serve as lower-cost primary care providers."

According to McHugh et al. (2008), "The nursing shortage is not only of total numbers but also of the level of nursing education" (p. 7). Over the last decade, nursing organizations have continued to lobby for legislative support to increase funding for nursing education at both the baccalaureate and graduate level. One legislative mechanism for funding is through the Nursing Workforce Development Programs (Title VIII of the Public Health

Service Act). Title VIII programs have been the largest source of federal funding for nursing education over the last 45 years. In the 1960s, nursing leaders lobbied Congress to enact legislation that would alleviate the nation's nursing shortage by funding nursing education. In 1964, President Lyndon Johnson signed the Nurse Training Act of 1964. In the years since its inception, Title VIII has expanded to include funding for advanced practice nursing education, for the education of disadvantaged and minority students, for nurse faculty loan programs, and for nurse education, practice, and retention grants (Nursing Community Consensus Document, 2008). Title VIII grants are an essential component for increasing the number of APRN graduates and for ensuring that medically underserved areas receive access to healthcare services. However, the level of funding is not guaranteed, and, despite the increased costs of education and inflation, the relative level of funding has remained unchanged. It is through the continued action of involved nurses that Title VIII funding consistently remains in the national budget and on the legislative agenda.

Along with a greater demand for nurses, the changing complexity of health care and healthcare systems requires that a greater number of advanced practice nurses and nursing faculty be prepared at the graduate level. APRNs must continue to monitor and support legislative issues that alleviate the nursing shortage by expanding funding for nursing education, promoting a favorable work environment, and eliminating barriers to practice.

Reimbursement

Although the complexity and changing nature of regulation make a detailed discussion of APRN reimbursement impractical for this venue, it is appropriate to discuss the fundamentals and historical background within the framework of advocating for APRN practice. It is imperative for the APRN provider to understand the challenges in achieving equality and to monitor for threats to APRN practice in the economic healthcare market within public policy. For over three decades, APRN groups have challenged our legislators to remove the financial barriers to practice (Sullivan-Marx, 2008).

For example, until 1989, all direct reimbursement for anesthesia services was limited to anesthesiologists. CRNAs were reimbursed from the money paid to the institution through Part A of Medicare. The disparity in the ability to directly bill for services created an inequality between providers delivering the same care. The Omnibus Reconciliation Act of 1987 required the federal Medicare program to create a separate payment plan for the anesthesia care delivered by a CRNA, which is now known as Medicare Part B. The change was budget neutral because responsibility for payment was moved from the Medicare Part A division to the Part B division (Broadston, 2001). The regulatory agency responsible for determining Medicare reimbursement was the Health Care Financing Administration (HCFA). When Medicare federal regulation changed, private insurance providers and state public health plans followed suit and opted to directly reimburse CRNAs for services provided (Broadston, 2001). It was essential during this time of legislative and regulatory change that CRNAs at all levels of the profession maintained close contact with Congress and the agencies responsible for transforming Medicare reimbursement.

During the 1970s and 1980s, as the number of nurse practitioners grew and diagnosis-related groups (DRGs) were created, nursing leaders in the American Nurses Association recognized the need for parity between physician and NP reimbursement. The ANA pressed for a mechanism to change Medicare rules through legislation (Sullivan-Marx, 2008). During this same time period, three policy reports were released supporting the role of NPs and the removal of barriers to reimbursement: the Graduate Medical Education National Advisory Council's (GMENAC) report, the Office of Technology Assessment's report to Congress, and the Physician Payment Review Commission's report (Sullivan-Marx, 2008). The reports cited barriers, including the lack of NP Medicare reimbursement. The GMENAC report concluded that direct reimbursement by Medicare and Medicaid would be necessary to facilitate full use of nurse practitioners and clinical nurse specialists (Sullivan-Marx, 2008, p. 122). Finally, with the passage of the 1990 Omnibus Budget Reconciliation Act, nurse practitioners and clinical nurse specialists in rural health clinics and in nursing homes were allowed to directly bill Medicare at 85% of the physician rate. Certified nurse midwives were allowed to bill at 65% of the physician rate (Sullivan-Marx, 2008). An additional seven years of encouraging legislators to act was required to include all NPs in direct reimbursement from Medicare. The Balanced Budget Act of 1997 granted NPs and CNSs the ability to bill Medicare in all geographic areas and settings, but still at only 85% of the prevailing physician rate (Abood & Franklin, 2000).

According to Abood and Franklin (2000), the ability to document and bill for APRN services creates transparency regarding which provider is actually performing the patient care. This documentation allows for connecting patient outcomes to healthcare providers and gives APRNs an additional tool to demonstrate their value to both the institution and policy makers. As we move forward with healthcare reform, through the knowledge gained during doctoral education and practice, APRNs can provide the skills necessary to analyze and engage in the discussion of cost-effectiveness, pay for performance, and reimbursement.

State Nurse Practice Acts and Scope of Practice

The first board of nursing and the first nurse practice act were created in 1903 in the state of North Carolina (Loversidge, 2008, p. 96). Initially, nurse practice acts (NPAs) focused on protecting the use of the title RN rather than defining the delivery of nursing care (Tobin, 2001). Following the 1971 report of the Department of Health, Education, and Welfare's Committee to Study Extended Roles for Nurses, state NPAs began to change to include regulations governing APRN practice (Tobin, 2001). The NPA is an example of an enabling law and contains the laws and regulations that credential and govern a profession (Loversidge, 2008). As noted in a previous section, boards of nursing and NPAs were created to protect the well-being of patients by ensuring consistent minimum standards of licensure and qualifications. Each state has a different nurse practice act, which defines the scope of practice for all nurses within that state and delineates the officers, staff, and powers of the state regulatory board (e.g., the board of nursing).

NPAs include language defining the roles and responsibilities of APRNs, including "accepting referrals from, consulting with, cooperating with, or referring to all other types of health care providers" and "must practice within a health care system that provides for consultation and collaborative management and referral as indicated by the health status of the patient" (Minnesota Board of Nursing, 2008). The evolution of the NPA is evident in the language regarding the roles of nurses. The initial ANA model definition of nursing practice in 1946 included the provision that the scope of practice for nursing is "not deemed to include acts of diagnosis or prescription of therapeutic or corrective measures" (Tobin, 2001). The ANA amended the model definition to allow for nurses to perform specific tasks (diagnosis and treatment) "under emergency or special conditions as are recognized by the medical and nursing professions" (Tobin, 2001). In 1996, the ANA revised the model practice definition to broaden the scope of practice of professional nursing, and a definition of APRN practice was explicitly included. The 2008 APRN Consensus Model grew out of the need for state NPAs to continue to evolve to meet the needs of the profession of nursing and the healthcare needs of the American public.

NPAs also include rules on delegation of duties to non-RN providers, continuing education requirements, and the administration of certain medications. CRNAs have opposed changes to state NPAs giving non–anesthesia providers the ability to administer Propofol as sedation in the nonintubated patient. To provide a basis for controlling the administration of Propofol, CRNAs used FDA labeling that requires that Propofol be administered by medical personnel experienced in general anesthesia. NPAs include the rules for prescriptive authority for APRNs. The authorization for APRNs to prescribe with or without a written collaborative agreement with a physician must be expressly written into the agreement. States differ in the authority for APRNs to prescribe controlled substances. CRNAs may be exempt from some of the prescriptive language requiring written collaboration in order to administer anesthetic agents and their adjuncts during the perioperative period.

Historically, APRNs have had to be diligent in monitoring proposed changes to a nurse practice act and to prevent other entities from attempting to supersede the power of the state board of nursing in defining APRN scope of practice. In 2005 the American Medical Association created the Scope of Practice Partnership (SOPP) and stated, in the report of the board of trustees, "[AMA] agreed that it was necessary to concentrate the resources of organized medicine to oppose scope of practice expansions by allied health professionals that would threaten the health and safety of the public" (American Medical Association, 2005). The SOPP objective is to fund studies refuting claims that APRNs were necessary to improve access to care in rural states and to create studies comparing the educational, training, and licensure requirements of physician and nonphysician providers. Just as nursing organizations should have no role in defining the practice of medicine, physician groups are in no position to define APRN practice, licensure, certification, or education. According to the Coalition for Patients' Rights, rather than creating division among healthcare professionals, the AMA and the allied health members of CPR should be working together to find solutions to the current healthcare challenges.

Any time a state nurse practice act is opened, whether the intent is to broaden scope of practice or not, the opportunity exists for language to be inserted increasing the need for supervision by a physician or removing prescriptive authority. State nursing organizations may be reluctant to open their nurse practice act for just those reasons. APRNs are responsible for remaining knowledgeable of the current status of the NPA in their state and for practicing within the limits of their scope of practice.

DNP graduates will be expected to not only exhibit the skills of advanced clinical practice and systems thinking but also to be accountable for driving the discussion that sustains nursing workforce development, maintains parity in reimbursement, and removes barriers to the full scope of practice for APRNs.

Integration of Policy with Ethics, Research, and Education

Ethics and Policy Making

Just as a vital link exists between policy and practice, so too the connection between policy and ethics is strong. The 2001 *Code of Ethics for Nurses with Interpretive Statements* (American Nurses Association, 2001) includes the following statement: "The profession of nursing, as represented by associations and their members, is responsible for articulating nursing values, for maintaining the integrity of the profession and its practice, and for shaping social policy."

Policy decisions are ethical decisions on many different levels, from choices made by professional organizations to prioritizing a legislative or regulatory agenda to the allocation of scarce resources. A political ethical conflict "occurs when what one is told to do (either covertly or overtly) by those having more power in the organization or what one feels compelled to do by the organization is in conflict with one's ethical belief structure" (Silva, 2002, p. 180). It becomes more of a challenge when the policy initially appears at odds with one's values, but upon further examination the eventual outcome of policy implementation does support the needs of the profession and public. For example, APRNs may have the ethical dilemma of supporting a legislator through PAC contributions who does not have the same values as organized nursing but sits in a position of power to influence legislation. Kent and Liaschenko (2004) examined the connection between nursing values and ANA PAC donations. They encouraged the ANA PAC to continue to evaluate the donation process for successful outcomes that are important to nursing while maintaining a connection with legislative leadership—Democratic or Republican (Kent & Liaschenko, 2004). As nursing continues to become more influential in the policy arena, it is important to develop partnerships on both sides of the legislative aisle. Regardless of the occasional differences in political viewpoints, it is necessary to ensure equal access when issues important to nursing arise.

Clinical APRNs are often the central decision makers in the allocation of resources, including laboratory and invasive testing, time spent in the delivery of patient care, medical equipment, and referrals for additional interventions (Aroskar, Moldow, & Good, 2004). This array of patient care concerns has the potential for both policy and ethical implications. Aroskar et al. (2004) used focus groups to examine the clinical nurse's perspective on changes in healthcare policy that affect patient care. Changes in legislative policy influence institutional policy, which in turn influences patient care. The most frequently noted themes included the policy implications of cost containment, the effects of policy on quality of care and patient education, and the overall effect on nurses and nursing (Aroskar et al., 2004). Medicare regulations may dictate where patients may receive care and how much care will be reimbursed. Legislation may influence the appropriate allocation of healthcare resources, as well as the decision makers who define "appropriate." Regulation regarding APRN licensure may affect quality-of-life and end-of-life matters if patients do not have access to all providers who can provide pain management and palliative care. However, although the researchers found that whereas all of the focus groups stressed the importance of nursing having a voice in policy development, the recognized need for "assertiveness does not always translate to advocacy for patients or participation in policy development" (Aroskar et al., 2004, p. 274).

APRNs educated and experienced in policy will have the ability to comprehend the ethical implications of policy development and implementation and be able to integrate both while achieving the ultimate goals of improving health and supporting the profession of nursing. According to Silva (2002), the solution to successful resolution of an ethical conflict between values and politics involves either integration or compromise. Integration includes the incorporation of all points of view into the policy, whereas compromise encourages all parties to forfeit something for the overall common good (Silva, 2002). Just as APRNs have a professional responsibility to be involved in policy, as noted by the ANA's Code of Ethics, they also have an ethical responsibility to the public to be engaged in healthcare policy.

Research and Policy Making

The initial link between nursing policy, practice, and research may have begun in the 1960s as nurse researchers sought federal funding and an equal playing field with medicine for research dollars (Milstead, 2008). Research and policy are connected in two interrelated ways: there is nursing research and policy research. Nursing research is used to supply the data and background information for creating policy. Policy research is the "analysis of a social problem to provide policy makers with alternative recommendations for future initiatives aimed at alleviating problems" (Nagelkirk & Henry, 1991, p. 20). During the process of restructuring health care in the United States, both types of research will be essential for creating an evidence-based plan that includes an examination of the alternatives. Nurse researchers have begun to realize that when using research to create policy, the largest challenge may originate from the inherent potential for ambiguous data to produce different interpretations and then different policies. In these situations, the successful APRN leader must shape the policy agenda such that the issue becomes defined as a problem backed by research requiring legislative or regulatory action. Often nursing research is "published by nurse academicians in the nursing literature but policymakers do not access their work" (Short, 2008, p. 266). APRNs can be the experts that bring the data to the legislator and discuss the outcomes and how they can be applied to public policy. Short (2008) encourages nurses to submit their research studies to journals outside of nursing and to include the potential policy implications of nursing research.

The media can be used to open a window of opportunity on an issue important to nursing. When the media started reporting the childhood obesity epidemic, nurse researchers were the content experts who used supporting data to influence public policy. Because of the favorable public impression of nurses, nurses have the ability to convey health-related information in a manner that is considered fact without a particular bias or slant. An institution's or organization's public relations staff can be used as a tool to stimulate public and legislator interest in nursing health policy research (Diers, 2002). Because research can be uninteresting or overwhelming to the lay public, the ability to translate research into powerful stories or anecdotes can serve as a catalyst for legislative activity.

Although the value of evidence-based research outcomes is not disputed, the ability of evidence to influence policy in the manner and to the degree expected by the researcher is still debated. Policy decisions are political decisions, and thus the rational, correct decision is not always made; instead, the decision may be a compromise between competing interests. Policy decisions must also be supported by the majority of citizens, who may have competing values at odds with the best policy evidence. The quality of the research or the research design may be less important than an understanding of the current political agenda or the agenda of special interest groups. In that case, the research may even be called into question despite solid methodology; or politicians and healthcare providers may use researched outcomes selectively to back an alternative course of action. APRNs educated in healthcare policy will be able to anticipate political trends, discover areas lacking in data, and design studies to seek out the answers.

Evidence-based practice data may be used to influence healthcare financing policy. Rather than focus on "this is the way we do it here," the impetus should instead be to focus on whether "the evidence support[s] the need for a procedure with increased cost without a proven benefit." According to P. R Orissa, former director of the Congressional Budget Office and currently the director of the Office of Management and Budget, when looking at the correlation between cost and quality, "the higher cost providers, the higher cost hospitals, the higher cost regions are not generating better health outcomes than the lower cost, more efficient providers" (Orszag, 2009, p. 74). Outcome-based research may be assisted by the use of information technology. With the increased emphasis on the use of electronic health records (EHRs), APRNs must be involved in the development of data entry points to support further research of outcomes relative to nursing care, including cost versus quality. Program evaluation is an integral part of policy research. Doctorally prepared APRNs are experts in program evaluation. As experts, APRNs must continue to use feedback to ensure that "old problems are being addressed, new problems are being identified and appropriate solutions are being considered" (Milstead, 2008, p. 21).

The political agenda is often shaped by cost, quality, and access to care. Research designed with that in mind can be used to a professional organization's benefit. In a May 2009 letter to the Senate Finance Committee answering a request for input into financing healthcare reform, Jackie Rowles, president of AANA, used data from a Government Accountability Office study (2007, p. 15) to communicate the financial incentive for including CRNAs in the blueprint for healthcare financing reform. President Rowles stated, "CRNAs predominate where there are more Medicare patients than average. CRNAs also predominate where private payment is lower than average, which is also where the gap between Medicare and private payment is less. Where anesthesiologists predominate, private payments are higher than average and the gap between Medicare and private payment is greater."

Clinical systems research, inherent in the final scholarly or capstone project of the DNP degree, is a useful means to provide an evidence-based approach to making policy changes within local, state, or federal health systems. Challenges within health care can often be traced back to a systems problem. APRNs with the clinical background and the education in evidence-based practice and policy will be able to frame the questions to search for the solutions. Is there a need to create policies that providers must follow to ensure delivery of evidence-based diabetes care or guarantee on-time immunizations? Why are some medical centers more efficient than others, and should their processes be emulated? How do we ensure access to care with a sustainable health policy?

Education, Practice, and Policy Making

According to Malone (2005), too often policy is not consistently emphasized as a part of nursing education despite the fact that policy can influence many aspects of patient care. When policy development has been included as part of nursing education, the primary focus has been on identifying and using an institution's policy manual (Malone, 2005). Policy-making skills are an integral part of doctoral education. Just as nurses learn the clinical skills necessary to care for patients, they are also compelled to learn the skills necessary for influencing policy. When new graduates have a sense of competency obtained through education and practical experience, they are more likely to become involved in the process. In the past, there were limited opportunities for formal policy education within nursing. Most skills were learned on the job through mentoring or self-directed education. With the increased complexity of health care and an increased need for nurses to become politically involved, the education process should now include a focused, systematic, consistent approach.

Maynard (1999) describes a four-dimensional intersecting model for teaching healthcare policy that includes information, commitment, initiative, and involvement. The first step is the responsibility that nurses have to remain informed and up to date about the health policy agenda. The second step is the commitment to act on an issue. Initiative, the third step, is the "power, ability, or instinct to begin or follow through with a plan or task" (p. 193). Although the model is not intended to be linear, the final step is involvement in the process of influencing policy. As the content of policy education is formalized within the curriculum of DNP programs, educators will need to be able to demonstrate the relevance of policy to practice. One approach to accomplish this is to instruct APRNs how to determine the basis of proposed policy changes.

An awareness of where legislation and regulation originate may be critical to understanding and influencing policy. Taft and Nanna (2008) stress the importance of educating nurses on the sources of healthcare policies that affect practice, including organizational, public, and professional sources. Examples of organizational sources are consumers of health care (patients), the media, and insurers. Patients who have experienced difficulties in the healthcare system are frequently an impetus for legislative change, for example, changes in insurance coverage for preventive exams. Public sources include the government at all levels and all branches, economic and demographic trends, and special interest groups (Taft & Nanna, 2008). Healthcare disciplines, including nursing, universities, and research-generating organizations, comprise the final type of source: professional sources. Professional APRN associations have played an integral role in proposing legislation that influences health care and have been involved in the regulatory role.

Nursing educators at all levels of entry to practice to nursing must serve as mentors by becoming role models for political activism, risk taking, and health policy advocacy. Experienced nurses can successfully communicate the connection between professional commitment and political responsibility. Rather than merely encouraging nurses to be politically involved, nursing faculty should equip students with the knowledge and skills to feel confident in their ability to influence policy. According to Rains and

Carroll (2000), "Health policy education at the graduate level has the potential to increase the political skills, involvement, and competence of nursing's future leaders" (p. 37). It is crucial during doctoral education that APRN students become actively involved in the process by lobbying on Capitol Hill, by serving as student representatives on professional organization committees, and by successfully demonstrating the ability to articulate the legislative and regulatory process. Policy-educated APRN clinicians should serve as role models to the next generations of baccalaureate- and graduate-prepared nurses. APRNs will be able to create a teaching environment that synthesizes didactic knowledge with the practice and work environments (Short, 2008). J. A. Milstead proposed that hospitals consider developing a "health policy/researcher" position to combine advanced clinical skills with the research skills necessary to influence health policy decisions within the organization and on a larger scale (Peters, 2002, p. 7).

Although all APRNs must participate in healthcare policy at some level, it is unrealistic to assume that all APRNs should become policy experts in addition to their roles in providing direct patient care. The extensive commitment of time and energy necessary to effectively perform all the duties of both roles may not be achievable. Instead, the future of advanced practice nursing may include the specialty of Health Policy APRN. As nurses become more adept and interested in policy, especially after doctoral education, they may choose to focus their career on influencing legislation and serving as a health policy expert. Nurses can gain practical experience by applying for policy fellowships in Washington, D.C. Perhaps the most well-known fellowship is the Robert Wood Johnson Foundation (RWJF) Health Policy Fellowship. Historically, nurses have not taken advantage of these opportunities. In the RWJF Fellowship's 33 years, 215 fellowships have been awarded, but only 23 nurses have been fellows (RWJF Health Policy Fellowships Program, n.d.). Health policy fellowships offer nurses an opportunity to brief legislators on healthcare issues, develop proposals, and staff conferences and hearings.

Although the relationship between policy and practice has focused on clinical care, nurse executives with a doctoral education foundation can play a critical role in influencing the policies that have a direct impact on patient care. Peters (2002) compares influencing policy to teaching an elephant to dance: difficult to do, but it can be accomplished if approached methodically. Administrators must be "committed to political activism;

stay informed through formal and informal channels; challenge the status quo; identify a base of support; and get the issues on the agenda" (Peters, 2002, pp. 5–7).

Phases of Policy Involvement

All APRNs have the responsibility to their patients to become involved in the political process at some level. Various authors have described levels of political involvement and emphasize that the focus is on finding a level at which the individual can be engaged and that is compatible with where the individual may be in his or her career. Boswell, Cannon, and Miller (2005) identified "three primary levels of commitment: survival, success, and significance" (p. 6). As APRNs become more engaged in the process, they may move through the levels or they may choose to stay at the level at which they are comfortable. At the survival level, the individual takes part in the voting process or may serve on a community board. At the next level, success, the individual "chooses to become influential in the policy arena" by becoming involved on the state or national level (Boswell et al., 2005, p. 6). Significance is the final level of involvement, whereby the individual is intensely involved in all aspects of healthcare policy, assuming leadership positions in influencing legislation at the state and national level.

Hewison (2008) describes nursing involvement in policy as a continuum from policy literacy to policy acumen to policy competence and finally to policy influence (p. 292). Rather than finding a level of engagement, Hewison (2008) applies the strategy to where individuals are in their careers, from novice to expert. Policy literacy may only involve reviewing the literature, defining the issues, and analysis of health policy research. This early stage provides a framework for the more experienced nurse to develop policy acumen. Policy acumen is "an awareness and understanding distilled from a policy analysis" that allows nurses to influence the manner in which health care is organized and delivered (Hewison, 2008, p. 293). APRNs who have come to understand the issues and can analyze policy that translates into action would be able to persuade policy leaders to make healthcare decisions that are favorable to nursing and to their patient population. They can make the transition from the introspective realm of acumen to the action of competence (Hewison, 2008). The final level of policy influence brings together all the elements of the previous levels. The APRN who has achieved this level integrates the issues with health policy research, formulates the agenda, and influences policy on the national and international scale.

Most authors agree that all nurses have the responsibility of becoming involved in the policy process (Boswell et al., 2005; Hewison, 2008; Peters, 2002). Although it may be an intimidating task for both the novice and the experienced APRN, there are opportunities for involvement at all levels and in all areas of interest to nursing, including legislation and regulation, research, ethics, and practice.

Conclusion

According to Peters (2002), nurses should start to look at policy as not just the legislative process but as a comprehensive method of identifying healthcare issues and then bringing those issues to the legislature and the American public. "Nurses will not be effective in politics or policy-making until they value their voices, develop policy agendas that embrace their core values, and learn the skills of policy making and influencing" (Mason et al., 2002, p. 12). Political expertise is essential for success. Nursing practice and health care must no longer be shaped by other dominant interest groups but instead by the inclusion of nurses using their education in policy combined with their unique understanding of the patient perspective.

Nurses must take advantage of positive public opinion and their pivotal position in the healthcare system as the largest group of providers. Patient advocacy should include policy advocacy, with APRNs increasing their knowledge of the issues and increasing political involvement. APRNs can be a crucial part of reforming health care by offering guidance and support to elected leaders. In the United States, APRNs have never been in a better position to influence health care as a whole, but it will require a group of "policy initiators who are willing to work toward eliminating the inequality of healthcare resources" (Peters, 2002, p. 5).

According to health policy expert Mary Wakefield (2008), "If nurses want to be sought out as health care resources and to have their views reflected in health policy, nurses have to get off the porch to run with the big dogs" (p. 86). It has been argued that clinically engaged APRNs already have a full daily agenda, so how can they take on the additional responsibility of influencing policy? A more vital question should be, How can we not? Political activism provides nurses with the means to promote overall health through passing supportive health policy legislation, using evidence-based policy to transform institutional and national health systems, and employing policy language that prevents discrimination in reimbursement and patient access to providers. The doctorally prepared advanced practice nurse is in the position to become this political advocate.

Acknowledgments

A special acknowledgment and thank you go out to my policy mentors: Laura Cohen, CRNA, and Brian R. Bullard, MBA, MPH, MA.

References

Abood, S., & Franklin, P. (2000). Why care about Medicare reimbursement? *American Journal of Nursing, 100*(6), 69–70, 72.

American Association of Colleges of Nursing. (2006). *The essentials of doctoral education for advanced nursing practice.* Retrieved from http://www.aacn.nche.edu/DNP/pdf/essentials.pdf

American Medical Association. (2005). *Scope of practice partnership.* Retrieved from http://www.ama-assn.org/ama1/pub/upload/mm/471/bot24A06.doc

American Nurses Association. (2001). *Code of ethics for nurses with interpretive statements.* Retrieved from http://nursingworld.org/ethics/code/protected_nwcoe813.htm

APRN Consensus Work Group & National Council of State Boards of Nursing. (2008, May 7). *Consensus model for APRN regulation: Licensure, accreditation, certification and education.* Retrieved from https://www.ncsbn.org/APRNJoint_Dia_report_May_08.pdf

Aroskar, M. A., Moldow, D. G., & Good, C. M. (2004). Nurses' voices: Policy, practice and ethics. *Nursing Ethics, 11*(3), 266–276.

Bankart, M. (1993). *Watchful care: A history of America's nurse anesthetists.* New York: Continuum.

Boswell, C., Cannon, S., & Miller, J. (2005). Nurses' political involvement: Responsibility versus privilege. *Journal of Professional Nursing, 21*(1), 5–8.

Broadston, L. S. (2001). Reimbursement for anesthesia services. In S. Foster & M. Faut-Callahan (Eds.), *A professional study and resource guide for the CRNA* (pp. 287–311). Park Ridge, IL: AANA Publishing.

Bureau of Labor Statistics. (2007). Registered nurses. In *Occupational outlook handbook, 2008–09 edition.* Retrieved from http://www.bls.gov/oco/ocos083.htm

Center for Responsive Politics. (2009). *Health professionals' PAC contributions to federal candidates, 2006–2008.* Retrieved from http://www.opensecrets.org/pacs/industry.php?txt=H01&cycle2008

Coalition for Patients' Rights. (n.d.). *About us.* Retrieved from http://www.patientsrightscoalition.org/about-us.aspx

Diers, D. (2002). Research as a political and policy tool. In D. J. Mason, J. K. Leavitt, & M. W. Chaffee (Eds.), *Policy and politics in nursing and healthcare* (pp. 141–156). St. Louis, MO: Saunders.

Ennen, K. A. (2001). Shaping the future of practice through political activity: How nurses can influence health care policy. *Journal of the American Association of Occupational Health Nurses, 49*(12), 557–569.

Federal Election Commission. (2009). *Quick answers to PAC questions.* Retrieved from http://www.fec.gov/ans/answers_pac.shtml

Government Accountability Office. (2007, July 27). *Medicare physician payments: Medicare and private payment differences for anesthesia services. Report to Subcommittee on Health, Committee on Ways and Means, US House of Representatives* (GAO Report GAO-07-463). Retrieved from http://www.gao.gov/new/items/d07463.pdf

Hamric, A. B., Spross, J. A., & Hanson, C. M. (2000). *Advanced practice nursing: An integrative approach* (3rd ed.). St. Louis, MO: Elsevier Saunders.

Health Resources and Services Administration. (2007). *The Registered Nurse population: Findings from the 2004 National Sample Survey of Registered Nurses.* Retrieved from http://bhpr.hrsa.gov/healthworkforce/rnsurvey04/default.htm

Hewison, A. (1999). The new public management and the new nursing: Related by rhetoric? Some reflections on the policy process and nursing. *Journal of Advanced Nursing, 29*(6), 1377–1384.

Hewison, A. (2008). Evidence-based policy: Implications for nursing and policy involvement. *Policy, Politics, and Nursing Practice, 9*(4), 288–298.

Institute of Medicine. (2001). *Crossing the quality chasm: A new health system for the 21st century.* Washington, DC: National Academies Press.

Interagency Collaborative on Nursing Statistics. (2006). *Home page.* Retrieved from http://www.iconsdata.org/index.htm

Jamelske, E. M., Johs-Artisensi, J. L., Taft, L. B., & German, K. A. (2009). A descriptive analysis of healthcare coverage and concerns in west central Wisconsin. *Policy, Politics, and Nursing Practice, 10*(1), 16–27.

Kent, R. L., & Liaschenko, J. (2004). Operationalizing professional values through PAC donations. *Policy, Politics, and Nursing Practice, 5*(4), 243–249.

Loversidge, J. M. (2008). Government regulation: Parallel and powerful. In J. A. Milstead (Ed.), *Health policy and politics: A nurse's guide* (pp. 91–127). Sudbury, MA: Jones and Bartlett.

Malone, R. E. (2005). Assessing the policy environment. *Policy, Politics, and Nursing, 6*(2), 135–143.

Mason, D. J., Leavitt, J. K., & Chaffee, M. W. (2002). *Policy and politics in nursing and healthcare* (4th ed.). St. Louis, MO: Saunders.

Maynard, C. A. (1999). Political influence: A model for advanced nursing education. *Clinical Nurse Specialist, 13*(4), 191–195.

McHugh, M. D., Aiken, L. H., Cooper, R. A., & Miller, P. (2008). The U.S. presidential election and health care workforce policy. *Policy, Politics, and Nursing, 9*(1), 6–14.

Milstead, J. A. (2003). Interweaving policy and diversity. *Online Journal of Issues in Nursing, 8*(1). Retrieved March 10, 2009.

Milstead, J. A. (2008). *Health policy and politics: A nurse's guide* (3rd ed.). Sudbury, MA: Jones and Bartlett.

Minnesota Board of Nursing. (2008). *Nurse Practice Act*. Retrieved from http://www.state.mn.us/mn/externalDocs/Nursing/Entire_Nurse_Practice_Act_042303011528_Nurse%20Practice%20Act.pdf

Nagelkerk, J. M., & Henry, B. (1991). Leadership through policy research. *Journal of Nursing Administration, 21*(5), 20–24.

National Council of State Boards of Nursing. (n.d.). *About NCSBN*. Retrieved from http://www.ncsbn.org/about.htm

National Health Security Plan. (1993). *Table of contents*. Retrieved from www.ibiblio.org/nhs/NHS-T-o-C.html

Nursing Community Consensus Document. (2008). *Reauthorization priorities for Title VIII Public Health Service Act (42U.S.C. 296 et seq.)*. Retrieved from www.apha.org/NR

Orszag, P. R. (2009). Beyond Economics 101: Insights into healthcare reform from the Congressional Budget Office. *Healthcare Financial Management, 63*(1), 70–75.

Patients' Access to Responsible Care Alliance. (n.d.). *Home page*. Retrieved from www.access-parca.com/home.html

Peters, R. M. (2002). Nurse administrators' role in health policy: Teaching the elephant to dance. *Nursing Administration Quarterly, 26*(4), 1–8.

Rains, J. W., & Carroll, K. L. (2000). The effect of health policy education on self-perceived political competence of graduate nursing students. *Journal of Nursing Education, 39*(1), 37–40.

Rice, R. (2002). Coalitions: A powerful political strategy. In D. J. Mason, J. K. Leavitt, & M. W. Chaffee (Eds.), *Policy and politics in nursing and healthcare* (pp. 121–140). St. Louis, MO: Saunders.

Robert Wood Johnson Foundation Health Policy Fellowships Program. (n.d.). *Alumni directory*. Retrieved from http://www.healthpolicyfellows.org/secure/alumni-search.php

Rowles, J. (2009). *Comments of the American Association of Nurse Anesthetists on financing healthcare reform to the Senate Finance Committee*. Park Ridge, IL: American Association of Nurse Anesthetists.

Rubotzky, A. M. (2000). Nursing participation in healthcare reform efforts 1993–1994: Advocating for the national community. *Advances in Nursing Science, 23*(2), 12–33.

Schroeder, S. A. (1993). The Clinton health care plan: Fundamental or incremental reform? *Annals of Internal Medicine, 119*(9), 945–947.

Senate Finance Committee. (2009). *Financing comprehensive health care reform: Proposed health system savings and revenue options*. Retrieved from http://www.finance.senate.gov/sitepages/leg/LEG%202009/051809%20Health%20Care%20Description%20of%20Policy%20Options.pdf

Short, N. M. (2008). Influencing health policy: Strategies for nursing education to partner with nursing practice. *Journal of Professional Nursing, 24*(5), 264–269.

Silva, M. C. (2002). Ethical issues in health care, public policy, and politics. In D. J. Mason, J. K. Leavitt, & M. W. Chaffee (Eds.), *Policy and politics in nursing and healthcare* (pp. 177–184). St. Louis, MO: Saunders.

Sudduth, A. L. (2008). Program evaluation. In J. A. Milstead (Ed.), *Health policy and politics: A nurse's guide* (pp. 171–196). Sudbury, MA: Jones and Bartlett.

Sullivan-Marx, E. M. (2008). Lessons learned from advanced practice nursing payment. *Policy, Politics, and Nursing Practice, 9*(2), 121–126.

Taft, S. H., & Nanna, K. M. (2008). What are the sources of health policy that influence nursing practice? *Policy, Politics and Nursing Practice, 9*(4), 274–287.

Tobin, M. (2001). State government regulation of nurse anesthesia practice. In S. Foster and & M. Faut-Callahan (Eds.), *A professional study and resource guide for the CRNA* (pp. 111–131). Park Ridge, IL: AANA Publishing.

Trotter Betts, V. (1996). Nursing's agenda for healthcare reform: Policy politics and power through professional leadership. *Nursing Administration Quarterly, 20*(3), 1–8.

Twedell, D. M., & Webb, J. A. (2007). The value of the political action committee: Dollars and influence for nurse leaders. *Nursing Administration Quarterly, 31*(4), 279–283.

Wakefield, M. K. (2008). Government response: Legislation. In J.A. Milstead (Ed.), *Health policy and politics: A nurse's guide* (pp. 65–90). Sudbury, MA: Jones and Bartlett.

Glossary

Caucus: A group of members of Congress or a political party created to support a defined political ideology or interest; in Congress, often votes en bloc.

Continuing resolution: A type of appropriations legislation that financially supports the government until a formal appropriations bill can be passed by Congress and signed into law.

Drop: Submitting the committee report concerning proposed legislation to the appropriate desk in the Senate or the House of Representatives.

Final rule: A regulation that has been published in the *Federal Register*. Includes the date on which the regulation goes into effect.

Grassroots lobbying: Occurs when nonpaid individuals contact their legislators to influence policy. May be very effective when coming from a legislator's constituency.

Hearing: A public meeting of a legislative committee or regulatory body held for the purpose of taking testimony concerning proposed legislation or regulation.

Jurisdiction: The authority or power granted to a legislative or regulatory body to allocate resources and approve, execute, and enforce laws. Typically has defined areas of responsibility.

Legislative assistant (LA): An employee of a senator or representative who keeps the legislator informed, meets with constituents, drafts reports, and so forth.

Mark up: A committee process that amends, debates, and rewrites proposed legislation.

Omnibus legislation: A single bill that is voted on once but contains diverse amendments to a variety of other laws. Notably used in spending bills.

Regulation: A principle, rule, or law designed to control or govern conduct.

Report out: The proposed legislation, along with the committee report, is sent out of committee to the floor of the House or Senate to be acted on.

Special interest group: A group of individuals who coordinate lobbying efforts around a common interest (e.g., nursing) and seek to influence policy makers.

Statute: A law that pertains to certain subject matters (e.g., tax code).

CHAPTER 6

Interprofessional Collaboration for Improving Patient and Population Health

Laurel Ash and Catherine Miller

The *Consensus Model for APRN Regulation* (2008), prepared by the APRN Consensus Work Group and the National Council of State Boards of Nursing APRN Advisory Committee and endorsed by numerous nursing organizations, defines APRN practice as nurses practicing in one of four recognized roles: certified nurse practitioners, certified nurse midwives, clinical nurse specialists, and certified registered nurse anesthetists. The primary focus of an APRN's practice includes provision of direct patient or population care. Conventionally, APRNs are prepared in accredited programs, sit for national certification, and meet regulatory requirements authorizing license to practice as an APRN. A number of nurses with advanced graduate preparation function in specialties that do not fall into these categories yet advance the health of an organization, population, or aggregate or provide indirect patient care. Such roles may include administration, informatics, education, and public health. Discussions are ongoing as to how these specialty practices fit into the traditional definition of APRN practice and subsequently the doctor of nursing practice (DNP) role. This chapter will use the term *APRN* to reflect all advanced roles of nursing practice.

Numerous research has well documented the impact APRNs have on health outcomes, including the ability to deliver excellent quality, cost-effective care with high levels of patient satisfaction (Cunningham, 2004; Dailey, 2005; Horrocks, Anderson, & Salisbury, 2002; Ingersoll, McIntosh, & Williams, 2000; Lambing, Adams, Fox, & Devine, 2004; Laurant et al., 2004; Miller, Snyder, & Lindeke, 2005; Mundinger et al., 2000). The world is changing, and APRNs must position themselves to be at the table with other disciplines and professionals to emphasize the influence of nursing care on the health of an individual or population. The complexity of the current healthcare delivery system, trends in patient demographics, epidemiological changes of disease and chronic conditions, economic challenges, the need for improved patient safety, and the call for a redesign or reform of the healthcare delivery system will challenge all professionals to envision health care in new ways.

Healthcare reform is a prominent issue for health professionals, policy makers, and the public. During the 2008 presidential campaign, President Obama announced a comprehensive healthcare reform proposal (Kaiser Family Foundation, 2008). This proposal outlines key points regarding restructuring our present system. As a foundation, all individuals and communities must be guaranteed a set of essential preventive care services. Reform must include measures to improve health outcomes and safeguard patients from preventable medical error. President Obama's platform supports programs that use collaborative teams as a means to deliver comprehensive, cost-effective, and safe care to persons with chronic conditions (Kaiser Family Foundation, 2008). Access to safe, effective, and affordable health care is a concern shared by the American public and rated of significant importance in a national poll conducted by researchers from the Kaiser Family Foundation and the Harvard School of Public Health released in January 2009.

The professions of nursing and medicine agree on the need to create organizational environments that promote interprofessional collaboration. The American Nurse's Association report *Nursing's Agenda for Health Care Reform* (2008) places particular emphasis on the role of collaboration in chronic disease management and patient safety. The American College of Physicians (ACP, 2009) also acknowledges that the future of healthcare delivery requires interprofessional teams who are prepared to meet the diverse, multifaceted health issues of the population. Providers, policy leaders, and health systems will need to shift their mind-set from traditional models of linear, disease-focused care to new delivery approaches. In a redesigned model, each discipline brings specialized skills and abilities, practices at the highest level of the individual provider's scope, assumes new roles, and participates in a collaborative manner with other professionals to provide high-quality, safe, cost-effective, patient-focused care. This call to action demands that APRNs perform at the highest level of clinical expertise, the Doctor of Nursing Practice, and collaborate interprofessionally to improve patient and population health outcomes.

Merriam-Webster's Collegiate Dictionary (2005) defines *collaborate* as "to labor together, to work jointly with others" (p. 224). Leaders in the business world further describe collaboration as a concept involving "strategic alliances" or "interpersonal networks" in an effort to accomplish a project (Ring, 2005). As healthcare professionals, we can learn from successful business and management practices and use the collaboration processes of communicating, cooperating, transferring knowledge, coordinating, problem solving, and negotiating to more effectively reach a healthcare goal or outcome. The ACP (2009) suggests that collaboration involves mutual acknowledgment, understanding, and respect for the complementary roles, skills, and abilities of the interprofessional team. Effective collaborative partnerships promote quality and cost-effective care through an intentional process that allows members to exchange pertinent knowledge and ideas and subsequently engage in a practice of shared decision making. The purpose of this chapter is to generate a better understanding of interprofessional collaboration, distinguish the elements DNPs must possess to successfully collaborate with other professionals to improve the health status of persons or groups, and provide an overview of models of interprofessional collaboration in the real world.

Improving Health Outcomes

The Institute of Medicine's (IOM) 2001 report, *Crossing the Quality Chasm: A New Health System for the 21st Century,* identifies four key issues contributing to poor quality of care and undesirable health outcomes: the complexity of the knowledge, skills, interventions, and treatments required to deliver care; the increase in chronic conditions; inefficient, disorganized delivery systems; and challenges to greater implementation of information technology. The report goes on to outline ten recommendations intended to improve health outcomes, one of which focuses on interprofessional collaboration. It emphasizes the need for providers and institutions to actively collaborate, exchange information, and make provisions for care coordination because the needs of any persons or population are beyond the expertise of any single health profession (IOM, 2001; Yeager, 2005). An earlier IOM report (1999), entitled *To Err Is Human: Building a Safer Health System,* addresses issues related to patient safety and errors in health care. This report articulates interprofessional communication and collaboration as primary measures to improve quality and reduce errors.

Accrediting and regulatory bodies such as the Joint Commission (2008) recognize interprofessional collaboration as an essential component of the prevention of medical error. This organization's mission is to continuously improve the safety and quality of care through the measure and evaluation of outcomes data. It has targeted improved communication and collaboration among providers, staff, and patients as a means to better protect patients from harm. Improved patient safety outcomes can additionally be facilitated through collaborative efforts such as development of interdisciplinary clinical guidelines and interprofessional curricula that incorporate proven strategies of team management and collaboration processes. Doctorally prepared APRNs are well positioned to participate and lead interprofessional collaborative teams in efforts to improve health outcomes of the individual patient or target population (American Association of Colleges of Nursing [AACN], 2006b).

Interprofessional Collaboration

The terms *interdisciplinary* and *interprofessional* are often interchanged in the literature about collaborative teams, but each has a slightly different connotation. Interprofessional collaboration describes the interactions among individual professionals who may represent a particular discipline or branch of knowledge, but who additionally bring their unique educational backgrounds, experiences, values, roles, and identities to the process. Each professional may possess some shared or overlapping knowledge, skills, abilities, and roles with other professionals with whom he or she collaborates. Hence, the term *interprofessional* offers a broader definition than *interdisciplinary*, which is more specific to the knowledge ascribed to a particular discipline. DNPs are suited to serve as effective collaborative team leaders and participants not only because of the scientific knowledge, skills, and abilities related to their distinctive advanced nursing practice disciplines, but also because of their comprehension of organizational and systems improvements, outcome evaluation processes, healthcare policy, and leadership. This new skill set will be critical for DNPs leading teams in the complex and ever-changing health arena. The AACN's *Essentials of Doctoral Education for Advanced Nursing Practice* (2006b) adds that collaborative teams must remain "fluid depending upon the needs of the patient (population) . . . and [DNPs] must be pre-

pared to play a central role in establishing interprofessional teams, participating in the work of the team and assuming leadership of the team when
appropriate" (p. 14).

The concept of interprofessional collaborations to improve health outcomes is not new; it has been and continues to be the cornerstone of public
health practice. Effective public health system collaborations are critical to
protect populations from disease and injury and to promote health. Public
health collaborations have involved not only vested professionals but also systems of communities, governmental agencies, nonprofit organizations, and
private-sector groups to address a common goal or complex health outcome
(Wilson & Bekemeir, 2004). DNPs can benefit from the experiences of public
health colleagues and expand the definition of interprofessional panel collaboration. This is particularly relevant when considering potential stakeholders and in assembling the team. Successful implementation of a system
or organizational improvement may require collaborations outside the typical healthcare team. The purpose or outcome of the project may dictate the
need to include patient or family representation in accordance with their
ability and willingness to participate, as well as professionals from information and technology, health policy, administration, governing boards,
and library science.

Interprofessional Healthcare Teams

Many healthcare practitioners indicate they practice within an interprofessional team. Often, this involves each professional addressing a particular
portion of patient or population care, working *independently* and in parallel
or in sequence to one another, with the physician frequently assuming the
role of team leader (Robert Wood Johnson Foundation [RWJF], 2008).
Drinka and Clark (2000) reinforce the need to function *interdependently* and
engage in collaborative problem solving. All too often competition exists
between roles, with each discipline holding to the belief that it is the most
qualified to manage the patient or problem, thus negatively influencing
the functioning of the team. In effective interprofessional teams, members
recognize and value dissimilar professional perspectives and overlapping
roles and share decision making and leadership to best meet the needs of
the patient or problem at hand (Drinka & Clark, 2000). To achieve optimal
health outcomes, it is essential for DNPs and other health professionals to
engage in true collaborative interprofessional practices. These types of

collaborative practices will be most successful when (1) the complexity of the problem is high, (2) the team shares a common goal or vision for the outcome, (3) members have distinctive roles, (4) members recognize the value of each other's positions, and (5) each offers unique contributions toward the improved patient or population outcome (ACP, 2009; Drinka & Clark, 2000; RWJF, 2008). This model for interprofessional healthcare teams will require DNPs to have a thorough understanding of effective collaboration, in addition to a firm grounding in effective communication, team processes, and leadership, to bring forth innovative strategies to improve health and health care.

Benefits of Collaboration

The literature of the past two decades well documents the numerous benefits of collaborative practices, including reduced error, decreased length of stays, improved health, better pain management, improved quality of life, and higher patient satisfaction (Brita-Rossi et al., 1996; Chung & Nguyen, 2005; Cowan et al., 2006; D'Amour & Oandasan, 2005; Drinka & Clark, 2000; Grady & Wojner, 1996; IOM, 1999; Joint Commission, 2008; Yeager, 2005). Nelson et al. (2002) and Sierchio (2003) note the additional benefits to healthcare systems of cost savings and healthy work environments. High-performing collaborative teams promote job satisfaction (D'Amour & Oandasan, 2005; Hall, Weaver, Gravelle, & Thibault, 2007; Sierchio, 2003), support a positive workplace atmosphere, and provide a sense of accomplishment while valuing the unique work and contributions of team members. These issues are particularly relevant to nursing practice. Addressing concerns of nursing shortages, improving working environments, and promoting measures to increase job satisfaction all have been found to correlate with lower rates of nurse burnout (Vahey, Aiken, Sloane, Clarke, & Vargas, 2004) and in turn indirectly influence nurse retention and recruitment.

The concept of "value added" has been discussed as an indirect benefit of effective collaboration (Dunevitz, 1997; Kleinpell et al., 2002). The term *value added* indicates the growth or improvement experienced in a group, project, or organization over a period, which yields an indirect "value" gained by a patient or population. Such value-added contributions may be the improvement to patient care delivery over time because of the rich professional interactions and exchanges that occur within an interprofessional team meeting. This enhanced communication would be more beneficial than the communication required from professionals working independent of one another. Value-added benefits may additionally be evident from the process itself, such as the creative problem solving that occurs during a brainstorming session designed to address a community health problem.

Barriers to and Drivers of Effective Collaboration in Interprofessional Healthcare Teams

Barriers

In spite of the mandates or recommendations by IOM, RWJF, the American Nurses Association (ANA), and the Joint Commission, effective interprofessional collaboration has yet to be adopted in any widespread form in the United States to improve patient or population outcomes. Literature from both Canada and Britain also makes recommendations for interprofessional collaboration to improve care (Oandason et al., 2004), along with current thinking as to why healthcare systems have not adopted interprofessional healthcare teams. Some of the barriers to interprofessional collaboration include (1) gender, power, socialization, education, status, and cultural differences between professions (Hall, 2005; Whitehead, 2007); (2) lack of a payment system and structures that reward interprofessional collaboration; (3) the misunderstanding of the scope and contribution of each profession; and (4) turf protection (Patterson, Grenny, McMillan, & Switzler, 2002). The DNP will need a comprehensive understanding of these barriers in order to provide fresh, creative thinking and leadership for the healthy development and sustainment of collaboration.

Nursing and medicine were and are often considered central players in healthcare teams; an examination of the issues related to these two professions is prudent. Nurse and physician role differences are easier to understand in light of the historical roles of gender. In the 19th century, nurses cared for patients in hospitals, while physicians cared for patients in their offices or patients' homes. According to Lynnaugh and Reverby's *Ordered to Care: The Dilemma of American Nursing 1850–1945* (1990), whereas physicians were "welcome visitors," hospitals were run by lay boards and often staffed by "live in" nurses (p. 26). That changed when medicine became more science oriented and realized hospitals were full of sick patients to whom they could apply their newly developed knowledge of science. Medicine soon controlled hospitals and defended this control with the argument that they owned "special knowledge" to diagnose and treat. Physicians were able to convince the public that nurses were not trustworthy enough to manage medications or capable of obtaining the "special knowledge" that physicians had (often due to the menstrual cycle). Nurses soon became handmaidens to physicians; they needed to be "self-less, knowledgeless and virtuous" (Gordon, 2005, p. 63).

Nursing education in the 20th century was designed to provide cheap labor for hospitals while educating its new workforce. Nurses came to view themselves as working for doctors, not patients. Nurses were valued for their virtue, not for their knowledge (Buresh & Gordon, 2006). Most nurse leaders either accepted this subjugated role or were unable to change it. As nursing lost power, medicine increased its social status by high-tech innovations in acute care (along with reimbursement for them). Healthcare delivery became fragmented based on physician specialty care for patients with acute care needs. Indeed, medicine dominated health care in the 20th century.

It can be argued that this physician-dominant, fragmented care has driven up healthcare costs, promoted polypharmacy, and encouraged "silo" practices. Wheatley (2005) compares organizations to the biological natural world. In the biological world, if a species becomes too dominant and loses its ability to work when the environment shifts, the entire system can collapse. According to *Healthy People 2010* (U.S. Department of Health and Human Services, 2000), the nation's healthcare system will be challenged to provide effective chronic disease prevention and treatment. The current system, which is based on episodic care, will not serve the needs of the population. To meet the needs of the early 21st century, DNPs will need to bring a full nursing perspective into the healthcare environment, along with the empowerment of other members of the team to improve the viability and strength of the healthcare system.

Physicians have also been closely aligned with the financial success of healthcare organizations (often hospitals) and therefore have often been designated leaders for any clinically based team. Even today, the American College of Physicians (2009) concludes that the "patient is best served by a multidisciplinary team where the clinical team is led by the physician" (p. 2). Although physicians may have the most training in diagnosis and treatment of disease, they may not always be the best choice to lead teams. Haas and Shaffir (1987) discuss the "cloak of competence" that is expected of physicians by society. Medical students eventually adopt this cloak in order to meet societal expectations, and may bring this "decisiveness" to the inter-professional arena. This may lead the physician to believe he or she must always make the final decision in the team, which may lead to a professional power imbalance whereby physicians have more power than other members of the team.

The issue of "disruptive behavior" in the workplace has been studied recently in light of the connection between poor communication and adverse events (Joint Commission, 2008). Rosenstein's (2002) qualitative study of physician–nurse relations found that almost all nurses in the study experienced some sort of "disruptive physician behavior," including verbal abuse. Rosenstein and O'Daniel (2008) repeated this work, expanded to include disruptive behavior by both nurses and physicians. This second report concluded that whereas "physician disruptive behavior is usually more direct and overt, nurse disruptive behaviors more frequently take the form of back-door undermining, clique formation, and other types of passive-aggressive behavior" (Rosenstein & O'Daniel, p. 467).

In its *Essentials of Doctoral Education for Advanced Nursing Practice,* the AACN (2006b) discusses the need for interprofessional healthcare teams to function as high-performance teams. High-performance teams are those that emphasize the skills, abilities, and unique perspective of each team member. If the nurses (or other team members) remain invisible, the overall effectiveness of the team will be impaired.

To work on interprofessional teams, nurses will need to articulate the role they play in improving patient care. The work that nurses perform is often not recognized by other healthcare professionals and reimbursement systems or found within the nomenclature of electronic health records. Many tasks that nurses perform are difficult to quantify, such as supporting a family through a crisis. A vital responsibility of the DNP (likely collaborating with other nursing PhD colleagues) is to articulate to the public, insurers, and policy makers the role nurses play in promoting positive patient and family outcomes.

Another key factor in empowering nurses in interprofessional collaboration is the importance of role identification and clarity. In the United States, there is confusion about the education and titling of nurses. Although many states protect the title of "nurse," the public (including other healthcare professionals) continues to be confused about just who nurses are. Nurses in administration may not identify themselves as nurses, whereas some medical assistants may call themselves "nurses." Although the work that medical assistants do with patients is valuable, it is not nursing. The first step to getting our voices heard is to identify who we are and call ourselves "nurses" at all levels. It is important that as nurses work to gain visibility and voice, they remain open to listening to other voices on the team.

Drivers

SUCCESSFUL TEAM DEVELOPMENT

What are the stages of development that transform groups of disparate professionals into high-performance teams? Tuckman and Jensen (1977) and many others believe that teams go through stages, including forming, storming, norming, performing, and adjourning. Amos, Hu, and Herrick (2005) recommend that nurses understand these developmental stages in order to promote the development of a successful team.

Forming is the stage when the team first comes together in order to serve a specific purpose. Team members come into the group as individuals and get to know each other while determining the mission of the team along with their roles and responsibilities. The development of trust is key in this stage. Davoli and Fine (2004) suggest incorporating activities that are designed to show the human side of each team member, such as "icebreakers" or "member check-in" (p. 269).

In an interdisciplinary team, it is likely there are members from diverse professions, which each have their own culture and language. An important first task of an interdisciplinary team is to discuss and understand the scope of each profession represented (Hall, 2005). It is likely there will be both overlap and diversity of function and skills among the professions. It is also important to develop a sense of shared language by reducing the use of professional jargon. Although it may be unintentional, jargon can prevent knowledge sharing, hinder communication, and promote power imbalances. Standardized tools such as SBAR (situation, background, assessment, and recommendation), developed and used by Kaiser Permanente, can be used by interprofessional teams for discussion and problem solving regarding patient situations (Leonard, Graham, & Bonacum, 2004).

In the *storming* stage, team members have not fully developed trust, and conflict inevitably arises. Within interprofessional teams, members come from diverse disciplines and worldviews. It is highly likely that there will be a wide range of opinions and thoughts related to the issues and work of the team. It is important to face this conflict directly, however, in order to move on to the next stage. During the storming stage, it is vital that members learn to listen to one another with tolerance and patience (Lee, 2008). If the team does not go through this stage successfully, differences between individuals will not be brought into the team process and outcome. Conflict resolution will be discussed at length later in this chapter.

Norming is the stage in which team members begin to develop a team identity. It is still important for the team to elicit differences of opinion in order to prevent "groupthink."

In the *performing* stage, team members work together to achieve team goals. Individual and professional turf needs will be set aside in order for the team to be effective in its mission. At this stage, the team members also learn to be flexible in tasks and roles in order to achieve the team's goals. Finally, the stage of *adjourning* concludes the formation of a team. The team evaluates its performance and progress by reviewing whether or not outcomes were met.

The following factors assist teams to progress through the stages of team development:

- Shared purpose, goal, and buy-in of members
- Reciprocal trust in team members
- Recognition and value of the unique role or skills each brings
- Functioning at the highest level of *skill*, ability, or practice
- Clear understanding of roles and the responsibilities of team members to meet goals
- Work culture and environment that embrace the collaborative process
- Collective cognitive responsibility and shared decision making

Shared Purpose

For a team to be effective, there must be a shared purpose or vision (Kouzes & Pozner, 2007). The purpose of the interprofessional healthcare team is based on improving some aspect of patient or population health outcomes. Competing needs of team members must be tabled in favor of the greater purpose. Turf wars and politicized thinking have no place in an effective interprofessional healthcare team. The leader must inspire this shared vision and elicit buy-in from each member. As Wheatley (2005) suggests, creativity is unleashed in people when they find "meaning" or purpose in "real" work. Meaningful teamwork can create synergistic solutions from members when the team has shared meaning or vision. Patterson et al. (2002) describe how free-flowing dialogue helps "fill the pool" of shared meaning. By allowing dialogue to be safe, more people can add their meaning to the "shared pool," giving the group a higher IQ. Learning to make dialogue safe is a skill that drives trust.

Team Members and Reciprocal Trust

An effective team must include the development of reciprocal trust between members. According to Kouzes and Pozner (2007), members of a high-trust team must continue to work to maintain interpersonal relationships with one another. In addition to the group mission and goals, the work of the group must also include getting to know one another. The leader or facilitator who is willing to trust others in the group enough to show vulnerability and give up control often begins a culture of trust. The leader needs to be self-confident enough to be willing to be the first to be transparent; because trust is contagious, others will likely follow. Team members and leaders need to listen intently and value the unique viewpoints of others in the group. If the group fails to develop trust or to listen and value each other, it is likely that group members will resist and sabotage the group's efforts (Wheatley, 2005). Many authors describe this aspect of team leadership as leading with the heart: looking at how the heart can help shape dialogue and goals (Kouzes & Pozner; Patterson et al., 2002).

Because of economic and time constraints, many teams meet in virtual formats. The question many have is, Are face-to-face encounters between team members vital to the development of trust building? Kouzes and Pozner (2007) propose that a group can only become a team when they have met face to face four to five times. These authors suggest that "virtual trust, like virtual reality, is one step removed from the real thing" (Kouzes & Pozner, p. 241). Other sources discuss the very real possibility of developing trust via virtual means (Grabowski & Roberts, 1999; Greenberg, Greenberg, & Antonucci, 2007). Because of the lack of eye contact and body language in virtual interactions, communication patterns should be more deliberate. Greenberg et al. propose that trust building in virtual teams intentionally includes activities that promote both cognitive and affective trust. Cognitive trust is implicated in the formation of "swift, but fragile trust" during the early development of the team (Greenberg et al., p. 325). For cognitive trust to develop, individual team members need to believe that group members have both ability (competence) and integrity. One action to promote a sense of competence in individual team members is to have the team leader introduce members and endorse their abilities and why they were chosen for the team. Another important asset for building the sense of integrity is for team members to keep deadlines and stay engaged in the process (no freeloading). Affective trust is essential during later stages of the team's development and is vital to the functioning of team members in order to complete the task. Development of affective trust is based on benevolence and relies on team members seeing the humanity in one another, with development of true caring and concern.

G. Boelhower (personal communication, April 10, 2009) recommends that virtual teams begin their time with "check in, story-telling, deep questioning and dialogue, and affirmation." He goes on to state that he "sees the level of trust develop regularly" in online groups when the human side of individuals is shared. As discussed earlier in this chapter, this type of sharing may be started with icebreakers, check-ins, and checkouts. DNPs will likely have experience with online relationship building during their education process and can continue to experiment with team building in face-to-face and virtual formats based on the current evidence.

Recognition and Value of Each Team Member

According to Burkhardt and Alvita (2008), "each person is a moral agent and must be recognized as worthy of dignity and respect" (p. 219). Without respect, the work of the group cannot move forward; dialogue is halted. Respect among team members is vital because, as Patterson et al. (2002) note, "Respect is like air. If it goes away, it is all people can think about" (p. 71). Each member's voice must be heard and respected whether he or she is the highest educated member or not. To do this, team members must recognize the moral agency of each member and his or her unique skills and abilities, often based on the individual's professional skill set.

Using structure in interprofessional team dialogue may be called for as a result of the entrenched perceived power and authority of individual members and the professions they represent. Such methods as the Indian talking stick and Johari window can be used proactively to be sure that all team members feel they have a voice, are understood, and are free to share their thoughts and feelings. The concept behind the talking stick is that only the person who is holding the stick may speak. When the person finishes speaking, the stick is passed to the next speaker. That next person may not argue or disagree with the former speaker, but is to restate what has been said.

This process allows for all team members to be and feel understood (Covey, 2004).

The Johari window is a tool developed in 1955 by Joseph Luft and Harry Ingham (Chapman, 2008). It is used to help build trust among group members by encouraging appropriate self-disclosure. The Johari window has four quadrants: the open area, the blind area, the hidden area, and the unknown area. The goal is to increase the open area so that team members can be more productive because communication is not hampered by "distractions, mistrust, confusion, conflict and misunderstanding" (Chapman, p. 4.) One team member (the subject) is given a list of 55 adjectives and is told to pick 5 or 6 that describe himself or herself. A team member is given the same list and also picks out 5 or 6 words that describe the subject. The adjectives are then placed in the four quadrants:

1. Both team members know the open area.
2. Only the subject, not the other team member, knows the hidden area.
3. Only the team member, not the subject, knows the blind spot.
4. The unknown area include adjectives not picked by either subject nor team member and may or may not be applicable to the subject. (Chapman, 2008)

The Johari tool can assist team members to learn about both themselves and each other. Appropriate and sensitive increases in the open area can be promoted by the use of team-building exercises and games, along with teams engaging in non-worktime activities.

Functioning at the Highest Level

American health care is expensive, but not always effective. There is pressure for innovative models of care that are cost effective and improve outcomes for patients. Many clinical systems have begun to use episodic treatment groups (ETGs) to measure patient outcomes and provider performance (Fortham, Dove, & Wooster, 2000). Examples of some of ETGs are those for chronic diseases such as diabetes, asthma, depression, and hypertension. Guideline development by such groups as the Institute for Clinical Systems Integration (ICSI) can provide evidence-based pathways of care for the various ETGs.

In the past, physicians have felt the need to perform all the primary care tasks for patients. Given the current complexity and expense of health care, it is not possible for one group to do it all. This realization has led to the concept of having all healthcare providers work to the top of their licenses. This involves a shifting of tasks, often with each discipline giving up some tasks that can be done by another care provider more cost effectively. An example of working to the top of one's license is for advanced practice nurses to take more responsibility for routine chronic and acute care and health mainte-nance, while physicians perform the diagnosing and treatment of more com-plex unstable patients, and RNs assume the role of care coordinator (including pre- and post-visit planning), coach, and educator. In this example, all disciplines may need to give up some tasks in order to be cost effective. An exemplar of a program that utilizes healthcare providers at the top of their licenses is the DIAMOND (Depression Improvement Across Minnesota, Offering a New Direction) project (ICSI, 2007). At the center of the DIA-MOND project is a case manager (typically an RN) who has 150 to 200 patients with depression in an outpatient setting. The case manager works with a consulting psychiatrist to review patients on a weekly basis (typically two hours per week). This has proven to be a cost-effective model that pro-vides better depression outcomes than standard care. The challenge is to provide a payment structure that rewards this type of innovative care.

Clear Understanding of Roles and Responsibilities

During the forming stage of the team (and beyond), it is vital that each team member understand his or her role and responsibilities. Role uncertainty can lead to conflict among team members and decrease team functioning (Baker, Baker, & Campbell, 2003). The leader should be certain that each team member has a clear understanding of his or her role by having the members restate their role to the team. This type of candid discussion can only occur if the team feels that open communication is safe. A clear under-standing of each team member's role helps to prevent role overlap as well as tasks falling through the cracks (Lewis, 2007).

Work Culture That Embraces Collaboration

Some of the components of a work culture that embraces collaboration are (1) providing psychological safety, (2) a flattened power differential (hier-archy), (3) administrative support and resultant resources allocated for col-laboration (Kelly, 2008), and (4) physical space design that promotes collaboration, such as rooms for interdisciplinary interaction (Lindeke & Sieckert, 2005).

According to Edmonson (2006), organizations that support "upward voice" promote a culture of psychological safety. She goes on to state that "upward voice is communication directed to someone higher in the organizational hierarchy with perceived power or authority to take action on the problem or suggestion" (Edmonson, p. 1). Some tangible evidence of this is leaders who walk around the organization and initiate conversation, suggestion boxes placed around the organization, and an open door policy. Individuals must have the sense that they can readily ask questions, try out new ideas and innovations, and ask for support from others.

Another way to promote psychological safety within an organization is employee confidence that there will not be a penalty for admitting to mistakes. Safety culture research is shifting from focusing on only the role of individuals in errors to the role of systems. Healthcare leaders have had to explore other industry successes that promote safety, such as aviation, where the focus of safety improvement is on the systems in which individuals operate (Feldman, 2008). Authors such as Snijders, Kollen, Van Lingen, Fetter, and Molendijik (2009) recommend a nonpunitive incident reporting system in order to improve safety standards. A nonpunitive incident reporting system helps ensure that issues are brought to the forefront so that improvements can be made. The Agency for Healthcare Research and Quality (2009) has developed evaluation tools for primary care offices, nursing homes, and hospitals with questions related to psychological safety and communication. DNPs will be required to provide leadership and recommend resources to champion the culture of both psychological and systems safety within the organizations they serve.

Collective Cognitive Responsibility and Shared Decision Making

As fundamental as it is for each team member to have a clear understanding of individual roles and responsibilities, it is also essential for high-performance teams to have a culture of shared decision making or collective cognitive responsibility. Scardamalia (2002) describes collective cognitive responsibility in terms of team members not only having responsibility for the outcome of the group but also for staying cognitively involved in the process as things unfold. She describes the functioning of a surgical team, in which members not only perform their assigned tasks but also keep involved in the entire process. The responsibility for the outcome lies not just with the leader of the surgical team, but with the entire team as a whole.

A key component of shared decision making is that it usually occurs at the point of service (Golanowski, Beaudry, Kruz, Laffey, & Hook, 2007; Porter-O'Grady, 1997). Porter-O'Grady states that "the point of decision making in the clinical delivery system is the place where patients and providers meet" (p. 41), which has implications for including patients as collaborators on the interprofessional team.

Healthcare systems, as complex adaptive systems, require flexibility and continuous participation, learning, and sharing (Begun, Zimmerman, & Dooley, 2003). All of the interprofessional healthcare team members must stay engaged in the process at the point of service in order for the outcome of care to be successful. Please see Chapter 11 for further discussion of team formation.

STRONG LEADERSHIP

There is no dispute that redesigning health care will require strong leadership. As opposed to "management," which seeks to control and manage, leaders seek to create and inspire change (Kotter, 1990). Leadership theories generally fall under the classifications of behavioral, contingency, contemporary, and Wheatley's "new leadership" approaches (Kelly, 2008). Behavioral theories posit that leadership style or behavior is the most important factor in the outcome desired. Behavioral approaches include autocratic, democratic, and laissez-faire, based on where the power or decision making occurs and the type of worker or task involved. Contingency theories recognize that there is more to leadership than the leader's behavior. One type of contingency theory is situational leadership, developed by Hershey and Blanchard, in which follower maturity is evaluated and determines the amount of direction, support, or delegation from the leader to the follower. Contemporary theories include transformational leadership, which IOM (2003) deemed vital to the achievement of the transformation of health care.

Transformational Leadership

The IOM (2003) report recommends transformational leadership in order to make the necessary changes to improve patient safety. Transformational leadership, developed first by Burns (1978), is based on the concept of empowering all team members (including the leader) to work together to achieve a shared goal. This fits with Covey's (2004) definition of leadership: "Leadership is communicating to people their worth and potential so clearly that they come to see it in themselves" (p. 98).

The transformational leader need not be in a formal position of administration, but can lead from any position within the organization and operates through an ethical and moral perspective. Transformational leaders lead with a clear vision and use coaching, inspiring, and mentoring to transform themselves, followers, and organizations (Burns, 1978; Kelly, 2008).

"New Leadership"

Wheatley (2005) describes a "new way" of leadership, which is contrary to the Western style of linear, hierarchical organizations. She bases her view of organizations on biology, which is self-organizing and complex. Instead of seeing change as negative, Wheatley views change as life itself. She states, "Nothing alive, including us, resists creative motions. However, all of life resists control. All of life reacts to any process that inhibits its freedom to create itself" (Wheatley, p. 28). She recommends that teams self-organize to build communities that are no longer ruled by "command and control" (Wheatley, 2005, p. 68). Instead of viewing organizations and workers as machines, Wheatley suggests that organizations model themselves after living systems, which are adaptive, creative, and depend on one another for growth and sustainability.

Leadership Versus Management

Whereas management is the coordination of resources to meet organizational goals, leadership is built on relationships. Kouzes and Pozner (2007), in their seminal book *The Leadership Challenge*, examined leaders over 25 years and determined that leadership is a relationship in which leaders do five things:

1. *Model the way.* The leader must be aware of his or her own values and live a life that expresses those values.
2. *Inspire a shared vision.* The leader must be able to imagine the future and inspire others to share that vision.
3. *Challenge the process.* Leaders are engaged in the processes of the team and continually looking for innovations. They are willing to take risks and learn from experiences.
4. *Enable others to act.* Leaders help to build trust in relationships through collaboration and competence.
5. *Encourage the heart.* Leaders identify the contributions of each individual team member and encourage celebration when victories occur.

Anyone can be a leader; a formal title is not necessary. Please see Chapter 3 for further discussion of leadership and systems thinking in advanced practice nursing.

EFFECTIVE COMMUNICATION

Remember not only to say the right thing in the right place, but far more difficult still, to leave unsaid the wrong thing at the tempting moment.
—Benjamin Franklin

All of the work of interprofessional collaborations involves communication. Success or failure of the team is dependent on the effectiveness of the communication processes. Communication is a complex process of transmitting a message between a sender and receiver. The sender must effectively deliver the content, and the receiver must in turn correctly interpret or decipher the message. Many sources of error can occur within this exchange, and skilled communicators must make a concerted effort to deliver clear, consistent messages to prevent misinterpretation and loss of meaning.

Communication is more than the exchange of verbal information; in fact, the majority of communication is nonverbal. The DNP must be accomplished not only in the art of verbal and written communication but also in the interpretation and effective use of nonverbal communiqués such as silence, gestures, facial expressions, body language, tone of voice, and space (Sullivan, 2004).

In addition to sending congruent verbal and nonverbal messages, it is vital for DNPs to employ strategies that enhance communication within the interprofessional team setting. Determining the timing and best medium for what, how, and when to deliver a message is a necessary skill (Sullivan, 2004). Appropriate timing of key messages increases the likelihood that the message will have the desired impact on the recipient. The message may be phrased well but rejected if the intended audience is not receptive. Consider the availability and state of mind of the recipient. Is there adequate time for the discussion? Is the recipient distracted, emotionally or physically? Are other issues more pressing now? Such factors may contribute to misinterpretation or lack of objectivity regarding the communication. Reflect as to whether an alternative time, venue, or medium may provide a more appropriate means by which to deliver the message. For instance, if the message is of a sensitive, confidential matter, face-to-face communication would be preferable to an e-mail, voicemail correspondence, or team discussion (Sullivan, 2004). In group settings, it is imperative to allow participants enough time to provide objective information and express thoughts, viewpoints, and opinions about the situation in order for meaningful collaboration to occur.

Buresh and Gordon, in their book *From Silence to Voice: What Nurses Know and Must Communicate to the Public* (2006), suggest use of the "voice of agency" when communicating the role of nursing to others. Within the collaborative team it is imperative that DNP members clearly communicate nursing's involvement in a patient care scenario or clinical project and, more important, articulate the level of clinical judgment and rationale required for such actions. It is important and necessary to embrace the opportunity to communicate to the team the role of the DNP in enhanced care delivery. This "voice of agency" is not boastful nor an attempt to be superior, but rather an accurate acknowledgment of the unique contributions, value added, and improved patient outcomes resulting from expert nursing care. Conversely, it may reflect the negative consequences or potential for error averted as a result of the expertise, skills, and knowledge of doctorally prepared nurses. Davoli and Fine (2004) offer a similar perspective and note, "Collaboration gives providers an opportunity to be introspective and solidify their role through the contributions they make. A successful collaborative process will enhance one's professional identity" (p. 268). Draye, Acker, and Zimmer (2006), in their article on the practice doctorate in nursing, propose that the educational preparation of DNPs include opportunity for the student to convene an interprofessional team. This experience allows the student to incorporate strategies to promote effective team functioning while communicating the unique contributions of nursing required for the improved health outcome.

Buresh and Gordon (2006) go on to discuss the role self-presentation plays in communicating information regarding the competency and credibility of the DNP to team members, patients, or the public. Attire and manner of address influence the perceptions of others. What does dress communicate if Mary wears teddy bear scrubs rather than street clothes and a lab coat to a committee meeting? How might the DNP's role be valued if she were introduced as Mary from Pediatrics versus Dr. Mary Jones, Pediatric Nurse Practitioner? How are physician colleagues addressed in similar workplace encounters? Introductions using one's full name and credentials convey professionalism, respect, and credibility on par with other healthcare professional colleagues (Buresh & Gordon, 2006).

Ineffective communication is a major obstacle in interprofessional collaboration, is directly related to quality of patient care, and contributes to adverse health outcomes (Clarin, 2007; IOM, 1999). Some barriers that lead to communication breakdowns are specific to interactions between the sender and receiver, whereas others relate to the organizational system. Defensiveness on the part of either participant can hamper communications (Sullivan, 2004). These behaviors may result from lack of self-confidence, a fear of rejection, or perceived threat to self-image or status. Defensiveness impedes communication by displacing anger via verbal aggression or conflict avoidance. Awareness of this mechanism and developing an approach to manage it in the context of the collaborative team are necessary attributes of an effective DNP leader.

As healthcare teams become more global and virtual, the potential for language and cultural communication barriers increases. Misreading body language or misinterpretation of the spoken or written message often results from a lack of understanding regarding language (especially in translation) and cultural differences (Sullivan, 2004). What one group finds acceptable another may consider offensive, such as eye contact, physical touch, or the use of space. Room for misinterpretation exists in translation. Language used by Western cultures typically is direct and explicit, in which the background is not necessarily required to interpret the meaning of the message. This may differ from cultures that use indirect communication, in which the intent of the message often relies upon the context in which it is used (Brett, Behfar, & Kern, 2006). DNPs and interprofessional colleagues have an obligation to increase their cultural competence and understanding of health issues and healthcare disparities to dispel any misconceptions, particularly if the team is composed of persons from diverse cultures.

Jargon is another "language" that can pose a barrier to understanding (Davoli & Fine, 2004; Sullivan, 2004). Unfamiliar terms can lead to confusion and error and should be avoided to prevent unfavorable outcomes. Although professional jargon may serve as a type of verbal shorthand among some group members, it can also be a form of intimidation or exclusion and contribute to an imbalance of knowledge or power within the team (Davoli & Fine, 2004). Lindeke and Block (2001) stress that collaborative teams communicate with a shared, inclusive (i.e., "we," "our") language to prevent this imbalance and promote participation of all members. Effective communication involves the use of a common, shared language that is understood by all members of the team.

Preconceived assumptions and biases prevent the listener from tuning in and focusing on the content (Sullivan, 2004). This hinders the communication process because the receiver has formulated a predetermined judgment or drawn a conclusion before all the information is shared or facts validated. Effective communicators need to suspend judgments until all viewpoints are shared.

Gender differences in style and approach to communication can also pose obstacles (Sullivan, 2004). Subtle differences exist in how men and women perceive the same message. In collaborative teams, women may strive for consensus whereas men may place emphasis on hierarchy and "leading the team." Differences exist in the use of questions and interruptions in communications. An appreciation and understanding of these dissimilarities can prepare the DNP to function more effectively in teams of mixed gender.

Organizations and systems may pose additional obstacles to effective interprofessional communications. Outdated, limited, or unavailable technologies, such as video conferencing, messaging or paging systems, or lack of electronic health record interoperability between systems, can significantly impair the ability of members to communicate on a timely basis. This can be of vital importance to patient safety when attempting to communicate critical changes in patient status, medications, or lab values. The system further contributes to communication problems when the roles and responsibilities of team members are unclear. Participants may be hesitant or resistant to engage in exchanges or knowledge sharing. Clear designation of roles is of particular importance in virtual organizations and teams (i.e., electronically linked providers). In these collaborative environments, risks can be mitigated if members have a clear understanding of what is expected of each other and have a preestablished path of communication (Grabowski & Roberts, 1999) (see Table 6-1).

CONFLICT RESOLUTION

As both leaders and members of interprofessional teams, DNPs will need to develop and continue to refine skills related to conflict resolution. Conflicts are inevitable, and are even vital for interprofessional team effectiveness. *Conflict* is defined in many ways, but generally includes disagreement, interference, and negative emotion (Barki & Hartwick, 2001). If conflict is disruptive or dysfunctional, team efforts can decrease communication and thus team functioning. On the other hand, conflict that is constructive leads to superior results by including the "shared pool of meaning" of all team members. According to Patterson et al. (2002), the "larger the shared pool, the smarter the decisions" (p. 21).

■ Table 6-1   Measures to Improve Communication

- Maintain eye contact: Convey interest, attentiveness. (U.S./Canada)

- Speak concisely: Avoid jargon.

- Use questions wisely: Clarify or elicit further information.

- Avoid qualifiers or tags (i.e., "sort of," "kind of," "I don't know if you would be interested"): These reduce the effectiveness of one's message.

- Be aware of gestures, facial expressions, posture: Send positive nonverbal signals (e.g., smiling conveys warmth, leaning forward indicates receptivity, and open-palm gestures suggest accessibility).

- Avoid defensiveness.

- Avoid responding emotionally: Never raise your voice, yell, or cry.

As stated earlier, nurses over the last century have often used passive-aggressive methods to resolve conflict, such as avoidance, withholding, smoothing over, and compromising (Feldman, 2008). These methods do not promote dialogue, the most central means to attain the shared pool of meaning of the entire team. DNPs need to lead nurses and other professionals in techniques that promote dialogue and thus collaboration between professionals. The purposes of collaborative conflict management are to promote win–win versus win–lose solutions. The skills for conflict resolution and improving dialogue can be learned. According to Patterson et al. (2002) in their book *Crucial Conversations*, conflict resolution includes such methods as starting with the heart, making conversation safe, staying in dialogue when emotions are high, using persuasion, and promoting positive actions. Most of the skills related to collaborative conflict management are intertwined with effective communication skills and the development of emotional intelligence.

Chinn (2008) offers suggestions that are foundational for the transformation of conflict into solidarity and diversity. These recommendations begin before there is any conflict in a group or team and include rotating leadership, practicing critical reflection, and adopting customs to value diversity. By rotating leadership, the team members all have a stake in the outcome of the team goals and processes. When a conflict arises, involved parties can step back while other members rise up to help lead the team. Critical reflection can be accomplished by incorporating a closing time at which all team members can share their thoughts and feelings about the team process. By practicing ways to value diversity, such as developing team processes during meetings that show appreciation and value for each individual, conflict can move from violence to peaceful recognition of the diversity of alternative views.

EMOTIONAL INTELLIGENCE

Emotional intelligence (EI) is yet another valuable attribute of successful interprofessional leadership. EI is the awareness of the role emotion plays in personal relationships and the purposeful use of emotion to communicate, build rapport, and motivate self and others. These characteristics have been found to play a far greater role than cognitive abilities in the success or failure of a leader (Goleman, Boyzatsis, & McKee, 2002).

Goleman et al. outline five realms of EI: self-awareness, self-regulation, motivation, empathy, and social skills. Self-awareness involves recognizing your own emotions and the effect your mood and confidence level have on persons. Maintaining your composure in high-emotion meetings or challenging clinical situations is an example of effectual self-regulation. Conflict is a natural process of interprofessional teamwork, which can lead to positive or negative group functioning, depending on leadership style. Emotionally intelligent leaders have the ability to adapt, withhold judgment, and exhibit self-control in emotionally charged situations. An optimistic attitude, passion, and commitment to pursuing the goals of the group and desire for excellence help provide the motivation factor of EI. Leaders who are sensitive and empathetic to the needs and perspectives of others encourage the group to carry on and perform to its best ability.

Drinka and Clark (2000) talk about the role of "reflective practice" in interprofessional team practice. This concept builds on the self-awareness and empathy qualities of EI: the understanding of how our professional cultures, preparations, and experiences shape how we function in teams, as well as the ability to appreciate the similar and dissimilar perspectives of other interprofessional team members.

A fifth element is that of social skill: The ability to build rapport, network, communicate, and facilitate change. As an effective leader, it is imperative to foster a system of open, timely communication, whether by face-to-face communication, phone, or electronic means, to meet the desired outcomes for the project, patient, or population successfully. Regularly practicing calming relaxation techniques and rehearsing responses prior to anticipated stressful encounters allow one to manage reactions in an emotionally intelligent manner. DNPs can develop these skills with regular practice, self-reflection, coaching, and feedback from colleagues, and can use "EQ" (emotional intelligence quotient) as a tool to gauge their performance as leaders.

McCallin and Bamford (2007) suggest that EI is integral to effective interdisciplinary team functioning. Healthcare providers may be highly skilled in practicing emotionally intelligent interactions with their patients and families but may receive little preparation in promoting emotionally intelligent, healthy communication and functioning *between* professionals. Miller et al. (2008) specifically explored the role of EI in nursing practice as it relates to interprofessional team functioning. In this qualitative study, the ability of the nurse to effectively collaborate on interprofessional teams was influenced by his or her degree of EI. Nurses who engaged in *esprit de corps* (significant role embracing to the exclusion of other professionals) were considerably less able to function successfully on the team, less able to have other members appreciate nursing's contribution to patient care, and generally less engaged in team processes. These researchers support the need to address not only the cognitive aspects of interprofessional teamwork but also the emotional aspects of optimal team functioning. DNP leaders versed in EI work are well suited to recognize individual and personality differences among team members and can build on them, mentor colleagues, and use EI to influence the effectiveness of the team and improve patient outcomes and satisfaction among interprofessional team members.

Necessities for Collaboration

Change Agent: Lewin's Model

The objective of interprofessional collaboration is, of course, to generate a practice or systems enhancement to improve the health of an individual or population. Whether implementing an evidence-based practice effort or a quality improvement initiative, some sort of change is required. Even what many group members view as a desirable change will inevitably encounter some reluctance or resistance. The ability to facilitate change or serve as an agent of change is a key function required for successful collaboration. DNPs must be versed in one or more theories of change to effectively motivate and move the collaborative team to the optimal goal.

Lewin's force field analysis model (1951) is a classic framework for understanding the process of change within a group, system, or health initiative. Lewin's theory recognizes change as a constant factor of life ensuing from a dynamic balance of driving and opposing forces. The desired change results from the addition of driving forces or the diminishing of opposing forces and progresses over a series of three stages: unfreezing, moving, and refreezing. Unfreezing necessitates assessing the need and preparing members to move from the status quo to an improved level of practice, whereas the movement phase involves the addition of driving forces to motivate and empower members to adopt the improved perspective while simultaneously minimizing restraining forces that pose barriers to the desired change (Lewin, 1951; Miller, 2008). Driving forces must outweigh opposing forces in order to shift the equilibrium in the direction of the desired change. The improvements must then be secured, or allowed to refreeze, in order to maintain the desired change (Lewin, 1951; Miller, 2008). Please see Chapter 11 for further discussion of models of change.

Continuous Reflective Learning

The drivers of effective interprofessional teams discussed in this chapter will evolve in teams over time. Knowing the drivers is the first step in the development of both personal and team skills, but individual team members and the team as a whole will need continuous reflection. Each leader and follower should develop habits that build in time for personal reflection and growth. Many find that reading sacred texts or poetry, listening to music, practicing yoga, praying, meditating, exercising, connecting with spiritual leaders, or being in nature allow for deep reflective thinking and learning. Covey (1991) calls this "sharpening the saw" (p. 38), and recommends that people proactively plan for daily time to renew themselves. The wholeness of each team member is vital for the best functioning of the entire team.

Teams within healthcare organizations in the 21st century will need to practice continuous reflective learning (developed by Senge, 1990) in order to adapt to the rapid changes taking place. Interprofessional teams can utilize the vast organizational behavior research on the significance of continuous reflective learning. Edmonson (1999) defines team learning as "the activities carried out by team members through which a team obtains and processes data that allow it to adapt and change" (p. 352). Spending some time on reflection regarding team functioning will be vital to learning. Structural practices that foster team learning include providing time during each meeting for reflection, leaving the worksite for retreats, conducting "critical incident" evaluations, discussing errors and failures, using patient satisfaction surveys and interviews, and celebrating successes.

The Patient and Family as Interprofessional Team Members

As health care reorganizes into interprofessional teams in which primary care is the hub of the system, central team members will be patients and their families. Patients and their families will need to be invited and supported into the interprofessional collaboration process through actions that promote meaningful dialogue, patient empowerment, self-efficacy, and activation (Hibbard, Stockard, Mahoney, & Tusler, 2004). Some tools the DNP may want to recommend include patient or family focus groups, satisfaction surveys, personal health records, decisional guides such as the *Ottawa Personal Decision Guide* (O'Connor, 2006), and advanced directives, along with ongoing patient education regarding the patients' and families' role in health care.

Models for Implementation: From Project to Practice

Value of Incorporating Collaborative Work into Educational Preparation Curricula

Although there is a growing body of evidence regarding the benefits of collaboration between disciplines in the delivery of optimal patient care, few healthcare professionals have received any formal training in this concept during their educational preparation. Students in health professional programs often are taught in both the classroom and clinical setting by faculty from the same professional background. They have little opportunity to learn about the work of other disciplines or participate in any shared learning experience. Brewer (2005) describes this pattern of education as "silo" preparation, in which each discipline believes it is best qualified to care for the patient. Without a formal structure and support for learning and practicing a team approach to care delivery in the educational setting, negative attitudes, prejudices, and misunderstanding of roles can occur. This contributes to an inability to collaborate effectively and consult with other providers as practicing professionals and may lead to discipline overlap and competition rather than collaboration for delivery of care.

A Cochrane systematic review of interprofessional education interventions (Reeves et al., 2008) examined six studies (four randomized control and two controlled before-and-after designs in a variety of settings). Interprofessional education was defined as any type of educational experience or learning opportunity in which interactive learning occurred between two or more health-related disciplines. Although a number of positive outcomes were noted, further rigorous studies are needed to draw conclusive evidence supporting core elements of interprofessional education and the subsequent impact of interprofessional collaborative education on health outcomes.

In an effort to increase the ability of health professional teams to deliver optimal patient care, RWJF funded educational programs (Partnerships for Quality Education [PQE]) designed to improve interprofessional collaboration, chronic disease management, systems-based care, and quality (RWJF, 2008). These initiatives were developed to provide nurse practitioners, physicians, and other allied healthcare providers with educational experiences, skills, and attitudes to deliver care that is of better quality than that which could be provided by any single discipline. One funded model was Collaborative Interprofessional Team Education (CITE); the objective of this program was to design collaborative clinical and educational interventions for health professional students from medicine, nursing, social work, and pharmacy (RWJF, 2008). The program did make some strides toward improvement in participants' understanding and attitudes toward other professions.

Whitehead (2007) offers some insight into the challenges of engaging medical students in interprofessional educational programs. Real and perceived power, high degree of status, professional socialization, and decision-making responsibility can limit the ability of physicians to collaborate with other members of the healthcare team unless efforts to change the culture, flatten hierarchy, and share responsibility are promoted. A number of additional obstacles prevented full implementation of the CITE initiative, including differing academic schedules and a lack of faculty practicing in teams to effectively mentor and model for students (RWJF, 2008).

The primary objective of Achieving Competence Today (ACT), another PQE initiative, was to promote interprofessional collaboration and quality improvement in the curriculum of healthcare professionals within two academic health centers (Ladden, Bednash, Stevens, & Moore, 2006; RWJF, 2008). Four disciplines worked jointly to plan and implement a quality improvement project. As a result, core competencies necessary for successful interprofessional teams were identified, and researchers suggested measures for incorporating these competencies into the educational preparation of future students as a means to improve quality and safety in health care.

DNP programs can build on concepts of interprofessional education by allowing and encouraging programs to use faculty from a variety of disciplines to prepare DNP students. Interprofessional faculty can add a depth and richness to the DNP curriculum by bringing and sharing skills, knowledge, and the highest level of expertise in areas of clinical practice—whether it be business and management, pharmacy, public policy, psychology, medicine, or informatics (AACN, 2006a). Educational experience related to interprofessional collaboration as a means to improve quality or promote safety should be highly visible within the scholarly DNP project.

Role of the Scholarly Project: Real Interdisciplinary Collaboration

The Essentials of Doctoral Education for Advanced Nursing Practice (AACN, 2006) refers to the final DNP scholarly project or capstone as a culminating, immersion experience that affords the opportunity to integrate and synthesize all elements of doctoral education competencies within an interprofessional work environment. DNP-led scholarly projects provide a venue for students to assume leadership roles for effective interprofessional collaboration to improve health care, patient outcomes, and healthcare systems.

The DNP project "Optimal Use of Individualized Asthma Action Plans in an Electronic Health Record" (Miller, 2008) involved a number of opportunities for interprofessional collaboration. This process improvement project involved a systems change designed to improve pediatric asthma care delivery in a regional health system. An asthma action plan tool built into the electronic health record of a multispecialty regional health system served as a vehicle for the delivery of evidence-based practice. Distinct DNP-led interprofessional teams collaborated during various stages of program planning, implementation, and evaluation. Collaboration with nursing professionals and professionals in the fields of informatics, information technology, statisticians, and management was active throughout the project, particularly during tool development and in the implementation phase. Key to ensuring effective communication within this group was the use of a common language and developing a clear understanding of each other's roles and contributions. A second opportunity for interprofessional collaboration occurred during the implementation phase. The members of the pediatric asthma team—the DNP, clinical nurse specialist, and physician—each came to the project with his or her own agendas and perspectives. Frequent revisiting of desired project outcomes, goals, and objectives was necessary early on in order to develop a cohesive, unified collaboration.

A third DNP-led collaboration took place at the pilot project site, a regional primary care clinic. This collaboration, which initially presented many challenges, involved physicians, nursing, administrative management, and administrative support. This site had recently been acquired by the parent organization. Previous quality improvement initiatives had been attempted and, due to a variety of factors, were not successfully implemented. A number of barriers to collaboration were anticipated at this site, including a sense of mistrust and resistance to change. Building trusting, nonthreatening relationships with staff and providers was a much-needed starting point. Issues of power were foreseeable between the physicians and the project manager. Initially, this group expressed hesitancy with the concept of anyone other than the physician being responsible for the optimal delivery of pediatric asthma care. It is important to acknowledge that providers might experience competing loyalties as they struggle to prioritize and balance the additional time needed to implement a project along with time required to see other patients or perform other duties. Avoiding these barriers requires mutual respect for each other's role, purpose, and workload. It is vital to continually clarify and communicate the shared vision of the collaborative project—in this case, it was improved asthma care for children. Building relationships, seeking team member input, and developing a shared vision play a critical role in negotiating hurdles for interprofessional collaboration and for effective project implementation and evaluation.

In the DNP project "Developing a Population-Focused Student Health Service" (Ash, 2005), interprofessional collaboration morphed from providers within the student health services (SHS) to a broad range of professionals. The ecologic approach (NASPA, 2004) was used in the final stages of the student DNP project, which broadened the stakeholders and thus the collaborating professionals. The ecologic perspective views the connections between health and learning within the campus setting (Sacher et al., 2005). The initial task force led by the DNP student included a project mentor who was an expert in group work as a result of his education and experience as a master of social work. His skills in the so-called softer side of team development molded the experience by bringing all the team members into the process. He was also continually willing to try new approaches and then evaluate the outcomes. He had direct access to the vice president of student affairs, who was also known to be innovative and skilled in human relationships due to his background in counseling.

Unlike many healthcare-related projects, there were no physicians on the interprofessional team. This may have changed the leadership and political issues that have plagued nurse–physician relationships in the past. The DNP student may have struggled to lead a team that included a physician. If, however, a physician was part of the team, increased efforts could have been conducted to develop reciprocal trust and to recognize and value each profession. Having a physician from outside the college may have afforded an opportunity for increased networking of the interprofessional team within the community in which the college is situated.

Some of the drivers of interprofessional team functioning (such as trust, recognition and value of team members, and a shared purpose) were already present on this team at some level. Team members knew each other and had passion for the team purpose: developing a culture that embraces health and well-being. The team members work within a college that espouses "Benedictine values" (College of St. Scholastica, 2009), which include community, hospitality, and stewardship. This emphasis on Benedictine values provided a work culture that embraced collaboration, which is a driver of interprofessional teams.

One of the barriers that plagued the team was that there was no clear understanding of roles and responsibilities. The team met and formed ideas that the team leader and mentor needed to follow through on. This team structure has changed since the end of the DNP project to four separate working groups focused on student health, faculty and staff health, marketing, and academic integration, respectively. The project, now entitled Well U, has been in full swing for over four years.

The use of Wheatley's "new leadership" approach helps account for the success of this project. The college campus, in relationship to health, could be seen as chaotic; once the relationships were formed between team members, however, information and ideas flowed. The team came to understand that all connections were vital to the development of a collegewide culture that embraced health and well-being. A long-term approach to building cultural change continues in this project. Table 6-2 shows interprofessional team members in the DNP project.

■ Table 6-2   Interprofessional Team Members

Initial Task Force	Final Multi-interprofessional Team
DNP student	DNP student
MSW mentor	MSW mentor
RN from SHS	RN from SHS
Student	Student
	Director of Institutional Research and Assessment
	VP for Enrollment Management
	Registrar
	Manager, Wellness Center
	International student advisor
	Department chair, Physical Therapy

Summary

Given their advanced preparation, DNPs are well positioned to participate and lead interprofessional teams. Recognizing obstacles and developing strategies to reduce such barriers are key functions of interprofessional team leadership. All members of the interprofessional team need to have preparation and opportunities to rehearse this new approach to patient care delivery. Incorporating shared interdisciplinary learning experiences in the educational preparation of healthcare professionals provides the foundation for forming partnerships rather than competition for patient care delivery. Further study is needed to demonstrate the most effective educational interventions to prepare healthcare providers for successful collaborative work.

Workforce and regulatory issues may present both challenges and opportunities for interprofessional collaborations. Shortages of physician primary care providers, particularly in rural settings, are likely to influence both the configuration and function of the interprofessional team (ACP, 2009; Minnesota Department of Health [MDH], 2009). DNP-prepared primary care providers can help to fill this gap, but must be allowed (regulatory wise) to practice at the top of their education and scope; this will necessitate that physician colleagues reexamine and relinquish some of the responsibilities and tasks traditionally "owned" by medicine. Nursing and medicine will need to work together to devise a vision for this new collaborative practice model to most efficiently and effectively address the needs of the population and improve the quality of care provided.

The American Academy of Pediatrics' concept of "medical home" suggests that all individuals, particularly those with complex or chronic health conditions, should receive a comprehensive, coordinated approach to health care and social services (MDH, 2009). The proposed Health Care Home initiatives expand the definition of primary care provider to include physicians, APRNs, and physician assistants (MDH, 2009). The primary care provider will lead and coordinate the efforts of the interprofessional team to best meet the needs of the patient. Nurse practice acts, regulations, and reimbursement issues must be reviewed and revised to support the ability of APRNs to assume this role and deliver comprehensive care. Continued research is needed to identify the full impact of workforce and regulatory issues on these collaborations as well as strategies to address these concerns. DNPs in both direct (CNP, CNS, CRNA, CNM) and indirect provider roles (health policy makers, administrators, informatics specialists, public health experts) must continue to effectively work with other members of the healthcare team to deliver comprehensive, patient-centered care. Interprofessional collaborations are an important facet of a reformed healthcare delivery system and a vital step toward improving health outcomes and reducing medical error.

References

Agency for Healthcare Research and Quality. (2009). *Patient safety culture surveys.* Retrieved from http://www.ahrq.gov/qual/patientsafetyculture/

American Association of Colleges of Nursing. (2006a). *DNP roadmap task force report, October 20, 2006.* Retrieved from http://www.aacn.nche.edu/DNP/pdf/DNProadmapreport.pdf

American Association of Colleges of Nursing. (2006b). *The essentials of doctoral education for advanced nursing practice.* Washington, DC: Author.

American College of Physicians. (2009). *Nurse practitioners in primary care* [Policy monograph]. Philadelphia: Author.

American Nurses Association. (2008, February). *Nursing's agenda for health care reform.* Silver Spring, MD: Author. Retrieved from http://www.nursingworld.org/MainMenuCategories/HealthcareandPolicyIssues/HSR/ANAsHealthSystemReformAgenda.aspx

Amos, M., Hu, J., & Herrick, C. (2005). The impact of team building on communication and job satisfaction of nursing staff. *Journal for Nurses in Staff Development, 21*(1), 10–16.

APRN Consensus Work Group & National Council of State Boards of Nursing APRN Advisory Committee. (2008, July). *Consensus model for APRN regulation: Licensure, accreditation, certification and education.* Retrieved from http://www.nonpf.com/Joint%20Dialogue%20ReportFinal0708.pdf

Ash, L. (2005). *Developing a population-focused student health service* (Unpublished doctoral project). Rush University, Chicago, IL.

Baker, S., Baker, K., & Campbell, M. (2003). *Complete idiot's guide to project management.* Indianapolis, IN: Alpha.

Barki, H., & Hartwick, J. (2001). Interpersonal conflict and its management in information system development. *MIS Quarterly, 25*(2), 195–228.

Begun, J., Zimmerman, B., & Dooley, K. (2003). Health care organizations as complex adaptive systems. In S. M. Mick & M. Wyttenbach (Eds.), *Advances in health care organization theory* (pp. 253–288). San Francisco: Jossey-Bass. Retrieved from http://www.change-ability.ca/Complex_Adaptive.pdf

Brett, J., Behfar, K., & Kern, M. (2006, November). Managing multicultural teams. *Harvard Business Review, 84*(11), 84–91. Retrieved from Business Source Premier database.

Brewer, C. (2005). The health care workforce. In A. Kovner & J. Knickman (Eds.), *Health care delivery in the United States* (pp. 320–326). New York: Springer.

Brita-Rossi, P., Adduci, D., Kaufman, J., Lipson, S. J., Totte, C., & Wasserman, K. (1996). Improving the process of care: The cost-quality value of interdisciplinary collaboration. *Journal of Nursing Care Quality, 10*(2), 10–16.

Buresh, B., & Gordon, S. (2006). *From silence to voice: What nurses know and must communicate to the public.* Ithaca, NY: Cornell University Press.

Burkhardt, M., & Alvita, K. (2008). *Ethics and issues in contemporary nursing.* Clifton Park, NY: Thomson Delmar Learning.

Burns, J. (1978). *Leadership.* New York: Harper and Row.

Chapman, A. (2008). *Johari window: Ingham and Luft's Johari window model diagrams and examples—for self-awareness, personal development, group development and understanding relationships.* Retrieved from www.businessballs.com/johariwindowmodel.htm

Chinn, P. (2008). *Peace and power.* Sudbury, MA: Jones and Bartlett.

Chung, H., & Nguyen, P. H. (2005). Changing unit culture: An interdisciplinary commitment to improve pain outcomes. *Journal for Healthcare Quality: Official Publication of the National Association for Healthcare Quality, 27*(2), 12–19.

Clarin, O. A. (2007). Strategies to overcome barriers to effective nurse practitioner and physician collaboration. *Journal for Nurse Practitioners, 3*(8), 538–548.

College of St. Scholastica. (2009). *Guiding documents.* Retrieved from http://www.css.edu/About/Leadership/Guiding-Documents.html

Covey, S. (1991). *Principle-centered leadership.* New York: Summit Books.

Covey, S. (2004). *The eighth habit: From effectiveness to greatness.* New York: Free Press.

Cowan, M. J., Shapiro, M., Hays, R. D., Afifi, A., Vazirani, S., Ward, C. R., et al. (2006). The effect of a multidisciplinary hospitalist/physician and advanced practice nurse collaboration on hospital costs. *Journal of Nursing Administration, 36*(2), 79–85.

Cunningham, R. (2004, March). Advanced practice nursing outcomes: A review of selected empirical literature. *Oncology Nursing Forum, 31*(2), 219–232. Retrieved from CINAHL Plus with Full Text database.

Dailey, M. (2005, April). Interdisciplinary collaboration: Essential for improved wound care outcomes and wound prevention in home care. *Home Health Care Management & Practice, 17*(3), 213–221. Retrieved from CINAHL Plus with Full Text database.

D'Amour, D., & Oandasan, I. (2005). Interprofessionality as the field of interprofessional practice and interprofessional education: An emerging concept. *Journal of Interprofessional Care, 19*, 8–20.

Davoli, G. W., & Fine, L. J. (2004). Stacking the deck for success in interprofessional collaboration. *Health Promotion Practice, 5*(3), 266–270.

Draye, M. A., Acker, M., & Zimmer, P. A. (2006). The practice doctorate in nursing: Approaches to transform nurse practitioner education and practice. *Nursing Outlook, 54*(3), 123–129.

Drinka, T., & Clark, P. (2000). *Health care teamwork: Interdisciplinary practice and teaching.* Westport, CT: Auburn House.

Dunevitz, B. (1997). Perspectives in ambulatory care. Collaboration—in a variety of ways—creates health care value. *Nursing Economics, 15*(4), 218–219.

Edmonson, A. (1999). Psychological safety and learning behavior in work teams. *Administrative Science Quarterly, 44*(2), 350–383.

Edmonson, A. (2006). Do I dare say something? Harvard Business School Working Knowledge. Retrieved from https://www.iterasi.net/openviewer.aspx?sqrlitid=j0ercd12deaukxst2bsbta

Feldman, H. (2008). *Nursing leadership: A concise encyclopedia.* New York: Springer.

Fortham, M., Dove, H., & Wooster, L. (2000). Episodic treatment groups (ETGs): A patient classification system for measuring outcomes performance by episode of care. *Topics in Healthcare Information Management, 21*(2), 51–61. Retrieved from http://www.thedeltagroup.com/Corporate/Pubs/ETGs.pdf

Golanowski, M., Beaudry, D., Kurz, L., Laffey, W., & Hook, M. (2007). Interdisciplinary shared decision-making: Taking shared governance to the next level. *Nursing Administration Quarterly, 31*(4), 341–353.

Goleman, D., Boyzatsis, R., & McKee, A. (2002). *Primal leadership: Realizing the power of emotional intelligence.* Boston: Harvard Business School Press.

Gordon, S. (2005). *Nursing against the odds.* Ithaca, NY: Cornell University Press.

Grabowski, M., & Roberts, K. (1999, November). Risk mitigation in virtual organizations. *Organization Science, 10*(6), 704–721. Retrieved from Business Source Premier database.

Grady, G. F., & Wojner, A. W. (1996). Collaborative practice teams: The infrastructure of outcomes management. *AACN Clinical Issues: Advanced Practice in Acute & Critical Care, 7*(1), 153–158.

Greenberg, P., Greenberg, R., & Antonucci, Y. (2007). Creating and sustaining trust in virtual teams. *Business Horizons, 50*(4), 325–333.

Haas, J., & Shaffir, W. (1987). Taking on the role of doctor. In D. Coburn, C. D'Arcy, & G. M. Torrance (Eds.), *Health and Canadian society.* Markham, Ontario, Canada: Fitzhenry & Whiteside.

Hall, P. (2005). Interprofessional teamwork: Professional cultures as barriers. *Journal of Interprofessional Care, 19*(Suppl. 1), 188–196.

Hall, P., Weaver, L., Gravelle, D., & Thibault, H. (2007). Developing collaborative person-centred practice: A pilot project on a palliative care unit. *Journal of Interprofessional Care, 21*(1), 69–81.

Hibbard, J. H., Stockard, J., Mahoney, E. R., & Tusler, M. (2004). Development of the patient activation measure (PAM): Conceptualizing and measuring activation in patient and consumers. *Health Services Research, 39*(4), 1005–1026.

Horrocks, S., Anderson, E., & Salisbury, C. (2002, April 6). Systematic review of whether nurse practitioners working in primary care can provide equivalent care to doctors. *BMJ: British Medical Journal, 324*(7341), 819–823. Retrieved from CINAHL Plus with Full Text database.

Ingersoll, G. L., McIntosh, E., & Williams, M. (2000). Nurse sensitive outcomes of advanced practice. *Journal of Advanced Nursing, 32*(5), 1272–1281.

Institute for Clinical Systems Integration. (2007). *DIAMOND initiative: Depression improvement across Minnesota: Offering a new direction.* Retrieved from http://www.icsi.org/colloquium-_2007/diamond_panel.html

Institute of Medicine. (1999). *To err is human: Building a safer health system.* Washington, DC: National Academies Press.

Institute of Medicine. (2001). *Crossing the quality chasm: A new health system for the 21st century.* Washington, DC: National Academies Press.

Institute of Medicine. (2003). *Health professions education: A bridge to quality.* Washington, DC: National Academies Press.

The Joint Commission. (2008). *Accreditation program: Ambulatory health care national patient safety goals.* Retrieved from http://www.jointcommission.org/NR/rdonlyres/979098FA-74FD-4F25-AF41-EDD48FBD300E/0/AHC_NPSG.pdf

Kaiser Family Foundation. (2008). *President-elect Barack Obama's health care reform proposal.* Retrieved from http://www.kff.org/uninsured/upload/Obama_Health_Care_Reform _Proposal.pdf

Kaiser Family Foundation/Harvard School of Public Health Survey. (2009). *The public's health care agenda for the new president and congress* (Publication No. 7853). Retrieved from http://www.kff.org/kaiserpolls/upload/7853.pdf

Kelly, P. (2008). *Nursing leadership and management.* Clifton Park, NY: Delmar.

Kleinpell, R. M., Faut-Callahan, M. M., Lauer, K., Kremer, M. J., Murphy, M., & Sperhac, A. (2002). Collaborative practice in advanced practice nursing in acute care. *Critical Care Nursing Clinics of North America, 14*(3), 307–313.

Kotter, J. (1990). What leaders really do. *Harvard Business Review, 68*, 104.

Kouzes, J., & Pozner, B. (2007). *The leadership challenge.* San Francisco: Wiley.

Ladden, M., Bednash, G., Stevens, D., & Moore, G. (2006). Educating interprofessional learners for quality, safety and systems improvement. *Journal of Interprofessional Care, 20*(5), 497–509.

Lambing, A., Adams, D., Fox, D., & Divine, G. (2004, August). Nurse practitioners' and physicians' care activities and clinical outcomes with an inpatient geriatric population. *Journal of the American Academy of Nurse Practitioners, 16*(8), 343–352. Retrieved from CINAHL Plus with Full Text database.

Laurant, M., Reeves, D., Hermens, R., Braspenning, J., Grol, R., & Sibbald, B. (2004, December). Substitution of doctors by nurses in primary care. *Cochrane Database of Systematic Reviews.* Retrieved from CINAHL Plus with Full Text database.

Lee, S. (2008). *The five stages of team development.* Retrieved from http://ezinearticles.com/?The-Five-Stages-of-Team-Development&id=1254894

Leonard, M., Graham, S., & Bonacum, D. (2004). The human factor: The critical importance of effective teamwork and communication in providing safe care. *Quality and Safety in Health Care, 13*(Supp. 1), 85–90.

Lewin, K. (1951). Frontiers in group dynamics. In D. Cartwright (Ed.), *Field Theory in Social Science* (pp. 188–237). New York: Harper.

Lewis, J. (2007). *Fundamentals of project management.* New York: AMACOM.

Lindeke, L. L., & Block, D. E. (2001). Interdisciplinary collaboration in the 21st century. *Minnesota Medicine, 84*(6), 42–45.

Lindeke, L. L., & Sieckert, A. M. (2005). Nurse-physician workplace collaboration. *Online Journal of Issues in Nursing, 10*(1). Retrieved from http://www.nursingworld.org/Main-MenuCategories/ANAMarketplace/ANAPeriodicals/OJIN/TableofContents/Volume 102005/No1Jan05/tpc26_416011.aspx

Lynnaugh, J., & Reverby, S. (1990). *Ordered to care: The dilemma of American nursing 1850–1945.* New York: Cambridge University Press.

McCallin, A., & Bamford, A. (2007). Interdisciplinary teamwork: Is the influence of emotional intelligence fully appreciated? *Journal of Nursing Management, 15*(4), 386–391.

Merriam-Webster's collegiate dictionary (11th ed.). (2005). Springfield, MA: Merriam Webster.

Miller, C. (2008). *Optimal use of individualized asthma action plans in an electronic health record* (Unpublished doctoral project). University of Minnesota, Minneapolis, MN.

Miller, K.-L., Reeves, S., Zwarenstein, M., Beales, J. D., Kenaszchuk, C., & Gotlib Conn, L. (2008). Nursing emotion work and interprofessional collaboration in general medicine wards: A qualitative study. *Journal of Advanced Nursing, 64*(4), 332–343.

Miller, M., Snyder, M., & Lindeke, L. (2005, September). Forces of change. Nurse practitioners: current status and future challenges. *Clinical Excellence for Nurse Practitioners, 9*(3), 162–169. Retrieved from CINAHL Plus with Full Text database.

Minnesota Department of Health. (2009). *Health workforce shortage study report: Report to the Minnesota legislature 2009.* St. Paul, MN: Author.

Mundinger, M., Kane, R., Lenz, E., Totten, A., Tsai, W., Cleary, P., et al. (2000). Primary care outcomes in patients treated by nurse practitioners or physicians: A randomized trial. *JAMA: Journal of the American Medical Association, 283*(1), 59–68. Retrieved from CINAHL Plus with Full Text database.

NASPA. (2004). *Leadership for a healthy campus: An ecological approach for student success.* Retrieved from *www.longwood.edu/Health/. . ./leadership_for_a_healthy_campus.pdf*

Nelson, E. C., Batalden, P. B., Huber, T. P., Mohr, J. J., Godfrey, M. M., Headrick, L. A., et al. (2002). Microsystems in health care: Part 1. Learning from high-performing front-line clinical units. *The Joint Commission Journal on Quality Improvement, 28*(9), 472–493.

Oandasan, I., D'Amour, D., Zwarenstein, M., Barker, K., Purden, M., Beaulieu, M.-D., et al. (2004). *Interprofessional education for collaborative patient-centred practice: An evolving framework* [Executive summary]. Retrieved from www.hc-sc.gc.ca/hcs-sss/hhr-rhs/strateg/interprof/summ-somm-eng.php

O'Connor, A. (2006). *Ottawa personal decision guide [Pamphlet].* University of Ottawa: Ottawa Health Research Institute.

Patterson, K., Grenny, J., McMillan, R., & Switzler, A. (2002). *Crucial conversations: Tools for talking when stakes are high.* New York: McGraw Hill.

Porter-O'Grady, T. (1997). *Whole systems shared governance.* Gaithersburg, MD: Aspen.

Reeves, S., Zwarenstein, M., Goldman, J., Barr, H., Freeth, D., Hammick, M., et al. (2008). Interprofessional education: Effects on professional practice and health care outcomes [Review]. *Cochrane Database of Systematic Reviews, 1,* CD002213. doi:10.1002/14651858.CD002213.pub2

Ring, P. (2005, January). Collaboration. In *Blackwell encyclopedic dictionary of organizational behavior*. Retrieved from Blackwell Encyclopedia of Management Library database.

Robert Wood Johnson Foundation. (2008, April). *Partnerships for quality education* (Robert Wood Johnson Grant Results Reports). Retrieved from http://www.rwjf.org/reports /npreports/pqe.htm

Rosenstein, A. (2002). The impact of nurse-physician relationships on nurse satisfaction and retention. *American Journal of Nursing, 102*(6), 26–34.

Rosenstein, A., & O'Daniel, M. (2008). A survey of the impacts of disruptive behaviors and communication defects on public safety. *The Joint Commission Journal on Quality and Patient Safety, 34*(8), 464–471.

Sacher, L., Moses, K., Fabiano, P., Haubenreiser, J., Grizzel, J., & Mart, S. (2005). *College health: Stretch your definitions of the core concepts, assumptions and practices*. American College Health Association. PowerPoint presentation at NASPA (Student Affairs Administration in Higher Education) session, March 22, 2005, Washington, DC.

Scardamalia, M. (2002). Collective cognitive responsibility for the advancement of knowledge. In B. Smith (Ed.), *Liberal education in a knowledge society* (pp. 67–98). Chicago: Open Court.

Senge, P. (1990). *The art and discipline of the learning organization*. New York: Doubleday.

Sierchio, G. P. (2003). A multidisciplinary approach for improving outcomes. *Journal of Infusion Nursing, 26*(1), 34–43.

Snijders, C., Kollen, B., Van Lingen, R., Fetter, W., & Molendijik, H. (2009). Which aspects of safety culture predict incident reporting behavior in neonatal intensive care units? A multilevel analysis. *Critical Care Medicine, 37*(1), 61–67.

Sullivan, E. J. (2004). *Becoming influential: A guide for nurses*. Upper Saddle River, NJ: Pearson Prentice Hall.

Tuckman, B. W., & Jensen, M. A. C. (1977). Stages of small-group development revisited. *Group & Organization Management, 2*(4), 419–427. doi:10.1177/105960117700200404

U.S. Department of Health and Human Services. (2000). *Healthy People 2010*. Rockville, MD: Author. Retrieved from http://www.healthypeople.gov/

Vahey, D. C., Aiken, L. H., Sloane, D. M., Clarke, S. P., & Vargas, D. (2004). Nurse burnout and patient satisfaction. *Medical Care, 42*(Suppl. 2), 1157–1166.

Wheatley, M. (2005). *Finding our way: Leadership for an uncertain time*. San Francisco: Berrett-Koehler.

Whitehead, C. (2007). The doctor dilemma in interprofessional education and care: How and why will physicians collaborate? *Medical Education, 41*(10), 1010–1016.

Wilson, J., & Bekemeir, B. (2004). Public health. In *Encyclopedia of leadership* (Vol. 3, pp. 1271–1274). Thousand Oaks, CA: Sage.

Yeager, S. (2005). Interdisciplinary collaboration: The heart and soul of healthcare. *Critical Care Nursing Clinics of North America, 17*(2), 143–148.

CHAPTER 7

Clinical Prevention and Population Health for Improving the Nation's Health

Diane Marie Schadewald

Introduction

The World Health Organization (WHO), in the preamble to its constitution, defines health as "a state of complete physical, mental and social well-being and not merely the absence of disease or infirmity" (2006, p. 1). The WHO constitution further advocates for the provision of measures that promote health and prevent disease in a population and notes that cooperation between the people of a nation and their governments in this endeavor is necessary for positive social and economic outcomes to occur within a nation as well as globally. To address health inequities and thereby promote health and prevent disease, WHO developed the Commission on Social Determinants of Health (CSDH) to identify social determinants of health, examine the impact of those determinants, and develop recommendations to address the determinants. Categories WHO identifies as social determinants of health include health behaviors, the physical and social environment, working conditions, healthcare coverage and infrastructure, and social protection. Recommendations developed by the CSDH to positively affect these social determinants include actions to address the following three principles:

1. Improve daily living conditions
2. Tackle the inequitable distribution of power, money, and resources
3. Measure and understand the problem and assess the impact of action (WHO, 2008, p. 2)

The U.S. Department of Health and Human Services (HHS) has proposed national goals for health each decade for the past three decades and is currently in the process of developing goals for the fourth time, for Healthy People 2020. The two overarching goals of Healthy People 2010 were to improve quality of health and longevity and eliminate health disparities (HHS, 2000). These goals have yet to be met (HHS, 2008). Social determinants of health that mirror those identified by WHO were included in the Healthy People 2010 report (Figure 7-1). Actualizing the WHO principles identified by the CSDH that address social determinants of health will help reach the goals of Healthy People 2010. Nursing leadership is needed in developing, implementing, and evaluating clinical prevention and population health interventions that address these social determinants of health. Reaching these goals is the ultimate aim of the seventh essential of DNP education.

Background of the Development of the Seventh Essential

The American Association of Colleges of Nursing (AACN), in *The Essentials of Doctoral Education for Advanced Nursing Practice* (2006), uses the definitions of Allan et al. (2004) for both *clinical prevention* and *population health*. The term *clinical prevention* is understood to mean "health promotion and risk reduction/illness prevention for individuals and families" (AACN, 2006, p. 15). The term *population health* encompasses "aggregate, community, environmental/

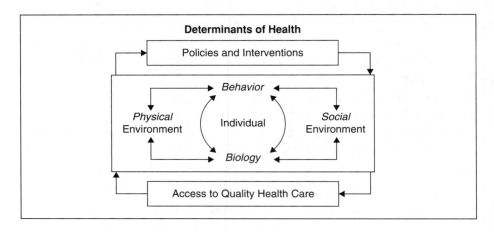

■ Figure 7-1   Social determinants of health.

Source: U.S. Department of Health and Human Services. (2000). *Healthy People 2010: Understanding and improving health* (2nd ed., p. 18). Washington, DC: U.S. Government Printing Office. Modified with permission.

occupational, and cultural/socioeconomic dimensions of health" (AACN, p. 15). Aggregates consist of a set of individuals with similarities. Examples of aggregate similarities could be similarities of age, diagnosis, or gender (AACN, 2006).

These definitions were developed by a task force made up of medical doctors, doctors of osteopathy, dentists, nurse practitioners, nurses, pharmacists, and physician assistants, who met to identify curriculum recommendations in order to meet the goal of increasing health promotion content in educational programs for these various professions as outlined in Healthy People 2010 (Allan et al., 2004; HHS, 2000). Development of the framework task force was proposed in 2000 by the Association of Teachers of Preventive Medicine and the Association of Academic Health Centers (Allan, Stanley, Crabtree, Werner, & Swenson, 2005), and the task force first met in 2002 as the Healthy People Curriculum Task Force (HPCT) (Fincham, 2008). This task force developed interdisciplinary curriculum recommendations to address the need for education about clinical prevention and population health that included four components: (1) evidence-base for practice, (2) clinical preventive services–health promotion, (3) health systems and health policy, and (4) community aspects of practice. The document developed by the HPCT that describes these curricular recommendations is the *Clinical Prevention and Population Health Curriculum Framework*. It is recommended that all disciplines use the terminology of clinical prevention and population health (CPPH) when discussing this area of curriculum to improve interdisciplinary communication regarding subjects covered within the curriculum framework (Allan et al., 2004; Riegelman, Evans, & Garr, 2004).

The Association of Teachers of Preventive Medicine has since changed its name to the Association for Prevention Teaching and Research (APTR) but remains a leader in the field of health promotion and disease prevention education and research. The CPPH framework curriculum recommendations were updated by the HPCT in January of 2008 and revised in January of 2009. The four components of the CPPH framework are now titled (1) evidence-based practice, (2) clinical preventive services and health promotion, (3) health systems and health policy, and (4) population health and community aspects of practice (APTR, 2009). These four components are further divided into a total of 19 domains distributed among the components. (See Table 7-1 for the complete framework.) The manner in which the CPPH framework recommendations are integrated into their curriculum is left to each discipline to decide.

■ Table 7-1 Clinical Prevention and Population Health Framework

Evidence-Based Practice
1. Problem Description: Descriptive Epidemiology
    - Burden of disease (e.g., morbidity and mortality)
    - Course of disease (e.g., incidence, prevalence, and case-fatality)
    - Determinants of health and disease (e.g., genetic, behavioral, socioeconomic, environmental, healthcare access and quality)
    - Distribution of disease (e.g., person, place, and time)
    - Sources of data (e.g., vital statistics, active and passive public health surveillance)
2. Etiology, Benefits and Harms: Evaluating Health Research
    - Study designs (e.g., surveys, observational studies, randomized clinical trials)
    - Estimation: magnitude of the association (e.g., relative risk/odds ratio, attributable risk percentage, number needed to treat, and population impact measures)
    - Inference (e.g., statistical significance test and confidence intervals)
    - Confounding and interaction: concepts and basic methods for addressing
    - Quality and presentation of data (e.g., accuracy, precision, and use of graphics)
3. Evidence-Based Recommendations
    - Assessing the quality of the evidence (e.g., types and quality of studies and relevance to target population)
    - Assessing the magnitude of the effect (i.e., incorporating benefits, harms, and values)
    - Grading of the recommendations (i.e., combining quality of the evidence and magnitude of the effect)
4. Implementation and Evaluation
    - Types of prevention (e.g., primary, secondary, tertiary)
    - At whom to direct intervention (e.g., individuals, high-risk groups, populations)
    - How to intervene (e.g., education, incentives for behavior change, laws and policies, engineering solutions)
    - Evaluation (e.g., quality improvement and patient safety, outcome assessment, reassessment of remaining problems)

Clinical Preventive Services and Health Promotion
1. Screening
    - Assessment of health risks (e.g., biopsychosocial, environment)
    - Approaches to testing and screening (e.g., range of normal, sensitivity, specificity, predictive value, target population)
    - Criteria for successful screening (e.g., effectiveness, benefits and harms, barriers, cost, acceptance by patient)
    - Clinician–patient communication (e.g., patient participation in decision making, informed consent, risk communication, advocacy, health literacy)

■ Table 7-1   Clinical Prevention and Population Health Framework (CONTINUED)

- Evidence-based recommendations
- Government requirements (e.g., newborn screening)

2. Counseling for Behavioral Change
   - Approaches to behavior change incorporating diverse patient perspectives (e.g., counseling skills training, motivational interviewing)
   - Clinician–patient communication (e.g., patient participation in decision making, informed consent, risk communication, advocacy, health literacy)
   - Criteria for successful counseling (e.g., effectiveness, benefits and harms, cost, acceptance by patient)
   - Evidence-based recommendations

3. Immunization
   - Approaches to vaccination (e.g., live vs. dead vaccine, pre vs. post exposure, boosters, techniques for administration, target population, population-based immunity)
   - Criteria for successful immunization (e.g., effectiveness, benefits and harms, cost, acceptance by patient)
   - Clinician–patient communication (e.g., patient participation in decision making, informed consent, risk communication, advocacy, health literacy)
   - Evidence-based recommendations
   - Government requirements

4. Preventive Medication
   - Approaches to chemoprevention (e.g., pre vs. post exposure, time limited vs. long term)
   - Criteria for successful chemoprevention (e.g., effectiveness, benefits and harms, barriers, cost, acceptance by patient)
   - Clinician–patient communication (e.g., patient participation in decision making, informed consent, risk communication, advocacy, health literacy)
   - Evidence-based recommendations

5. Other Preventive Interventions
   - Approaches to prevention (e.g., diet, exercise, smoking cessation)
   - Criteria for successful preventive interventions (e.g., effectiveness, benefits and harms, barriers, cost, acceptance by patient)
   - Clinician–patient communication (e.g., patient participation in decision making, informed consent, risk communication, advocacy, health literacy)
   - Evidence-based recommendations

Health Systems and Health Policy

1. Organization of Clinical and Public Health Systems
   - Clinical health services (e.g., continuum of care—ambulatory, home, hospital, long-term care)
   - Public health responsibilities (e.g., public health functions [IOM]; ten essential services of public health)

(continues)

■ Table 7-1   Clinical Prevention and Population Health Framework (CONTINUED)

- Relationships between clinical practice and public health (e.g., individual and population needs)
- Structure of public health systems

2. Health Services Financing
   - Clinical services coverage and reimbursement (e.g., Medicare, Medicaid, employment based, the uninsured)
   - Methods for financing healthcare institutions (e.g., hospitals vs. long-term care facilities vs. community health centers)
   - Methods for financing public health services
   - Other models (e.g., international comparisons)
   - Ethical frameworks for healthcare financing

3. Health Workforce
   - Methods of regulation of health professionals and healthcare institutions (e.g., certification, licensure, institutional accreditation)
   - Discipline-specific history, philosophy, roles and responsibilities
   - Racial/ethnic workforce composition, including underrepresented minorities
   - Interdisciplinary health professional relationships
   - Legal and ethical responsibilities of healthcare professionals (e.g., malpractice, HIPAA, confidentiality)
   - The role of public health professionals
   - Interprofessional activities

4. Health Policy Process
   - Process of health policy making (e.g., local, state, federal government)
   - Methods for participation in the policy process (e.g., advocacy, advisory processes, opportunities and strategies to impact policy)
   - Impact of policies on health care and health outcomes, including impacts on vulnerable populations and eliminating health disparities
   - Consequences of being uninsured or underinsured
   - Ethical frameworks for public health decision making

Population Health and Community Aspects of Practice

1. Communicating and Sharing Health Information with the Public
   - Methods of assessing community needs/strengths and options for intervention (e.g., community-oriented primary care)
   - Media communications (e.g., strategies for using mass media, risk communication)
   - Evaluation of health information (e.g., websites; mass media; patient information, including literacy level and cultural appropriateness)

2. Environmental Health
   - Sources, media, and routes of exposure to environmental contaminants (e.g., air, water, food)
   - Environmental health risk assessment and risk management (e.g., genetic, prenatal)
   - Environmental disease prevention focusing on susceptible populations

▪ **Table 7-1** Clinical Prevention and Population Health Framework (CONTINUED)

3. Occupational Health
   - Employment-based risks and injuries
   - Methods for prevention and control of occupational exposures and injuries
   - Exposure and prevention in healthcare settings
4. Global Health Issues
   - Roles of international organizations (e.g., WHO, UNAIDS, NGOs, private foundations)
   - Disease and population patterns in other countries (e.g., burden of disease, population growth, health and development)
   - Effects of globalization on health (e.g., emerging and reemerging diseases/conditions, food and water supply)
   - Socioeconomic impacts on health in developed and developing countries
5. Cultural Dimensions of Practice
   - Cultural influences on clinicians' delivery of health services
   - Cultural influences on individuals and communities (e.g., health status, health services, health beliefs)
   - Culturally appropriate and sensitive health care
6. Community Services
   - Methods of facilitating access to and partnerships for physical and mental health care services, including a broad network of community-based organizations
   - Evidence-based recommendations for community preventive services
   - Public health preparedness (e.g., terrorism, natural disasters, injury prevention)
   - Strategies for building community capacity

Source: Association for Prevention Teaching and Research. (2009, January). *Clinical prevention and population health curriculum framework.* Retrieved from http://www.atpm.org/resources/pdfs/Revised_CPPH_Framework_2009.pdf. Modified with permission.

Exploration of the Terminology Used for This Essential

One might ask why the term *clinical prevention* is used in the title of the framework. Did the interdisciplinary nature of this task force possibly influence the terminology used? Actually, the original title planned for the framework was "Health Promotion–Disease Prevention" (Allan et al., 2005). It is arguable that the term *health promotion* is inclusive of all interventions focused on avoidance of health risks or illness as well as improvement of current and future health status. The term *clinical prevention* seems so clinical. The term implies a power differential, with the dominant power belonging to the healthcare provider. This implied power delegation clashes with the nursing paradigm of patient-centered care, in which the nurse and the patient are equal partners in care activities.

Furthermore, the term *clinical prevention* is not yet included as a subject heading in either the Cumulative Index to Nursing and Allied Health Literature (CINAHL) or Medline, whereas *health promotion* is included as a subject heading in both of these databases. CINAHL defines the subject heading of health promotion as "the process of fostering awareness, influencing attitudes, and identifying alternatives so that individuals can make informed choices and change their behavior to achieve an optimum level of physical and mental health and improve their physical and social environment." Medline defines the subject heading of health promotion as "encouraging consumer behaviors most likely to optimize health potentials (physical and psychosocial) through health information, preventive programs, and access to medical care." Nola Pender, a pioneer in health promotion theory, differentiates health promotion from disease prevention by equating health promotion with the desire to reach or maintain high-level wellness and by equating disease prevention with desire to avoid illness, discover it in early stages, or manage illness well (Pender, Murdaugh, & Parsons, 2006). Thus, health promotion, by conventional understanding, tends to have an individual focus that could limit its application to populations, and disease prevention is not a subset of health promotion by definition.

On the other hand, clinical preventive services are considered to include interventions such as immunizations, screenings, counseling for behavioral change, and chemoprevention (Fletcher & Fletcher, 2005). All of these interventions are domains included under the component of clinical preventive services and health promotion within the CPPH curriculum framework. These domains are also consistent with the manner in which the U.S. Preventive Services Task Force (USPSTF) organizes its recommendations (Allan et al., 2004, 2005). *Clinical prevention* is also the terminology used in Institute of Medicine reports (Allan et al., 2005). The term *clinical preventive services* has versatility in application, because these services can be focused on an individual or a population or both. Likewise, population health is inclusive of interventions focused on an individual or a population or both. Therefore, the term *clinical prevention* was purposefully chosen for these reasons (Allan et al., 2004, 2005; Riegelman, Evans, & Garr, 2004). Nevertheless, the term doesn't seem to fit the science of nursing well in all circumstances, and within this chapter there may be times when the term *health promotion* will be substituted for *clinical prevention*.

Population health as it relates to nursing has also been defined by Radzyminski (2007), who describes population health as inclusive of the socioeconomic, cultural, and physical environments and their impact on health. Individual behaviors, beliefs, health policy, and media communications are all components factored into a nursing assessment that is based on a population health model. Concepts of both public health nursing and community health nursing are included within this definition of population health nursing. In performing an assessment, the nurse practicing within a population health perspective looks for factors that are antecedent to the development of a problem and develops health promotion interventions to address the problem at that level for the population at large as well as treating the problem on the individual level (Radzyminski, 2007).

Educational Focus for This Essential

Health promotion has been an essential component of nursing education since the days of Florence Nightingale, the founder of modern nursing. Educational focus on prevention in order to improve health diminished with the rise of the use of technology in medicine and the accompanying increased emphasis on diagnosis and treatment of disease in order to improve health (Allan et al., 2005; Radzyminski, 2007). Nevertheless, nursing continued to include education on health promotion and disease prevention within its curriculum at all educational levels, with the depth of knowledge and expected degree of performance increasing for those with advanced degrees (AACN, 1996, 2006, 2008; Allan et al., 2005). What has been missing to this point in many nursing educational programs is a population health perspective regarding health promotion (Radzyminski, 2007; Zahner & Block, 2006). Exceptions to this deficiency may have been master's-prepared advanced practice registered nurses (APRNs) educated at the community health level (AACN, 1996). The combination of the concept of clinical prevention, which includes health promotion and disease prevention, and the concept of population health in this essential addresses this curricular deficiency. The concept of population-focused nursing is also included in the most recent AACN baccalaureate essentials (AACN, 2008).

In *The Essentials of Baccalaureate Education for Professional Nursing Practice* (2008), the AACN lists the seventh educational essential for baccalaureate nursing education as "Clinical Prevention and Population Health" (p. 23). The baccalaureate-prepared nurse has developed fundamental knowledge of concepts of prevention, causation, and risk reduction while also being prepared to assess individuals, families, groups, communities, and populations utilizing appropriate psychosocial and cultural theories in order to collaborate in development and implementation of plans of care. The baccalaureate-prepared RN also can utilize evaluative data related to health promotion and disease prevention in care delivery, use of resources, and policy development. The educational outcomes for this essential are as follows:

1. Assess protective and predictive factors, including genetics, which influence the health of individuals, families, groups, communities, and populations.
2. Conduct a health history, including environmental exposure and a family history that recognizes genetic risks, to identify current and future health problems.
3. Assess health/illness beliefs, values, attitudes, and practices of individuals, families, groups, communities, and populations.
4. Use behavioral change techniques to promote health and manage illness.
5. Use evidence-based practices to guide health teaching, health counseling, screening, outreach, disease and outbreak investigation, referral, and follow-up throughout the lifespan.
6. Use information and communication technologies in preventive care.
7. Collaborate with other healthcare professionals and patients to provide spiritually and culturally appropriate health promotion and disease and injury prevention interventions.
8. Assess the health, healthcare, and emergency preparedness needs of a defined population.
9. Use clinical judgment and decision making skills in appropriate, timely nursing care during disaster, mass casualty, and other emergency situations.
10. Collaborate with others to develop an intervention plan that takes into account determinants of health, available resources, and the range of activities that contribute to health and the prevention of illness, injury, disability, and premature death.
11. Participate in clinical prevention and population-focused interventions with attention to effectiveness, efficiency, cost-effectiveness, and equity.
12. Advocate for social justice, including a commitment to the health of vulnerable populations and the elimination of health disparities.
13. Use evaluation results to influence the delivery of care, deployment of resources, and to provide input into the development of policies to promote health and prevent disease. (AACN, 2008, pp. 23–25)

In *The Essentials of Master's Education for Advanced Practice Nursing* (1996), the AACN listed the seventh educational essential of APRN programs as "Health Promotion and Disease Prevention" (p. 11). Of note is the use of the term *health promotion* in this essential rather than *clinical prevention*. These essentials were in the process of being updated in 2009, and the seventh essential will most likely have its title changed to the CPPH terminology for consistency in titling. The educational outcomes for this essential as of 1996 were as follows:

1. Use epidemiological, social, and environmental data to draw inferences regarding the health status of client populations, i.e., individuals, families, groups, and communities;
2. develop and monitor comprehensive, holistic plans of care that address the health promotion and disease prevention needs of client populations;
3. incorporate theories and research in generating teaching and counseling strategies to promote and preserve health and healthy lifestyles in client populations;
4. foster a multidisciplinary approach to discuss strategies and garner multifaceted resources to empower client populations in attaining and maintaining maximal functional wellness;
5. influence regulatory, legislative, and public policy in private and public arenas to promote and preserve healthy communities. (AACN, 1996, pp. 11–12)

New essentials for APRN education were developed for doctorate of nursing practice (DNP) programs. The AACN (2006) lists the seventh essential of DNP education as the title of this chapter: "Clinical Prevention and Population Health for Improving the Nation's Health" (p. 15). According to the AACN, the graduate of a DNP educational program meets this essential by being able to do the following:

1. Analyze epidemiological, biostatistical, environmental, and other appropriate scientific data related to individual, aggregate, and population health.
2. Synthesize concepts, including psychosocial dimensions and cultural diversity, related to clinical prevention and population health in developing, implementing, and evaluating interventions to address health promotion/disease prevention efforts, improve health status, access patterns, and/or address gaps in care of individuals, aggregates, or populations.
3. Evaluate care delivery models and/or strategies using concepts related to community, environmental and occupational health, and cultural and socioeconomic dimensions of health. (AACN, 2006, p. 16)

Analysis of Data

Nursing's Use of Data Analysis Historically

Analysis of data is not new to the nursing profession. Florence Nightingale was in the vanguard regarding use of statistical models to improve health by improving sanitation. Her wedge diagram illustrating cause of death of soldiers in the Crimean War was a relatively new method for presentation of statistical information, and her report is famous for changing the way British soldiers were housed, with the result being a decrease in illness and death among this population (Dossey, 2000). This may well have been the first clinical prevention intervention by a nurse. Nightingale continued to expand use of statistics to develop recommendations for a uniform method of collection of hospital and surgical data, analysis of which led to changes in hospital design and surgical practices (Dossey, 2000). Data analysis did not routinely continue to be seen as an important part of the education of nurses or in the practice of nursing, despite calls for the need for nursing research to be recognized (Henderson, 1991). Also, much of nursing research in the middle years of the past century focused on the process of nursing and the methods of nursing education rather than the outcomes of nursing practice (Cullum, Ciliska, Marks, & Haynes, 2008; Henderson, 1991).

This paucity in nursing research changed around the 1980s, but analysis of raw data to improve health continued not to be emphasized in nursing education at the baccalaureate-prepared RN level or at the master's-prepared APRN level (Henderson, 1991). Baccalaureate nursing programs include classes on nursing research focused on educating the graduate to have beginning skill in reading and critiquing research articles. Educational programs for master's-prepared APRNs include classes in statistics and nursing research to prepare the graduate to understand and participate in nursing research activities, therefore assisting with the development of nursing knowledge. But emphasis on the analysis of data, beyond a rudimentary understanding of basic statistics, was not generally a concern at the baccalaureate or the master's level. This type of education was reserved for the doctorally prepared nurse. Also, few programs required any classes in epidemiology, in which analysis of health data and its impact on populations is learned. Epidemiological concepts have been included within classes at the baccalaureate level, especially classes on community or public health nursing. Otherwise, the most notable exceptions to lack of specific coursework in epidemiology may be master's-level programs on population health nursing (Frisch, George, Giovoni, Jennings-Sanders, & McCahon, 2003).

The need for greater knowledge of data regarding the impact of the environment on health and the need for health promotion and disease prevention activities related to the data available regarding environmental risks led to the formation of the Alliance of Nurses for Healthy Environments (ANHE) in

December of 2008. This alliance has a website that links to up-to-date information about the impact of the environment on health (ANHE, 2008). Another nursing organization, the American Association of Occupational Health Nurses (AAOHN), identifies itself as the professional organization for occupational and environmental health nurses (AAOHN, n.d.). The AAOHN focuses on environmental health in the workplace, whereas the newly formed ANHE has a broader focus for its environmental health efforts. Both of these organizations have a role for the baccalaureate-prepared RN and the master's-prepared APRN in clinical prevention efforts regarding environmental effects on health.

According to AACN educational essentials, the baccalaureate-prepared RN has been educated to gather data and assess for risk, whereas the master's-prepared APRN has been educated to use data to draw inferences regarding the health status of client populations or aggregates, but not to analyze data, for which the DNP is prepared. According to the *Oxford American Dictionary* (2006), to assess is to "evaluate or estimate the nature, ability, or quality of" something. Inference is "a conclusion reached on the basis of evidence and reasoning." To analyze is to "examine methodically and in detail the constitution or structure of [something, esp. information], typically for purposes of explanation and interpretation." By these definitions, it is clear that the DNP will look more deeply at various aspects of available data than the baccalaureate-prepared RN or the master's-prepared APRN has been prepared to do in order to explain and interpret the data. The DNP will use this comprehensive data analysis in performing a holistic assessment to identify appropriate health promotion or disease prevention interventions.

Data Analysis and the DNP

Courses on biostatistics and epidemiology are to be included as part of the DNP curriculum, therefore preparing the graduate to meet the first goal of this essential. An understanding of biostatistical and epidemiological methods prepares the DNP to analyze environmental and other scientific data. That is, the DNP will be able to analyze census data, morbidity and mortality reports, data from the National Center for Health Statistics (NCHS), and other sources of public health data in relationship to population health. The DNP has knowledge of how to perform rate adjustments, determine number needed to treat (NNT), and interpret confidence intervals. Knowledge of epidemiological principles of risk is also vital when considering prevention activities. An understanding of the difference between relative risk and attributable risk is necessary when working on the population health level in order to develop appropriate interventions and decrease any potential for causing harm by inappropriate prevention activities (Gévas, Starfield, & Heath, 2008). The DNP graduate is well prepared to do this. Data regarding the negative impact of environmental changes and toxins on health are becoming more prevalent, and analysis of these data may provide the basis for prevention interventions developed for use by the DNP in program project planning (Ashton & Green, 2008; Hall, Robinson, & Broyles, 2007).

The DNP's ability to perform analysis of data is further enhanced by developing proficiency in the practice of evidence-based nursing. DiCenso, Guyatt, and Ciliska (2005) have provided a framework for utilization of evidence-based nursing in a text on implementation of evidence-based nursing in clinical practice. Of course, development of any nursing intervention always begins with assessment. In order to practice evidence-based nursing, however, it is also necessary to develop a properly formulated question about the patient population, the intervention, a comparison, and outcome (PICO) to facilitate gathering the available evidence. The addition to question formulation of the element of time (PICOT), if indicated by the condition or population of interest, has been suggested by others (Fineout-Overholt & Johnston, 2005; Flemming, 2008). Next, the evidence gathered in answer to these questions needs to be analyzed to determine whether it is appropriate to use for the particular population of interest. This is where additional background from coursework in statistics and epidemiology is so vital for the DNP graduate. By developing skill in these areas, all DNP graduates will be prepared to analyze data at individual, aggregate, and population health levels in order to use such data appropriately when developing interventions.

Psychosocial Dimensions and Cultural Diversity in Clinical Prevention and Population Health

Role of the Baccalaureate-Level RN and the Master's-Level APRN in Health Promotion and Disease Prevention

Education for both baccalaureate-level RNs and master's-level APRNs has included an emphasis on health promotion via patient education focused on behavioral counseling in such areas as diet (e.g., caloric intake, fiber, and vitamins), exercise, stress reduction, and measures to avoid tobacco, alcohol, and drug abuse, to name a few. The baccalaureate-level RN also gathers health assessment data to identify risks and collaborates with others regarding various other health promotion and disease prevention activities. In addition, master's-level APRN educational programs regarding health promotion focus on developing knowledge of when to implement recommended screenings. Familiarity with recommended screenings, such as those developed by the USPSTF, is expected. The USPSTF published its first recommendations about preventive services in 1989. An update to these recommendations was made in 1996; since then, guidelines have been updated annually, with the pocket guide released in 2008 containing 65 clinical preventive services recommendations (Agency for Healthcare Research and Quality [AHRQ], n.d.). The pocket guide is available free upon request from the AHRQ. These recommendations are also available online at http://www.ahrq.gov/clinic/prevenix.htm.

The master's-level APRN has also been expected to have competence in clinical prevention regarding immunization schedules recommended by the Centers for Disease Control and Prevention (CDC). In addition, USPSTF recommendations include clinical prevention guidelines regarding chemoprevention, such as use of aspirin for cardioprotective benefit for those at risk for heart attack, that the master's-level APRN utilizes. Other professional specialty organizations, such as the American Cancer Society (ACS), the American College of Obstetrics and Gynecology (ACOG), the American Academy of Pediatricians (AAP), and the Academy of Family Physicians (AFP), also have guidelines regarding clinical prevention that the master's-level APRN utilizes in planning patient-specific care interventions.

The master's-level APRN develops and monitors plans of care focused on health promotion and disease prevention, whereas the baccalaureate-level RN collaborates with others in the development and monitoring of such plans. Clinical prevention services can be focused on the primary, secondary, or tertiary level of prevention. Primary prevention activities are focused on prevention of illness and can be done in many settings, including the local community, such as providing a class on hand washing for kindergartners, or setting up an immunization clinic. Primary prevention by the master's-level APRN in a hospital setting would include implementation of wound care protocols aimed at preventing wound infection, with the baccalaureate-level RN utilizing such implemented protocols.

Secondary prevention activities have the focus of early detection of illness and traditionally can be done in a clinic setting by the master's-level APRN. Secondary prevention activities center on implementation of USPSTF screening recommendations. Tertiary prevention activities are those done to prevent worsening of a condition that is already present and traditionally have been delivered by the baccalaureate-level RN or the master's-level APRN in a clinic or a hospital setting (Aschengrau & Seage, 2008; Fletcher & Fletcher, 2005). Tertiary prevention activities, such as diabetes education classes, have been done at the individual or group level based on patient need. Both secondary and tertiary prevention activities have been moving into the community setting, such as screenings at health fairs or in the work setting and home care services focused on prevention of complications from chronic illness (McEwen & Nies, 2007).

Baccalaureate-Level RN and Master's-Level APRNs and the Use of Psychosocial Dimensions

Identification of psychosocial dimensions that may affect care regarding health promotion has been incorporated into baccalaureate-level RN educational programs. As mentioned previously, basic health promotion has been a focus of nursing practice for many years. But understanding how psychosocial dimensions affect health promotion practice has been in the forefront since Nola Pender began developing her nursing theory of health promotion (Pender, 1975). The first version of her health promotion model (HPM) was published in 1982 (Pender et al., 2006). The model was revised in 1996. The HPM is described as a theory that "integrates a number of constructs from expectancy-value theory and social cognitive theory" (Pender et al., 2006, p. 50). The theory incorporates personal biologic, psychological, and sociocultural considerations within factors that need to be taken into account for success in planning health promotion activities (Figure 7-2). Her middle-range nursing theory has been used in many master's-level APRN educational programs as an introduction to the health promotion theory needed for planning and providing care in the clinical setting. The master's-level APRN uses this theory to assess a patient's readiness to engage in health-promoting behaviors and to plan where to intervene in the model to affect health behaviors.

Another assessment model for use in planning health promotion activities that master's-level APRNs working in public health, community health, and population health may be familiar with is the PRECEDE-PROCEED model, which was developed by Green and Kreuter for use in planning public health activities. The Cleveland State University uses this model for its master's-level population health nursing program (Frisch et al., 2003). The dimension of health promotion was added to this model in 1999 (Green & Kreuter, 1999).

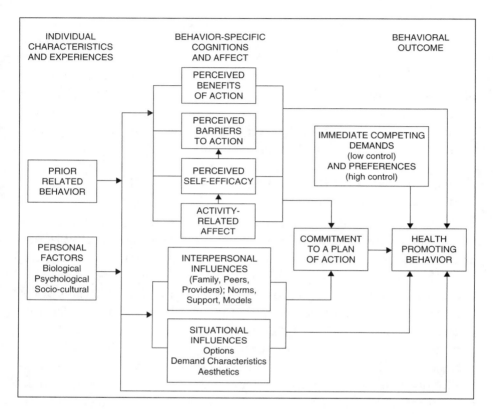

■ Figure 7-2   Nola Pender's health promotion model.

Source: Courtesy of Nola Pender, PhD, RN, FAAN. Reprinted with permission.

Knowledge about change theory is included in baccalaureate-level RN and master's-level APRN educational programs because readiness to change is an important concept to understand when developing plans of care for health promotion that include behavioral change. In assessing readiness to change, one of the theories both the baccalaureate-level RN and the master's-level APRN may use is the transtheoretical model of change (TTM). This theory was developed by DiClemente and Prochaska and is based on identification of stages of readiness to change (Prochaska, Norcross, & DiClemente, 1994). The stages are pre-contemplation, contemplation, preparation, action, maintenance, and relapse (Geraci, 2004). Assessment regarding the stage that the target population is in is used to help direct intervention. Please see Chapter 11 for further discussion of change theories.

In addition to the previously discussed theories, the baccalaureate-level RN and the master's-level APRN may have used various other middle-range nursing theories in planning health promotion activities, such as the health belief model, modeling and role-modeling, self-efficacy theory, and the theory of planned behavior (Frisch et al., 2003; Peterson & Bredow, 2004). In using these theories, master's-level APRNs, with the exception of those educated in population health, focus on the level of individuals, families, groups, and communities and not at the level of population health.

Baccalaureate-Level RNs and Master's-Level APRNs and Cultural Competence

The AACN educational recommendation at the APRN master's level does not address cultural competence explicitly as a goal for the seventh essential. The cultural competence goal for the seventh essential for the baccalaureate-level RN is to collaborate with other healthcare professionals in planning culturally appropriate health promotion interventions. Nevertheless, some degree of cultural competence is expected at all levels of nursing. Nursing theorist Madeleine Leininger (1981) was the first to introduce nursing to the concept of the need for transcultural understanding in the provision of patient care and is considered the founder of transcultural nursing. Her sunrise model (Figure 7-3) depicts how her theory can be used for assessment in order to develop culturally congruent interventions (Leininger & McFarland, 2006). Nursing education has included a focus on the need for cultural competence for development and provision of patient care since that time at all educational levels.

The master's-level APRN may also be familiar with a cultural assessment model developed by another nursing leader, Larry Purnell. Purnell developed a model for use in assessing culture in order to develop culturally acceptable healthcare interventions. The Purnell model for cultural competence (Figure 7-4) is made up of 12 domains that need to be assessed: overview/heritage, communications, family roles and organization, workforce issues, biocultural ecology, high-risk health behaviors, nutrition, pregnancy, death rituals, spirituality, healthcare practices, and healthcare practitioners (Purnell, 2002; Purnell & Paulanka, 2005). Purnell and Paulanka (2005) have developed a handbook for use by healthcare providers that contains information about each of these domains for various religious and ethnic groups.

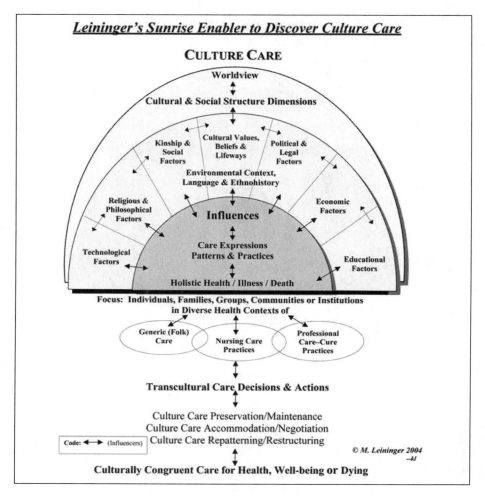

Figure 7-3   Madeleine Leininger's sunrise model.

Source: Leininger, M. M., and McFarland, M. (2006). *Culture care diversity and universality: A worldwide nursing theory* (2nd ed., p. 25). Sudbury, MA: Jones and Bartlett.

The question could be asked as to whether cultural considerations are really vital to planning appropriate health promotion interventions. Anne Fadiman, author of *The Spirit Catches You and You Fall Down,* the famous account of an adverse healthcare outcome that occurred when aspects of Hmong culture were not considered during care provision, addressed this question in a lecture at the University of Minnesota (personal communication, March 2,

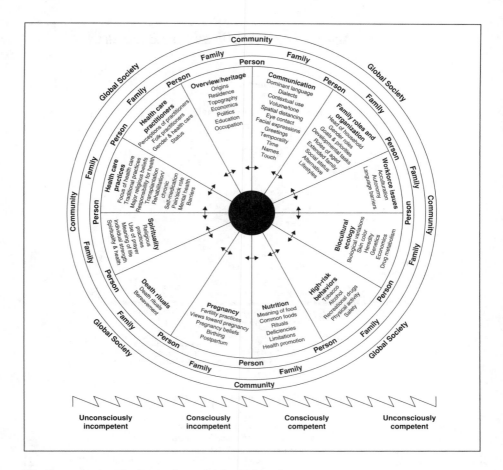

■ Figure 7-4   The Purnell model for cultural competence.

Source: Purnell, L. (2002). The Purnell model for cultural competence. *Journal of Transcultural Nursing, 13*(3), 194. Reproduced with permission.

2009). She recommended that cultural competence be considered an assessment tool, like an otoscope, that healthcare providers need to develop the ability to use. This recommendation was made secondary to concern that the concept of being culturally competent may be devalued as the "politically correct" manner of behavior or a fad, rather then being recognized as an important assessment tool that needs to be used routinely in order to develop expertise in its use and to provide proper care.

Role of the DNP in Health Promotion and Disease Prevention

Individual-based interventions for health promotion and disease prevention performed by the DNP continue to be guided by the USPSTF recommendations. The DNP also may find *The Guide to Community Preventive Services*, an online resource (www.thecommunityguide.org), useful in planning health promotion and disease prevention activity for population health–based interventions (Briss, Brownson, Fielding, & Zaza, 2004). Knowledge of materials in national and state health planning documents has also been recommended as essential for planning of population health–related activity (Zahner & Block, 2006). When using these guides and documents, the DNP will also be aware of the need to synthesize psychosocial and cultural dimensions of the target population into the planning of any clinical prevention and population health interventions and can provide leadership in this area of project planning.

DNP-Level Synthesis of Psychosocial Dimensions and Cultural Diversity

The DNP-prepared APRN will be able to synthesize the various theoretical concepts and models described previously in this chapter when planning any health promotion intervention. Coursework in the DNP curriculum enables the DNP to synthesize the body of knowledge regarding the impact of psychosocial and cultural factors on health promotion and disease prevention in a way not previously promoted in master's-level APRN education. Knowledge of the impact of health policy on access to health care and the intersection of these factors with cultural diversity and psychosocial dimensions allows the DNP to perform a more in-depth analysis than the master's-level APRN for guidance regarding how to develop and implement health promotion and disease prevention interventions appropriately for individuals and groups in the target population. In developing interventions, the DNP will also integrate concepts of change theory and leadership theory determined by analysis to be appropriate for the target population. The DNP develops familiarity with concepts of program planning and evaluation that are missing from the curriculum of many master's-level APRN programs. Use of these concepts is vital in order to plan programs and properly evaluate outcomes of program interventions. All of these abilities are actualized in DNP capstone or scholarly projects. Please see Chapter 11 for further discussion of the DNP scholarly project.

Another strength the DNP brings to the development of clinical prevention interventions is an increased depth of knowledge regarding how to implement programs. As discussed previously in this chapter, whether clinical prevention would be best delivered at the individual or the population level or simultaneously at both levels is a question that the DNP is able to assess. In performing a needs assessment while planning a project, the DNP is prepared to identify stakeholders and examine threats and barriers to planned project intervention. Such information will help determine the appropriate level for intervention. The DNP is also aware that planning for evaluation of the process of implementation of an intervention is also vital in order to understand what went wrong if a program is not successful (Issel, 2004).

Health promotion and disease prevention interventions can be focused on an individual level, an aggregate level, or a population level and at the primary, secondary, or tertiary level. Psychosocial and cultural diversity factors will be considered by the DNP when planning what level or levels on which to provide intervention for a particular health need. Pender's HPM or Green and Kreutzer's PRECEDE-PROCEED model (Figure 7-5) are examples of models that can be used as a theoretical basis for individual, aggregate, or population assessment regarding clinical prevention and population health project interventions planned and implemented by the DNP. Data on cultural diversity factors that already exist in the literature (for example, Monsen, 2009; Purnell & Paulanka, 2005) may be used in developing interventions. However, the DNP will also gather data on cultural diversity factors that are unique to the population of interest while performing a needs assessment as one of the initial steps in project planning.

The following are examples of some questions that may be considered in a needs assessment: Will the need respond to an educational intervention? If so, is the intervention best delivered on an individual level during a routine health maintenance visit, on an aggregate level such as by providing a diabetes class in the clinic or the community, or on a population level by print media or broadcast media for the particular need and the population of interest? Is the population of interest of varied cultures? If so, are different approaches to intervention delivery needed in order to reach all population group members? Are there socioeconomic factors that would necessitate modifications in intervention plans?

In planning health promotion interventions, the DNP will also synthesize theoretical concepts related to the readiness of the target audience to

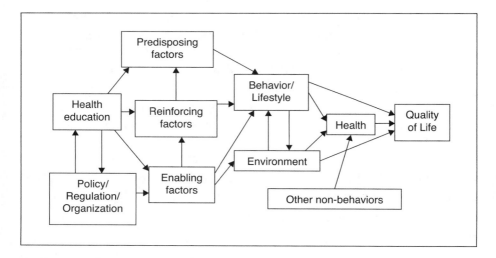

■ Figure 7-5   The PRECEDE-PROCEED model as used for development of health promotion planning.

Source: Wilson and Kolander (2011). Adapted from L. W. Green and M. W. Kreuter, *Health promotion planning: An educational ansd environmental approach.* Mayfield Publishing Company, 1991.

change. The DNP has become familiar with many change theories in his or her previous coursework and will learn more about how to use these theories appropriately. For example, Lewin's change theory is one such theory that may be applicable for use by the DNP when planning health promotion activities. Three processes that occur during any change are included in Lewin's theory: unfreezing, moving, and refreezing (Geraci, 2004; Lewin, 1951, 1975). When performing a needs assessment, the DNP may assess driving and restraining factors to change and will need to overcome restraining forces first in order to unfreeze the situation and implement change. Many of the questions presented earlier integrate Lewin's concepts. In assessing readiness to change, the DNP may also use the TTM theory discussed previously in this chapter (Geraci, 2004).

Another change theory the DNP may use in health promotion project planning takes into consideration factors that might influence the rate of change to expect in response to an intervention and provides information as to how best to promote the intervention. Everett Rogers's (2002, 2003) diffusion of innovation theory addresses how the process of change is influenced by the rate of acceptance of change. He categorizes population groups responding to change as consisting of innovators, early adopters, early majority, late majority, and laggards. This theory was used in development of the STOP AIDS program in San Francisco in the 1980s (Rogers, 2003), therefore demonstrating proven utility for health promotion intervention in a population. It has been recommended that the focus of initial promotion in a community be on the innovators in an attempt to use this population to accelerate the change within the community of interest (Haider & Kreps, 2004). Please see Chapter 11 for further discussion of change theories.

Focus of DNPs' Health Promotion and Disease Prevention Interventions

IMPROVEMENT IN HEALTH STATUS

Evaluation of the impact of socioeconomic factors and cultural beliefs on health status is necessary in order to formulate an intervention that will be successful for the target population. The DNP will synthesize concepts from the theories discussed previously while formulating these interventions. For example, if while using Pender's HPM it is discovered that the population of interest is not able to attend a class because of lack of transportation, then provision of transportation may be the first step needed in order to improve health status for this population. The DNP will also assess for antecedent factors that contribute to the lack of transportation for this population and develop interventions to address the problem at that level. Likewise, if while performing a cultural assessment using Leininger's sunrise model it is discovered that a cultural belief that factors in life are predetermined and nothing can be done to change one's fate exists, then the first step in intervening to improve health status for this population will need to be focused on how to work within this belief. Leadership in addressing social determinants of health that are adversely affecting improvement in health status in the areas of health promotion and disease prevention is another way in which the DNP will improve health status.

ACCESS PATTERNS

One factor that is recognized as a contributor to limitation of access to care is limitation in the supply of providers (Chang, 2001). In recent years there has been a steady decrease in the number of primary care providers (Walker, 2006). This decrease has occurred because fewer and fewer medical students are choosing family practice, internal medicine, and pediatrics as specialties because of the decreased potential for income in this type of practice. One solution the medical community has proposed to deal with this is for primary providers to charge patients an extra fee in order to make primary care practice more lucrative and therefore attract an increased number of medical school graduates to the field (Walker, 2006). Unfortunately, this proposed solution will do nothing to meet the needs of the underserved and uninsured and lacks focus on the needs of the patient.

DNPs can improve access by direct care provision of preventive services on the individual level in the primary care setting. Mundinger et al. (2000), in a randomized trial performed in the 1990s, provided evidence that care delivered by nurse practitioners was equivalent to care provided by physicians. Pohl, Barkauskas, Benkert, Breer, and Bostrom (2006) went one better, as far as promotion of use of nurse practitioners as primary care providers is concerned, with findings that academic nurse-managed centers (ANMCs) produced a quality of care that was seen by patients as superior to care provided by physicians. This superiority was related to care being perceived by patients as secondary to the following care characteristics: "health (not just medical) care, comprehensive care and follow-through with problems and concerns, prevention, teaching, and listening" (Pohl et al., 2006, p. 273). The fact that patients included provision of information on prevention in a list of characteristics that defined the superior care received in ANMCs highlights the importance patients place on preventive services.

Academic nurse-managed centers that serve underprivileged populations have been around since the 1970s, but they rarely have been able to function without an outside funding source and usually have operated in the red, therefore making it difficult to expand such services (Barkauskas et al., 2004). Improvement in access to care for the underprivileged continues to be necessary. The American College of Physicians' (ACP) 2009 policy statement on care provision by nurse practitioners advocated for inclusion of nurse-managed demonstration projects for the "medical home" model for primary care services (called "health care homes" in Minnesota), yet they maintained that physician management of such primary care services would most likely prove to be the better model (ACP, 2009). If these nurse-managed demonstration projects prove successful, as historical information suggests would be the case, then nurse-managed clinics should increase in number and success and provide an intervention that will improve access to care for underserved populations.

Nursing has a long history of patient-centered care delivery, and the DNP is poised to fill this gap in primary care. However, improving access to preventive service care by expansion of ANMCs may not be fully realized unless current restrictions on reimbursement for APRNs are dealt with legislatively (Barkauskas et al., 2004; Hansen-Turton, Ritter, Rothman, & Valdez, 2006). There is hope this will occur soon, because nurse-managed health centers (NMHCs) have been acknowledged as a possible vehicle to improve access for underserved populations by the Senate Committee of Appropriations in 2005 (Newland, 2006). Familiarity with how health policy is developed and how best to influence policy will be crucial for the DNP in this instance. Inclusion of health policy in the curriculum framework for clinical prevention and population health is part of HPCT recommendations, but is not included as part of the AACN goals for this DNP essential. Instead, the AACN made health policy advocacy a separate essential. Nevertheless, these two essentials intersect, and a change in health policy to improve access to NMHCs is one way in which the DNP can improve access to health care.

GAPS IN CARE

In recent years a gap in care for the underinsured and uninsured has been partially met by a new type of healthcare entity in the form of the retail-based clinic. These clinics have become financially successful, and their numbers have grown (Hansen-Turton, Ryan, Miller, Counts, & Nash, 2007; Nelson, 2007). These clinics not only provide easy access to care, since they function as a walk-in form of service, but also have become useful to provide care to the uninsured for at least a limited number of minor acute illnesses, therefore providing a form of tertiary prevention by decreasing risk for complications from untreated illness. These clinics also administer primary prevention services by providing immunizations for a reasonably affordable fee. Retail clinics have been staffed mainly with nurse practitioners and will be well served by the leadership expertise of the DNP.

Evaluate Care Delivery Models

Role of the Baccalaureate-Level RN and the Master's-Level APRN Regarding Evaluation of Care Delivery Models

Evaluation is the last step of the nursing process of assessment, diagnosis, planning, implementation, and evaluation of intervention outcomes. It is done to determine whether modification of the planned intervention is needed because a desired outcome was not met. However, as far as evaluation of care delivery models is concerned, the role defined by the goals for the seventh AACN essential for the baccalaureate-level RN is to use available evaluation results to affect delivery of care, use of resources, and development of policy (AACN, 2008). Evaluation of care delivery models is likewise not specifically included in the goals for the seventh AACN essential for the master's-level APRN (AACN, 1996). The master's-level APRN was to function in development and monitoring of plans of care but was not charged with evaluating models of care. Nevertheless, master's-level APRNs have done assessment of factors related to the concepts of community, environmental and occupational health, and cultural and socioeconomic dimensions of health, which the DNP is charged to use in evaluation of care delivery models.

Identification of factors related to the concepts of socioeconomic risk has been performed at the master's level by APRNs working in clinics on the individual level when obtaining health histories and in the public health arena when performing community assessments. Assessment of social, political, environmental, and economic factors that lead to illness have also been done by master's-level APRNs who work in the fields of community, environmental, and occupational health with use of various assessment tools and strategies. Based on these assessments, interventional plans of care that may affect care delivery models have been developed by master's-level APRNs (Nies & McEwen, 2007; Stanhope & Lancaster, 2008).

ROLE OF THE BACCALAUREATE-LEVEL RN AND THE MASTER'S-LEVEL APRN IN COMMUNITY HEALTH NURSING

Community and public health nurses at the baccalaureate level (RNs) and the master's level (APRNs) keep in focus the following three main functional concepts of community and public health nursing while performing assessments and planning interventions: assessment, policy development, and assurance (Allender, Rector, & Warner, 2010; Keller, Strohschein, Lia-Hoagberg, & Schaffer, 1998; Nies & McEwen, 2007; Stanhope & Lancaster, 2008). The function of assessment can be done at the individual, community, or population level. Policy development is performed by ensuring that developed policies are evidence based and community focused. Finally, the function of assurance is to determine that access exists for essential services and that personnel are available to provide services (Stanhope & Lancaster, 2008).

Interventions developed based on assessments can be primary, secondary, or tertiary in focus and usually address all three of the main functional concepts.

Also, interventions can be delivered at the individual, community, or systems level (Keller et al., 1998). Models have been developed to illustrate how community and public health nurses plan and develop interventions (see Figure 7-6 for diagrams of two such models). Community and public health nursing can include work with a focus on many different public health problems. The following are examples of areas of focus: communicable disease, violence, substance abuse, home hospice care, and disasters (both man-made and natural). The community health nurse is an activist, is resourceful, prioritizes prevention, considers the client as an equal partner, is population focused, works collaboratively, and bases interventions on the concept of the greatest good (Allender, Rector, & Warner, 2010).

ROLE OF THE BACCALAUREATE-LEVEL RN AND THE MASTER'S-LEVEL APRN IN OCCUPATIONAL AND ENVIRONMENTAL HEALTH NURSING

The occupational health nurse (OHN), depending on the scope of practice regulations in the individual state, provides health surveillance in the workplace and is responsible for ensuring maintenance of Occupational Safety and Health Administration (OSHA) mandates in regard to the monitoring and reporting of hazard exposures (American Association of Occupational Health Nurses [AAOHN], 2004). The level of RN education required for the OHN may vary from state to state, but in general the OHN is prepared at the master's level or doctoral level (AAOHN, 2004; Stanhope & Lancaster, 2008). The certifying agency for occupational health nurses, the American Board of Occupational Health Nurses (ABOHN), however, allows the associate-degree RN to take a certification exam and will bestow the credential of certified occupational health nurse (COHN) at this educational level. Nurses taking the certifying exam with a baccalaureate degree or higher are eligible to take another certifying exam and will be certified as a specialist in occupation health nursing with the credential COHN-S (ABOHN, n.d.).

The focus of the OHN is promotion of health and recovery from illness, injury and illness prevention, and hazard protection. The AAOHN promotes the OHN as one who role models healthy behavior, encourages employees to self-manage health, promotes employee accountability for health by making disease management and health promotion programs and services available, and is a health advocate and expert within the company and the community (AAOHN, 2004). The OHN may plan for work-related disasters, plan prevention strategies regarding violence in the workplace, and plan wellness programs and other health promotion activities in the workplace involving all three levels of prevention. The master's-

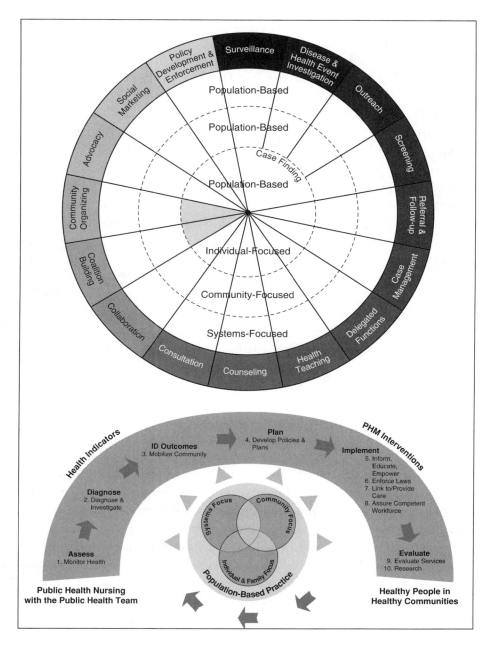

■ Figure 7-6   (a) Minnesota's public health intervention wheel. (b) Los Angeles County's public health nursing practice model.

Source: (a) Minnesota Department of Health, Division of Community Health Services, Public Health Nursing Section. (b) Los Angeles County Department of Health. Copyright 2007 by Los Angeles Country DPH Public Health Nursing.

prepared APRN working in occupational health may also provide primary care services in the workplace (AAOHN, 2004; Stanhope & Lancaster, 2008).

Occupational and environmental health nursing, as mentioned earlier in the chapter, have been linked in the past. However, the health promotion and disease prevention objectives for Healthy People 2010 included, among many other objectives, specific separate objectives for occupational health nursing and environmental health nursing (Table 7-2). The National Institute of Environmental Health Sciences, the Agency for Toxic Substances and Disease Registry (ATSDR), and the National Institute for Nursing Research met in August of 2002 to consider measures to increase involvement of nurses in environmental health (O'Fallon, 2003). Environmental health nursing seems poised to become a specialty of its own, but no nursing certifying organization currently offers certification in this area as a specialty for either the baccalaureate-level RN or the master's-level APRN. Graduate-level education in environmental health nursing is available at several universities. However, the nurse working in environmental health who wants to become certified would need to seek certification in occupational and environmental health nursing from the ABOHN at this point in time.

Nevertheless, nurses have done environmental risk assessments for many years. Knowledge of the exposure risks of toxic chemical substances and other environmental factors was generally not stressed in nursing education until the end of the last century, despite the fact that the writings of nursing pioneers, such as Florence Nightingale and Lillian Wald, include multiple references to the importance of the environment to health (Stanhope & Lancaster, 2008). For a number of years, assessment for environmental risk for exposures of children to lead has been done in pediatrics, but it is now recommended that nursing assessments for environmental exposures be broadened beyond lead and beyond pediatrics. The mnemonic I PREPARE is used for an assessment tool that has been recommended by the ATSDR for use by nurses in order to perform an appropriate environmental assessment (Figure 7-7) (Centers for Disease Control and Prevention, n.d.; Stanhope & Lancaster, 2008). Beyond risk assessment, other roles suggested for the environmental health nurse are "community involvement/public participation, risk communication, epidemiological investigations, and policy development" (Stanhope & Lancaster, 2008, p. 236).

■ Table 7-2   Healthy People 2010 Objectives

Occupational Health

20-1.   Reduce deaths from work-related injuries.
20-2.   Reduce work-related injuries resulting in medical treatment, lost time from work, or restricted work activity.
20-3.   Reduce the rate of injury and illness cases involving days away from work due to overexertion or repetitive motion.
20-4.   Reduce pneumoconiosis deaths.
20-5.   Reduce deaths from work-related homicides.
20-6.   Reduce work-related assaults.
20-7.   Reduce the number of persons who have elevated blood lead concentrations from work exposures.
20-8.   Reduce occupational skin diseases or disorders among full-time workers.
20-9.   Increase the proportion of worksites employing 50 or more persons that provide programs to prevent or reduce employee stress.
20-10. Reduce occupational needle-stick injuries among health care workers.

Environmental Health

8-1.   Reduce the proportion of persons exposed to air that does not meet the U.S. Environmental Protection Agency's health-based standards for harmful air pollutants.
8-2.   Increase use of alternative modes of transportation to reduce motor vehicle emissions and improve the Nation's air quality.
8-3.   Improve the Nation's air quality by increasing the use of cleaner alternative fuels.
8-4.   Reduce air toxic emissions to decrease the risk of adverse health effects caused by airborne toxics.
8-5.   Increase the proportion of persons served by community water systems who receive a supply of drinking water that meets the regulations of the Safe Drinking Water Act.
8-6.   Reduce waterborne disease outbreaks arising from water intended for drinking among persons served by community water systems.
8-7.   Reduce per capita domestic water withdrawals.
*
8-11.   Eliminate elevated blood lead levels in children.
8-12.   Minimize the risks to human health and the environment posed by hazardous sites.
8-13.   Reduce pesticide exposures that result in visits to a health care facility.
8-15.   Increase recycling of municipal solid waste.
8-16.   Reduce indoor allergen levels.
8-18.   Increase the proportion of persons who live in homes tested for radon concentrations.
8-19.   Increase the number of new homes constructed to be radon resistant.
*

(continues)

■ Table 7-2   Healthy People 2010 Objectives (CONTINUED)

8-22.   Increase the proportion of persons living in pre-1950s housing that has been tested for the presence of lead-based paint.

8-23.   Reduce the proportion of occupied housing units that are substandard.

8-24.   Reduce exposure to pesticides as measured by urine concentrations of metabolites.

*

8-27.   Increase or maintain the number of Territories, Tribes, and States, and the District of Columbia that monitor diseases or conditions that can be caused by exposure to environmental hazards.

*

8-29.   Reduce the global burden of disease due to poor water quality, sanitation, and personal and domestic hygiene.

8-30.   Increase the proportion of the population in the U.S.–Mexico border region that have adequate drinking water and sanitation facilities.

* Objectives at developmental stage not listed.

Source: U.S. Department of Health and Human Services. (2000). *Healthy People 2010 national health promotion and disease prevention objectives.* Washington, DC: U.S. Government Printing Office.

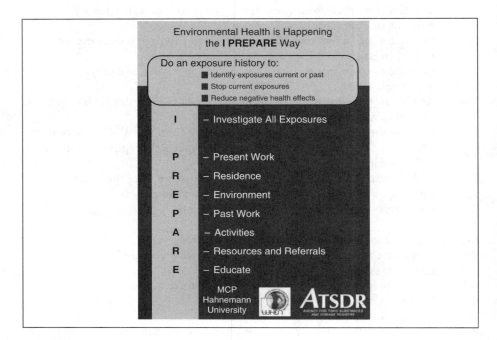

■ Figure 7-7   Environmental assessment tool: I PREPARE.

Source: Centers for Disease Control and Prevention. (n.d.). *I PREPARE.* Retrieved from http://www2a.cdc.gov/phtn/envhealth/pdf-files/CARDFRNT.pdf.

The Role of the DNP Regarding Evaluation of Care Delivery Models

The DNP will identify strategies that lead to good outcomes within care delivery models. An unsatisfactory outcome may be the impetus for such an evaluation. More in-depth preparation in program planning and evaluation methods makes the DNP better able to perform evaluation of a care delivery model than the master's-prepared APRN. While performing this evaluation, the DNP may use concepts from the field of quality improvement in addition to psychosocial and cultural concepts. Concepts from community, environmental, and occupational health, such as the primacy of prevention, surveillance for exposures, and need for the greatest good, may also be used in evaluation of care delivery models and strategies.

One theory that can be used for outcomes assessment is the theory of quality assessment developed by Avedis Donabedian (1966, 1980). Donabedian provides an easy-to-use framework for evaluation of care delivery outcomes that consists of three concepts: structure, process, and outcome. According to Donabedian, when evaluating an outcome, the structure of an organization must be examined. The structure includes available finances, staff, and resources. The process also needs to be examined in order to formulate an intervention to affect outcome. In his theory, process includes such factors as utilization of care and timeliness of care (Donabedian, 1980). This simple but elegant theory can provide a framework for evaluation of the organizational aspects of care delivery models.

The DNP might also use the PRECEDE-PROCEED model. Green and Kreuter's PRECEDE-PROCEED model was developed for program planning and evaluation in the community health arena. The model assesses behavioral, social, and environmental factors influencing health. The PROCEED portion of this model is where evaluation of the implemented program occurs. The model guides evaluation of the process of implementation of interventions, the impact of interventions, and the outcomes from interventions. It is an excellent model for the DNP to use in evaluation of care delivery models or strategies and has been used for evaluation of many health promotion programs (Green & Mercer, 2006).

Familiarity with evidence-based practice and the economics of health care also helps prepare the DNP to evaluate care delivery models or strategies. Knowledge regarding the strength of evidence at each level is necessary to evaluate the suitability of the level of evidence for a given care delivery model. The DNP is prepared to identify the appropriateness of the evidence for the population of interest or the appropriateness of any evidence-based intervention chosen to improve an existing care delivery model. Consideration of the economic dimensions of cost-effectiveness, cost-utility and cost-benefit ratios, cost minimization, and cost consequences of the continued use of or proposed change to a current delivery model is also a necessary component for thorough evaluation.

In their capstone projects, DNP students at the University of Minnesota have evaluated care delivery models, identified needed change in these models, and developed interventions to change these care delivery models. Interventions developed have improved care delivery or strategies in the following areas: access to care for truckers, continuity of care for those using retail clinics, patient flow patterns in an emergency room, timeliness in reporting of abnormal test results to patients, and immunization rates in healthcare providers. These projects have incorporated concepts of community health as well as cultural and socioeconomic factors. Also, the project that focused on implementing a new delivery strategy to improve immunization rates for healthcare providers addressed an important concept of occupational health.

Conclusions

Future Roles for DNPs in Clinical Prevention and Population Health

The acronym DNP, doctor of nursing practice, means that the practice of nursing, regardless of setting, has been brought to the doctoral level of expertise. There are vast opportunities for leadership and service for each individual DNP. The DNP graduate should be well prepared to lead in the development, implementation, and evaluation of interventions to meet the goals of Healthy People 2020. The proposed goals are as follows:

- Eliminate preventable disease, disability, injury, and premature death.
- Achieve health equity, eliminate disparities, and improve the health of all groups.
- Create social and physical environments that promote good health for all.
- Promote healthy development and healthy behaviors across every stage of life. (U.S. Department of Health and Human Services, 2008, p. 6)

The advisory committee for Healthy People 2020 developed a model to illustrate how these goals can be addressed (Figure 7-8). For each example, the population level of intervention is also identified.

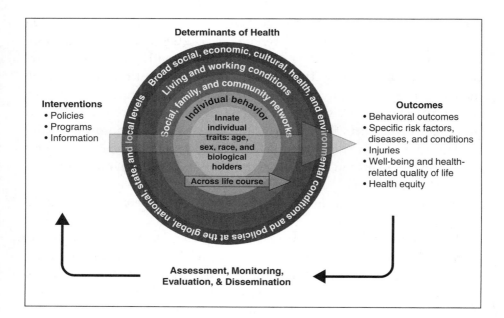

Determinants of Health

Interventions
- Policies
- Programs
- Information

Broad social, economic, cultural, health,
and working conditions
Living and community networks
Social, family, and
Individual behavior
Innate
individual
traits: age,
sex, race, and
biological
holders

Across life course

and environmental conditions
Institutions, state, and local levels
and policies at the global, national,

Outcomes
- Behavioral outcomes
- Specific risk factors,
  diseases, and conditions
- Injuries
- Well-being and health-
  related quality of life
- Health equity

**Assessment, Monitoring,
Evaluation, & Dissemination**

■ Figure 7-8   Action model to achieve the overarching goals of Healthy People 2020.

Source: U.S. Department of Health and Human Services, Secretary's Advisory Committee on Health Promotion and Disease Prevention Objectives for 2020. (2008). *Phase I report: Recommendations for the framework
and format of Healthy People 2020* (p. 8). Retrieved from http://www.healthypeople.gov/hp2020/
advisory/PhaseI/PhaseI.pdf

INDIVIDUAL LEVEL

The DNP as the expert provider in the area of health promotion and disease
prevention is a role proposed by Burman et al. (2009). These authors maintain that "disease prevention has always been the soul of nursing, while
health promotion has been its heart" (p. 14) and that the nursing educational curriculum for the DNP should focus on the fields of health promotion and disease prevention rather then just borrowing much of its
curriculum from the medical field. In the view of Burman et al., this borrowing of curriculum model from medicine has contributed to the view of
the APRN as a "substitute for a physician" with titles such as *physician extender*
or *mid-level provider*. Titles such as these may contribute to an impression of
an accompanying need for dependent practice rather than visualization of
an independent unique profession with ability to practice on its own right.
This proposed change in the focus of education for the DNP graduate to
one of health promotion and disease prevention would produce providers of

care that are fundamentally different than medical providers, would lead to improved patient satisfaction (see Pohl et al., 2006), and would provide patients with a much-needed type of care that is currently missing. Of course, Burman et al. acknowledge that each profession will continue to have some intersection regarding care provided, but each will also have its unique focus that is reflected in its educational preparation. Prevention of disease and promotion of health are key to decreasing healthcare costs, improving quality of life, and increasing longevity. Having a provider whose focus of care and educational preparation is devoted to prevention of disease and health promotion could enhance the potential for these outcomes to be realized. This role would promote healthy development and healthy behaviors across the life span.

This proposed change in curriculum focus works in parallel with this essential but may not be welcomed by all APRNs or medical providers, because both may perceive the recommendation as limiting their respective roles in some manner. APRNs may see the proposed change as taking away from their ability to provide independent primary care services, whereas primary care medical providers may be reluctant to be limited in providing health promotion services.

AGGREGATE LEVEL

The Human Genome Project, completed in 2003, holds promise to provide new opportunities for clinical prevention. The project, in addition to identifying all the genes that make up the human genome, also made possible identification of gene defects that may indicate disease or disease risk. Unfortunately, merely testing for the presence of a gene defect is not sufficient in many cases to develop disease preventive interventions because the presence or absence of a defect is not diagnostic of the presence or absence of future risk for disease or diagnostic of current disease condition (Janssens et al., 2008; Monsen, 2009; Tranin, 2006).

Because of this ambiguity and the potential for psychosocial and cultural stressors for the patient considering genetic testing, Tranin, in her 2006 Oncology Nursing Society Clinical Lectureship, advised that counseling regarding genetic testing is best done by nurses. Tranin's reasoning for why counseling would be best done by nurses is that nurses take a holistic view of a patient, have a wealth of experience in communicating with patients and their families, and know how to access the resources a patient might need to deal with the test results. Provision of genetic counseling is within the scope of practice of the APRN certified in oncology nursing who has also obtained specialty training in genetics and genomics (Oncology Nursing Society, 2009). This is a role in which the educational preparation of the DNP in analysis of data, synthesis of psychosocial and cultural diversity concepts, and evaluation of care strategies can be well utilized. This role for the DNP would also help meet a Healthy People 2020 goal, since the goal of genetic testing and counseling is to eliminate preventable disease, disability, injury, and premature death.

POPULATION LEVEL

With the importance of the environment to health recently coming to the forefront in nursing practice, the field of environmental health nursing holds much opportunity for the DNP to provide leadership in planning and evaluation of care delivery models or strategies that will decrease adverse health outcomes at the population level related to environmental risks. Possibly the greatest area of opportunity and need in environmental health nursing at the population level exists in the area of climate change. Environmental risks related to climate change threaten everyone in the population, and population health–focused interventions will need to be developed to address these risks. Climate change health risks that have been identified by the Environmental Protection Agency (EPA) include extreme heat waves, other extreme weather events, increases in climate-sensitive diseases, air pollution, and adverse effects on agricultural production (EPA, 2007). Barbara Sattler, in a presentation on global warming, identified the following factors that will contribute to increased health risks: increased sea levels, increased storms, problems with food security secondary to agricultural changes, fires related to increased episodes of drought, heat waves, problems with access to potable water, refugees created by climate change, and resulting increases in morbidity and mortality rates (Sattler, 2008). The DNP with nursing's holistic focus, knowledge of and grounding in community and public health concepts, consideration for psychosocial and cultural dimensions when planning interventions, and strong background in provision of health promotion education and interventions is best suited for the task of addressing these risks to populations that threaten to arise from climate change. If they were alive today, this may be the area of nursing on which Nightingale and Wald would be focusing.

DNP Outcome Potentials Related to Improving the Nation's Health

Broad dissemination of knowledge regarding effective health promotion and disease prevention measures is needed to reach the goal of improving the nation's health. The APTR provides all healthcare providers interested in prevention education, including the DNP, with the potential to communicate easily within an interdisciplinary healthcare community about clinical prevention and population health interventions and programs with its Web-based resource called the Prevention Education Resource Center (PERC). The PERC website (www.teachingprevention.org) is a place where registered members can submit prevention-related educational material, access materials submitted by others, and evaluate the quality of these materials (Fincham, 2008). This site holds much promise for improvement in population health by serving as a portal for speedy and broad dissemination of information to the prevention education and research community. The DNP graduate could submit any prevention-related capstone project to this site to be used as a resource for others who may be dealing with similar problems. The potential for others to more quickly benefit from broader use of successful health promotion interventions through the PERC website provides a positive impetus toward reaching the goal of improving the nation's health.

Proof as to whether DNP graduates will exceed the abilities of master's-prepared APRNs in practice has yet to be determined, and opinion as to whether improvement in practice ability will result from the additional coursework provided to the DNP graduate is mixed (Dreher, 2009; Ford, 2009; Kaplan & Brown, 2009). But consideration of the expanded potential the DNP brings for improvements in outcomes related to clinical prevention and population health interventions as discussed in this chapter leads to the conclusion that the DNP will help propel the nursing profession to new horizons while promoting improvement in the nation's health.

Clinical prevention interventions developed, implemented, and evaluated by the DNP and directed at the levels of individual, aggregate, and population health hold much promise to improve health status at all of these levels and may reach beyond improvements in health status. The World Health Organization's agenda includes six points focused on improvement of population health: "promoting development; fostering health security; strengthening health systems; harnessing research, information, and evidence; enhancing partnerships; and improving performance" (WHO, n.d.). Within the description of the goal of "promoting development" is the need for access to health-promoting interventions in order to ensure the health of populations. This WHO goal is parallel to a portion of one of the AACN educational goals of this essential. The DNP is prepared to develop health promotion interventions focused on improving access patterns for health care. The WHO also closely ties good health to the socioeconomic development of nations; that is, good health is needed for a worker to be productive. If large portions of the population of a nation are in poor health, it will be difficult for that nation to improve its socioeconomic status because of the lack of capable workforce. This is a concept well known to occupational health nurses. Ill health leads to absenteeism and increased risk for workplace injury. By meeting the goals of this essential, the DNP may hold promise to not only improve the nation's health but also improve the socioeconomic status of this nation. Truly, the potential for contribution by the DNP to improvement in the health of individuals, families, communities, and beyond is enormous for this nation as a whole.

References

Agency for Healthcare Research and Quality. (n.d.). *U.S. Preventive Services Task Force: About the USPSTF*. Retrieved from http://www.ahrq.gov/clinic/uspstfab.htm

Allan, J., Barwick, T. A., Cashman, S., Cawley, J. F., Day, C., Douglass, C. W., et al. (2004). Clinical prevention and population health: Curriculum framework for health professions. *American Journal of Preventive Medicine, 27*(5), 471–476.

Allan, J. D., Stanley, J., Crabtree, M. K., Werner, K. E., & Swenson, M. (2005). Clinical prevention and population health curriculum framework: The nursing perspective. *Journal of Professional Nursing, 21*(5), 259–267.

Allender, J. A., Rector, C., & Warner, K. D. (2010). *Community health nursing: Promoting and protecting the public's health* (7th ed.). Philadelphia: Lippincott Williams & Wilkins.

Alliance of Nurses for Healthy Environments. (2008). *About ANHE*. Retrieved from http://e-commons.org/anhe/about-the-e-commons

American Association of Colleges of Nursing. (1996). *The essentials of master's education for advance practice nursing*. Retrieved from http://www.aacn.nche.edu/education/pdf/MasEssentials96.pdf

American Association of Colleges of Nursing. (2006). *Essentials of doctoral education for advanced nursing practice*. Retrieved from http://www.aacn.nche.edu/DNP/pdf/Essentials.pdf

American Association of Colleges of Nursing. (2008). *The essentials of baccalaureate education for professional nursing practice*. Retrieved from http://www.aacn.nche.edu/education/pdf/BaccEssentials08.pdf

American Association of Occupational Health Nurses. (n.d.). *About AAOHN*. Retrieved from http://www.aaohn.org/about/index.cfm

American Association of Occupational Health Nurses. (2004). *Position statements*. Retrieved from http://www.aaohn.org/practice/positions/index.cfm

American Board of Occupational Health Nursing. (n.d.). *Certification*. Retrieved from http://www.abohn.org

American College of Physicians. (2009). *Nurse practitioners in primary care* [Policy monograph]. Philadelphia: Author.

Aschengrau, A. & Seage, G. R. (2008). Screening in public health practice. In A. Aschengrau & G. R. Seage III, *Essentials of epidemiology in public health* (2nd ed., pp. 411–438). Sudbury, MA: Jones and Bartlett.

Ashton, K. & Green, E. S. (2008). *The toxic consumer: Living healthy in a hazardous world.* New York: Sterling.

Association for Prevention Teaching and Research. (2007). *About APTR.* Retrieved from http://www.atpm.org/about/index.html

Association for Prevention Teaching and Research. (2008, January). *Clinical prevention and population health curriculum framework.* Retrieved from http://www.atpm.org/resources/pdfs /Official_CPPH_Framework_2008.pdf

Association for Prevention Teaching and Research. (2009, January). *Clinical prevention and population health curriculum framework.* Retrieved from http://www.atpm.org/resources/pdfs /Revised_CPPH_Framework_2009.pdf

Barkauskas, V. H., Pohl, J., Breer, L., Tanner, C., Bostrom, A. C., Benkert, R., et al. (2004). Academic nurse-managed centers: Approaches to evaluation. *Outcomes Management, 8*(1), 57–66.

Briss, P. A., Brownson, R. C., Fielding, J. E., & Zaza, S. (2004). Developing and using the *Guide to Community Preventive Services:* Lessons learned about evidence-based public health. *Annual Review of Public Health, 24,* 281–302.

Burman, M. E., Hart, A. M., Conley, V., Brown, J., Sherard, P., & Clarke, P. N. (2009). Reconceptualizing the core of nurse practitioner education and practice. *Journal of the American Academy of Nurse Practitioners, 21,* 11–17.

Centers for Disease Control and Prevention. (n.d.). *I PREPARE.* Retrieved from http://www2a.cdc.gov/phtn/envhealth/pdf-files/CARDFRNT.PDF

Chang, C. F. (2001). Access to health care. In C. F. Chang, S. A. Price, & S. K. Pfoutz (Eds.), *Economics and nursing: Critical professional issues* (pp. 335–363). Philadelphia: F. A. Davis.

Cullum, N., Ciliska, D., Marks, S., & Haynes, B. (2008). An introduction to evidence-based nursing. In *Evidence-based nursing: An introduction* (pp. 1–8). Hong Kong: Blackwell Publishing.

DiCenso, A., Guyatt, G., & Ciliska, D. (2005). *Evidenced-based nursing: A guide to clinical practice.* St. Louis, MO: Elsevier Mosby.

Donabedian, A. (1966). Evaluating the quality of medical care. *Milbank Quarterly, 44*(3), 166–203.

Donabedian, A. (1980). *Explorations in quality assessment and monitoring: The definition of quality and approaches to its assessment* (Vol. I). Ann Arbor, MI: Health Administration Press.

Dossey, B. M. (2000). *Florence Nightingale: Mystic, visionary, healer.* Springhouse, PA: Springhouse Corporation.

Dreher, H. M. (2009). Education for advanced practice. In L. A. Joel (Ed.), *Advanced practice nursing: Essentials for role development* (2nd ed., pp. 58–71). Philadelphia: F.A. Davis.

Environmental Protection Agency. (2007). *Climate change: Health and environmental effects.* Retrieved from http://www.epa.gov/climatechange/effects/health.html

Fincham, J. E. (2008). Clinical prevention and population health enabled through the prevention education resource center. *Journal of Public Health Management Practice, 14*(4), 396–399.

Fineout-Overholt, E., & Johnston, L. (2005). Teaching EBP: Asking searchable, answerable clinical questions. *Worldviews on Evidence Based Nursing, 2,* 157–160.

Flemming, K. (2008). Asking answerable questions. In N. Cullum, D. Ciliska, R. B. Haynes, & S. Marks (Eds.), *Evidence-based nursing: An introduction* (pp. 18–23). Hong Kong: Blackwell Publishing.

Fletcher, R. W., & Fletcher, S. W. (2005). Prevention. In *Clinical epidemiology: The Essentials* (4th ed., pp. 147–167). Baltimore: Lippincott Williams & Wilkins.

Ford, J. (2009). The doctorate of nursing practice: Coming into focus. *Advance for Nurse Practitioners, 17*(1), 31–38.

Frisch, N. C., George, V., Giovoni, A. L., Jennings-Sanders, A., & McCahon, C. P. (2003). Teaching nurses to focus on the health needs for populations: A master's degree program in population health nursing. *Nurse Educator, 28*(5), 212–216.

Geraci, E. P. (2004). Planned change. In S. J. Peterson & T. S. Bredow (Eds.), *Middle range theories: Application to nursing research* (pp. 323–340). Philadelphia: Lippincott Williams & Wilkins.

Gévas, J., Starfield, B., & Heath, I. (2008). Is clinical prevention better than cure? *Lancet, 372,* 1997–1999.

Green, L. W., & Kreuter, M. W. (1999). *Health promotion planning: An educational and ecological approach* (3rd ed.). Mountain View, CA: Mayfield.

Green, L. W., & Mercer, S. L. (2006). Precede-Proceed model. In L. Breslow & G. Cengage (Eds.), *Encyclopedia of public health*. Retrieved from http://www.enotes.com/public-health-encyclopedia/precede-proceed-model

Haider, M., & Kreps, G. L. (2004). Forty year of diffusion on innovations: Utility and value in public health. *Journal of Health Communication, 9,* 3–11.

Hall, J. M., Robinson, C. H., & Broyles, T. J. (2007). Environmental health. In M. McEwen & M. A. Nies, *Community/public health nursing: Promoting the health of populations* (4th ed., pp. 236–260). St. Louis, MO: Saunders Elsevier.

Hansen-Turton, T., Ritter, A., Rothman, N., & Valdez, B. (2006). Insurer policies create barriers to health care access and consumer choice. *Nursing Economics, 24*(4), 204–211.

Hansen-Turton, T., Ryan, S., Miller, K., Counts, M., & Nash, D. B. (2007). Convenient care clinics: The future of accessible health care. *Disease Management, 10*(2), 61–73.

Henderson, V. A. (1991). *The nature of nursing: Reflections after 25 years.* New York: National League for Nursing.

Issel, L. M. (2004). *Health program planning and evaluation: A practical, systematic approach for community health.* Sudbury, MA: Jones and Bartlett.

Janssens, A. C., Gwinn, M., Bradley, L. A., Oostra, B. A., van Duijn, C. M., & Khoury, M. J. (2008). A critical appraisal of the scientific basis of commercial genomic profiles used to assess health risks and personalize health intervention. *American Journal of Human Genetics, 82,* 593–599.

Kaplan, L., & Brown, M. (2009). Proud to be a pioneer: Perspectives of a first cohort of DNP students. *American Journal for Nurse Practitioners, 13*(3), 10–20.

Keller, L. O., Strohschein, S., Lia-Hoagberg, B., & Schaffer, M. (1998). Population-based public health nursing interventions: A model from practice. *Public Health Nursing, 15*(3), 207–215.

Leininger, M. (1981). Transcultural nursing: Its progress and its future. *Nursing and Health Care, 2*(7), 365–371.

Leininger, M., & McFarland, M. R. (2006). *Culture care diversity and universality: A worldwide nursing theory* (2nd ed.) Sudbury, MA: Jones and Bartlett.

Lewin, K. (1951). *Field theory in social science.* London: Harper Row.

Lewin, K. (1975). *Field theory in social science.* Westport, CT: Greenwood Press.

McEwen, M., & Nies, M. A. (2007). Health: A community view. In *Community/public health nursing: Promoting the health of populations* (4th ed., pp. 2–18). St. Louis, MO: Saunders Elsevier.

Monsen, R. B. (2009). *Genetics and ethics in health care: New questions in the age of genomic health.* Silver Spring, MD: American Nurses Association.

Mundinger, M. O., Kane, R. L., Lenz, E. R., Totten, A. M., Tsai, W., Cleary, P. D., et al. (2000). Primary care outcomes in patients treated by nurse practitioners or physicians: A randomized trial. *Journal of the American Medical Association, 283*(1), 59–68.

Nelson, R. (2007). Retail health clinics on the rise. *American Journal of Nursing, 107*(7), 25–26.

Newland, J. (2006). Nurse managed health centers: Strengthening the healthcare safety net. *The Nurse Practitioner, 31*(2), 5.

Nies, M. A. & McEwen, M. (Eds.), (2007). *Community/public health nursing: Promoting the health of populations.* St. Louis, MO: Saunders Elsevier.

O'Fallon, L. (2003). NIEHS extramural update: Nursing and environmental health roundtable. *Environmental Health Perspectives, 111*(2). Retrieved from http://www.ehponline.org/docs/2003/111-2/extram-speaking.html

Oncology Nursing Society. (2009). *The role of the oncology nurse in cancer genetic counseling.* Retrieved from http://www.ons.org/publications/positions/documents/pdfs/CancerGenetic.pdf

Pender, N. J. (1975). A conceptual model for preventive health behavior. *Nursing Outlook, 23,* 385–390.

Pender, N. J., Murdaugh, C. L., & Parsons, M. A. (2006). Introduction. In *Health Promotion in Nursing Practice* (5th ed., pp. 1–12). Upper Saddle River, NJ: Pearson Prentice Hall.

Peterson, S. J., & Bredow, T. S. (Eds.). (2004). *Middle range theories: Application to nursing research.* Philadelphia: Lippincott Williams & Wilkins.

Pohl, J. M., Barkauskas, V. H., Benkert, R., Breer, L., & Bostrom A. (2007). Impact of academic nurse-managed centers on communities served. *Journal of the American Academy of Nurse Practitioners, 19,* 268–275.

Prochaska, J. O., Norcross, J. C., & DiClemente, C. C. (1994). *Changing for good: The revolutionary program that explains the six stages of change and teaches you how to free yourself from bad habits.* New York: William Morrow.

Purnell, L. (2002). The Purnell model for cultural competence. *Journal of Transcultural Nursing, 13*(3), 193–196.

Purnell, L., & Paulanka, B. J. (2005). *Guide to culturally competent health care*. Philadelphia: F. A. Davis.

Radzyminski, S. (2007). The concept of population health within the nursing profession. *Journal of Professional Nursing, 23*(1), 37–46.

Riegelman, R. K., Evans, C. H., & Garr, D. R. (2004). Why a clinical prevention and population health curriculum framework? *American Journal of Preventive Medicine, 27*(5), 477.

Rogers, E. M. (2002). The nature of technology transfer. *Science Communication, 23,* 323–341.

Rogers, E. M. (2003). *Diffusion of innovations* (5th ed.). New York: Free Press.

Sattler, B. (2008). *Global warming and public health*. Presented at the 136th APHA Annual Meeting and Exposition, San Diego, CA.

Stanhope, M., & Lancaster, J. (2008). *Public health nursing: Population-centered health care in the community* (7th ed.). St. Louis, MO: Mosby Elsevier.

Tranin, A. S. (2006). The bridge from genomic discoveries to disease prevention. *Oncology Nursing Forum, 33*(5), 891–900.

U.S. Department of Health and Human Services. (2000). *Healthy People 2010: Understanding and improving health* (2nd ed.). Washington, DC: U.S. Government Printing Office.

U.S. Department of Health and Human Services, Secretary's Advisory Committee on Health Promotion and Disease Prevention Objectives for 2020. (2008). *Phase I report: Recommendations for the framework and format of Healthy People 2020*. Retrieved from http://www.healthypeople.gov/hp2020/advisory/PhaseI/PhaseI.pdf

Walker, H. K. (2006). Primary care is dying in the United States: *mutatis mutandis. Medical Education, 40,* 9–11.

Wilson, R. W., & Kolander, C. A. (2011). *Drug abuse prevention: A school and community partnership* (3rd ed.). Sudbury, MA: Jones and Bartlett.

World Health Organization. (n.d.). *The WHO agenda*. Retrieved from http://www.who.int/about/agenda/en/index.html

World Health Organization. (2006). *Constitution of the World Health Organization, basic documents* (45th ed., Supplement). Retrieved from http://www.who.int/governance/eb/who_constitution_en.pdf

World Health Organization. (2008). *Closing the gap in a generation: Health equity by action on the social determinants of health*. Retrieved from http://www.who.int/social_determinants/en

Zahner, S. J., & Block, D. E. (2006). The road to population health: Using *Healthy People 2010* in nursing education. *Journal of Nursing Education, 45*(3), 105–108.

CHAPTER 8

Ethics

Kathryn Waud White, Mary E. Zaccagnini, Katherine H. Casey, and Marcia K. Britain

Ethics, too, are nothing but reverence for life. This is what gives me the fundamental principle of morality, namely, that good consists in maintaining, promoting, and enhancing life, and that destroying, injuring, and limiting life are evil.
—ALBERT SCHWEITZER, *CIVILIZATION AND ETHICS*

We are at the nexus of cataclysmic changes in both the healthcare environment and nursing practice. Because of the complexity of the issues in health care and in society, the growth in communication and emerging technologies, and the sheer amount of information available, advanced practice nurses (APNs) must not only incorporate ethics into practice but into their professional identity as well. We are not only aware of worldwide issues, we can affect world issues and are affected by them. We now understand that our healthcare environment is interrelated to the issues of the world, not just to our own individual practice and community. For example, hunger is a local, national, and world issue that could affect our practice. Where does nursing stand on these issues? Are we our brother's keeper? Now that we are aware of these issues as a result of advances in technology and communication, where do our responsibilities lie? With the homeless shelter down the street? With the Salvation Army in national disaster areas? Or with Nurses Without Borders? Are our ethical obligations limited to our practice of nursing or should they be incorporated into our person?

The Doctor of Nursing Practice (DNP) graduate must thoroughly understand the ethical aspects of the issues in health care and the world. DNP graduates are prepared not only to identify ethical issues but also to lead discussions and formulate approaches to resolve ethical dilemmas (American Association of Colleges of Nursing [AACN], 2006). The public looks up to nurses, and nurses hold the public trust. For seven years running, nurses have been at the top of the list in the annual Gallup survey of the perceived honesty and ethics of professions ("Nurses Top Honesty List," 2009). This trust emerges from a number of different sources, such as the development of nursing as a profession that is rich in religious tradition and founded in strong ethical statements from our professional practice associations. Nevertheless, as holders of public trust, nurses also bear the responsibility for understanding and acting on ethical issues at a local, national, and global level.

This chapter presents a brief overview of ethical principles and nursing standards. It is by no means a comprehensive review of normative ethics; rather, it is intended to refresh the memory of the reader and precipitate discussion of ethical issues. The chapter also presents a framework for understanding how nurse leaders develop competency in ethical decision making. The chapter was written in an effort to promote discussion and to pose difficult and provocative questions related to compelling ethical issues confronting advanced practice nursing so that the reader can further develop and hone leadership competencies in ethical decision making. The chapter has a special emphasis on issues that are particularly salient to nurse leaders prepared with the Doctor of Nursing Practice degree.

Overview of Ethical Principles

To care for anyone else enough to make their problems one's own, is ever the beginning of one's real ethical development.

—FELIX ADLER

History

Modern healthcare ethics is built on a history of medical malfeasance in research using human subjects. In 1947, the Nuremberg Code was written in response to the trial of physicians who performed medical experimentation on prisoners during World War II in Nazi Germany (Mitscherlich & Mielke, 1949). This code forms the basis of our modern understanding of medical ethics. It outlines ten standards that must be present in order to conduct research on human subjects. It includes the concepts of informed consent, the right of the individual to self-determination, the thoughtful evaluation of risks and benefits, discussion of risks and benefits with the subject before enrollment in the research, and the avoidance of harm to the person. This code is accepted internationally. In 1964, the World Medical Association took these ethical principles and developed the Helsinki Declaration, which made recommendations for physicians involved in human experimentation. The Declaration has undergone many revisions and is now reflected in the Good Clinical Practices document promulgated by the World Medical Association.

The Tuskegee Syphilis Study was conducted by the U.S. Public Health Service in Alabama from 1932 to 1972, although it was originally designed to last only six months. The study followed the progression of untreated syphilis in poor black sharecroppers in Tuskegee, Alabama. The intent was to secure funding for syphilis treatment programs in this population. In 1947, penicillin was demonstrated to be a curative agent for syphilis. Nevertheless, this efficacious treatment was withheld from the study participants. Intense public outcry followed an investigative report from the Associated Press in 1972. The Assistant Secretary for Health and Scientific Affairs appointed an investigative panel. The panel revealed that the men in the study did not give informed consent, did not get proper treatment for their condition following the discovery that penicillin was curative, were not informed of this cure, and were not informed that they could quit the study. In response to the ethical shortcomings unearthed by investigation into the Tuskegee Syphilis Study, Congress passed the National Research Act in 1974. This act produced the National Commission for the Protection of Human Subjects of Biomedical and Behavioral Research, and this commission in turn produced the Belmont Report (Centers for Disease Control and Prevention [CDC], 2009).

The Belmont Report is a landmark document that laid the ethical foundation for research in the United States. It identifies three major ethical principles: respect for persons, beneficence, and justice (National Commission for the Protection of Human Subjects of Biomedical and Behavioral Research, 1979). In 1981, the Food and Drug Administration and the Department of Health and Human Services issued federal regulations based on the Belmont Report. In 1991, the Department of Health and Human Services regulations were formally adopted by other federal departments and agencies that conduct human experimentation. Today, these regulations are known as the Common Rule.

Other well-publicized medical ethical issues (Table 8-1) that have formed our current discussion include the ethics related to the transplantation of organs, Karen Ann Quinlan and end-of-life issues, Jack Kevorkian and physician-assisted suicide, the Human Genome Project, stem cell research, and cloning.

■ Table 8-1 Medical Ethical Issues That Have Caused Debate

Date	Case	Ethical Issue
1932–1972	Tuskegee Syphilis Study	Lack of consent; withholding treatment and education
1949	Nuremberg Trial	Horrific medical experimentation without consent
1954	First kidney transplant	Organ transplantation guidelines emerged
1954–present	Organ transplantation	Distribution of organs
1960	Cardiopulmonary resuscitation	Prolonging life versus limited resources
1973	Roe v. Wade	Abortion legalized in United States
1985	Karen Ann Quinlan	Unlawful killing versus withdrawal of care
1986	Baby M	Surrogate motherhood
1990	Jack Kevorkian	Physician-assisted suicide found to be outside the law
1996	Dolly the Sheep	First cloned mammal
2003	Human Genome Project	Use of genetic material in research
2006	Evans' request for frozen embryo	European Court of Human Rights rules against embryo's independent right to life
2009	Suleman octuplets	In vitro fertilization
Present	Stem cell research	Origin of stem cells for research

Basic Principles

Beauchamp and Childress (2001), who are leaders in the United States in the area of medical ethics education, expanded on the Belmont Report's principles as they relate to professional nursing practice. Their four guiding ethical principles are respect for autonomy, nonmaleficence, beneficence, and justice.

RESPECT FOR AUTONOMY

Autonomy: Self-directed freedom, especially moral independence

The principle of respect for autonomy is at the heart of informed consent or refusal. Two philosophers, Immanuel Kant and John Mills, formed the modern concept of respect for autonomy: Mills believed that individuals have the right to develop according to their potential and that societal controls should not be exercised unless others are at risk of harm (Beauchamp & Childress, 2009). An example of this is the individual who drinks and drives. Although society does not completely forbid drinking and driving, individuals may place other people at risk when they do so. Therefore, to limit the risk of harm to others, society has developed laws and constraints on how much alcohol any individual can legally have in his or her system while driving a vehicle.

Kant believed that each person has inherent worth and the right to make his or her own decisions. To make decisions related to one's health, patients must be fully informed as to the risks, benefits, and alternatives. It is the APN's ethical obligation to give full disclosure of all facts relevant to the provision of care in such a manner that patients can understand. The APN must be respectful of individuals' choices when this information is given to them, even when the practitioner disagrees with a patient's decision. The APN must also be respectful of those whose decisions are guided by outside influences such as religious beliefs or cultural customs. In this context, an individual may choose to refuse a blood transfusion in accordance with his or her religious traditions, but must be fully informed of the risk of doing so. Autonomy can also include an individual transferring decisional authority to another person. In some cultures this may mean giving information to a third party who will then make a decision related to the health care of the individual. As DNPs enter into the current debate on healthcare reform in America, they must be informed of the debate about policy changes so that the principle of respect for autonomy is maintained.

NONMALEFICENCE

Nonmaleficence: Avoidance of harm

"It may seem a strange principle to enunciate as the very first requirement in a Hospital that it should do the sick no harm." This quote from Florence Nightingale over 100 years ago points to the ethical principle of nonmaleficence, which is as relevant today as it was then. We have only to think of the number of patients harmed through poor handwashing practices throughout the years to understand how healing professionals have unintentionally inflicted harm. The principle of not inflicting harm encompasses more than simply not hurting someone. In most instances, it is a matter of a risk–benefit analysis. For example, is it inflicting harm to surgically remove a breast for cancer even though the person's life is spared? Is it acceptable to inflict harm if the ultimate goal is to save life? The role of the APN is to assist the patient through this risk–benefit analysis with information and patience and without imposing his or her personal values on the patient. Risk–benefit analysis is inherent in most healthcare decisions or recommendations.

BENEFICENCE

Beneficence: An action that is done for the benefit of others

Nonmaleficence and beneficence are intertwined in many instances. The most common ethical dilemma for the APN is balancing beneficence and nonmaleficence (Pantilat, 2008). The rapid expansion of technologies has sometimes created situations in which treatment can inflict harm. Many end-of-life ethical issues are related to beneficence, weighing the risk of the intervention against the comfort and wishes of the patient or surrogate decision maker. The issue of allowing natural death to occur versus actively giving medications that would hasten the patient's death is relevant to these principles. If a patient is at the end of life, allowing natural death to occur while providing measures to increase comfort and quality of life is an act of beneficence. Actively assisting a patient to die is killing, and although it may end suffering, euthanasia is in contradiction to the principle of nonmaleficence (American Nurses Association [ANA], 2001, p. 8).

On a more global scale, if we as nurses are aware of global atrocities such as famine, genocide, or injustices and do not speak out against them to prevent harm from coming to that population, are we ignoring the ethical principles of nonmaleficence and beneficence? What are our obligations in these situations as individuals and as a profession?

JUSTICE

Justice: The quality of being just, impartial, or fair

> *Where justice is denied, where poverty is enforced, where ignorance prevails, and where any one class is made to feel that society is an organized conspiracy to oppress, rob and degrade them, neither persons nor property will be safe.*
> —FREDERICK DOUGLASS

The most fundamental principle of justice is that "Equals should be treated equally and unequals should be treated unequally" (Aristotle). Justice is often a question of distribution of resources. One of the current debates in health-care reform centers on equal access to health care. It is well established that many Americans do not have healthcare insurance and thus do not have access to the health care they need. In addition, not all healthcare plans are created equal. Some insurance policies may not provide the same level of protection from financial harm or the same level of benefits as others. In rural areas, people may not have access to specialized treatment that they require. How do we position resources so that the most good comes from the limited resources of healthcare professionals? Given the current inequities, the doctorally prepared nurse should adhere to the principle of justice through advocating for equal access to health care for all citizens.

Framework for Developing Ethical Competency

Never ascribe to malice that which can adequately be explained by incompetence.
—NAPOLEON BONAPARTE

Three of the AACN's essentials for doctoral education have ethical compo-nents to them. Essential II states that "DNP graduates have the ability to organize care to address emerging practice problems and the ethical dilemmas that emerge as new diagnostic and therapeutic technologies evolve. Accordingly, DNP graduates are able to assess risk and collaborate with others to manage risks ethically, based on professional standards" (AACN, 2006, p. 11). Thus, the DNP graduate should exhibit advanced skills in eth-ical decision making. Competence in identification and resolution of ethical dilemmas does not come simply by reading books and articles. Like most skills, it needs to be processed and practiced before the practitioner can become fully competent.

Hamric and Delgado (2009) suggest that there are four phases of devel-opment of competency in ethical decision making. Phase 1 is *knowledge devel-opment:* learning the language, theories, and professional guidelines that enable the new professional to develop sensitivity about ethical problems. This phase includes clarification of one's own ethical values. It is appropriate in this phase to gather information about ethics and professional codes of ethics. Typically, this starts in the nurse's undergraduate education. In the graduate school curriculum, knowledge is further developed through reading of classical works and professional codes and through discussions. This prepares the nurse for the next phase of competency development, *knowledge application:* application of the learned theories and ethical decision-making frameworks to clinical ethical dilemmas, often in consultation with other healthcare professionals. The APN is able to identify ethical dilemmas when they occur but may need help in processing the dilemma and selecting a course of action to resolve the dilemma. As the skill of the APN increases in this arena, he or she is ready for phase 3: *creating a moral environment.* The APN takes on the role of mentor or role model within the practice environment to create systems change. As practitioners mature into these mentoring relationships, their skill in identification and resolution of ethical dilemmas grows. This may include participation on ethics committees and eventually chairing institution-wide ethics committees. Phase 4 is *promoting social justice within the healthcare system.* This is the life work of the doctorally prepared nurse: creating lasting change in healthcare systems large and small (Hamric & Delgado, 2009). AACN Essential II implies a far larger application of ethics than just the immediate practice environment.

Ethics is cited specifically as a part of the competencies expected from the DNP graduate in two additional sections within the *Essentials* document. Essential I states that DNP educational programs will prepare the graduate to "[i]ntegrate nursing science with knowledge from ethics, the biophysical, psychosocial, analytical, and organizational sciences as the basis of the highest level of nursing" (AACN, 2006, p. 9). Essential V states that the DNP graduate will have the skills to "[a]dvocate for social justice, equity, and ethical policies within all healthcare arenas" (AACN, 2006, p. 14). It is clear from these three essentials that the vision of the DNP held by the champions of the clinical doctorate in nursing is that each graduate will be an advocate for change within the entire healthcare system and the nation. That change has an ethical dimension to it and demands a clear understanding of ethical principles coupled with the ability to apply those principles to real-life situations.

Ethical Codes of Nursing

The American Nurses Association's Code of Ethics

Relativity applies to physics, not ethics.

—ALBERT EINSTEIN

Nursing has a written set of ethical standards for practice known as the Code of Ethics for Nurses (Table 8-2) (ANA, 2001). The American Nurses Association has developed, promulgated, and promoted these standards. The history of the development of these standards mirrors the development of nursing into a profession. The first code was the "Nightingale Pledge," which was written by Mrs. Lystra E. Gretter for the graduating class of nursing students at Farrand Training School for Nurses in Detroit, Michigan, in 1893 (ANA, n.d.). The most recent version of the code was adopted by the ANA in 2001. It took a 12-member task force five years to produce the document, reflecting the complexity of the ethical issues nurses face. The code is the guiding document for daily practice, a concise statement of the ethical

■ **Table 8-2   ANA's Code of Ethics for Nurses**

---

1) The nurse, in all professional relationships, practices with compassion and respect for the inherent dignity, worth, and uniqueness of every individual, unrestricted by considerations of social or economic status, personal attributes, or the nature of health problems.

2) The nurse's primary commitment is to the patient, whether an individual, family, group, or community.

3) The nurse promotes, advocates for, and strives to protect the health, safety, and rights of the patient.

4) The nurse is responsible and accountable for individual nursing practice and determines the appropriate delegation of tasks consistent with the nurse's obligation to provide optimum patient care.

5) The nurse owes the same duties to self as to others, including the responsibility to preserve integrity and safety, to maintain competence, and to continue personal and professional growth.

6) The nurse participates in establishment, maintaining, and improving health environments and conditions of employment conducive to the provision of quality health care and consistent with the values of the profession through individual and collective action.

7) The nurse participates in the advancement of the profession through contributions to practice, education, administration, and knowledge development.

8) The nurse collaborates with other health care professionals and the public in promoting community, national, and international efforts to meet health needs.

9) The profession of nursing, as represented by associations and their members, is responsible for articulating nursing values, for maintaining the integrity of the profession and its practice, and for shaping social policy.

Source: American Nurses Association. (2001). *Code of ethics for nurses with interpretive statements.* Washington, DC: Author. Reprinted with permission.

responsibilities of individual nurses, the "nonnegotiable" ethical standard of the profession, and an expression of the nursing profession's understanding of its ethical commitment to society (ANA, 2001).

It is the recommendation of the chapter authors that every nurse have a copy of the Code of Ethics at hand. The Code of Ethics can be obtained from the American Nurses Association. The ANA task force deconstructed each provision with interpretive statements. The first three provisions affirm what has been described as nursing's fundamental values (White, 2001). The first provision names "compassion and respect for the inherent dignity, worth, and uniqueness of every individual" (ANA, 2001, p. 7) as values central to the practice of nursing. The second provision reaffirms that "the nurse's primary commitment is to the patient, whether that be one person, a family or an entire community" (p. 9). It discusses concepts relevant to conflict of interest and professional boundaries in the context of our primary commitment to the patient. The third provision states that the nurse will "promote, advocate for and strive to protect the health, safety, and rights of patients" (p. 12). This provision covers the topics of confidentiality, human research subjects, standards of practice, incompetence, and impaired providers in the context of protecting patients (ANA, 2001). Because the American Association of Nurses has articulated this Code of Ethics, it has earned the right for nursing to participate in ethical discussions at all levels. These three foundational ethical principles earn nursing the right to a seat at the table when discussions about issues of health care occur on a local, state, national, and international level.

The next three provisions describe the boundaries of nursing practice and duty (ANA, 2001; White, 2001). The fourth provision states, "The nurse is responsible and accountable for individual nursing practice and determines the appropriate delegation of tasks consistent with the nurse's obligation to provide optimal patient care" (ANA, 2001, p. 16). Concepts of accountability, responsibility, and delegation of tasks are discussed. Provision 5 notes that the nurse has the same ethical duties to himself or herself as to others. In that context, professional growth, maintenance of competence, character, and professional integrity are discussed. The code supports a nurse's right to decline to participate in activities (either in direct patient care or institutional decisions about patient care) that breach ethical boundaries. In fact, the nurse is obligated to bring those situations to the attention of the appropriate committee or body without abandoning the patient. In the last provision of this series, provision 6, the nurse is to participate in creating healthcare environments that lend themselves to the provision of quality patient care. This provision supports respectful communication, habits of excellence, and the development of practice environments that foster ethical practices (ANA, 2001).

The final three provisions describe the duties of the nurse beyond the individual practice (ANA, 2001; White, 2001). Provision 7 describes participation in the advancement of the profession itself. Provision 8 describes collaboration with other health professionals to improve the health of the community, the nation, and the world (ANA, 2001). Now that technology and improved communication have made us aware of international issues, where do our obligations lie—with the clinic for homeless veterans down the street or with international aid relief programs? Are our ethical obligations limited to our practice or should they be incorporated into our professional identity?

The ninth provision outlines the ethical obligations of our professional associations and societies, asserting that the professional associations articulate the values of the profession and that our collective wisdom on this is representative of the profession. It describes the contract with society that nursing holds, the integrity of the profession, and the role of the profession in social reform (ANA, 2001). In the end, this provision upholds the notion that nursing is a distinctive profession, different from other types of healthcare providers; with that notion come responsibilities regarding the microcosm of health care in our own practices and the macrocosm of health care in the world. These final three provisions support the doctoral education of advanced practice nurses in that the AACN *Essentials* (2006) speak very specifically about systems leadership (Essential II), healthcare policy advocacy (Essential V), interprofessional collaboration for improving patient and population outcomes (Essential VI), and clinical prevention and population health for improving the nation's health (Essential VII). All of these elements of the expected competencies of the DNP graduate speak to this broader picture of the macrocosm of the nation's health.

The ANA's Standards of Nursing Practice

Art, like morality, consists of drawing the line somewhere.

—G. K. CHESTERTON

The American Nurses Association, as one of the primary professional associations of nurses, has the responsibility to develop, promote, and articulate the standards of nursing practice (ANA, 2004). These standards represent the profession's self-described standard of practice. Because the standards were developed by the professional association and its membership, they reflect the profession's ideals, values, and agenda. They represent a baseline competency, not excellence in practice. Nevertheless, because they are written in measurable terms, the standards delineate nursing's accountability to the public as a profession and as individual practitioners (ANA, 2004). Standard of Professional Practice 12 is the practice standard concerning ethics. It simply states, "The registered nurse integrates ethical provisions in all areas of practice" (p. 39). The measurement criteria are as follows.

The registered nurse:

- Uses Code of Ethics for Nurses with Interpretive Statements (ANA, 2001) to guide practice.
- Delivers care in a manner that preserves and protects patient autonomy, dignity, and rights.
- Maintains patient confidentiality within legal and regulatory parameters.
- Serves as a patient advocate assisting patients in developing skills for self advocacy.
- Maintains a therapeutic and professional patient-nurse relationship with appropriate professional role boundaries.
- Demonstrates a commitment to practicing self-care, managing stress, and connecting with self and others.
- Contributes to resolving ethical issues of patients, colleagues, or systems as evidenced in such activities as participation on ethics committees.
- Reports illegal, incompetent, or impaired practices. (ANA, 2004, p. 39)

The ANA recognizes the additional ethical obligations of advanced practice nurses with additional measurement criteria.

The advanced practice nurse:

- Informs the patient of the risks, benefits, and outcomes of healthcare regimens.
- Participates in interdisciplinary teams that address ethical risks, benefits, and outcomes. (ANA, 2004, p. 39)

The ANA includes statements that reflect the complexity of specialty roles through additional measurement criteria for this group as well.

The registered nurse in a nursing role specialty:

- Participates on multidisciplinary and interdisciplinary teams that address ethical risks, benefits, and outcomes.
- Informs administrators or others of the risks, benefits, and outcomes of programs and decisions that affect healthcare delivery. (ANA, 2004, p. 39)

The Doctor of Nursing Practice program fits into both additional statements. Not only is the program of study intended to educate advanced practice nurses at the highest level of clinical practice, but also it intentionally adds advocacy, economics, population health, and other courses that are foundational to the emerging specialty roles such as quality improvement, administration, education, and informatics and other roles that are a blend of traditional nursing and other knowledge areas.

The International Council of Nurses' Code of Ethics for Nurses

The first step in the evolution of ethics is a sense of solidarity with other human beings.

—ALBERT SCHWEITZER

The International Council of Nurses (ICN) represents nurses in 120 nations around the world. The ICN adopted a code of ethics in 1953. Most recently the code was appraised for relevancy to practice and revised in 2006 (ICN, 2006). The code outlines four basic responsibilities of nurses: health promotion, disease prevention, health restoration, and alleviation of suffering (Table 8-3). The ICN's code also describes four principle elements that it believes define standards of ethical conduct.

The ICN gives examples of applications of the elements for nurses in different roles (see Appendix 8-1). The ICN tools apply to practice as an advanced practice nurse as well. The DNP-prepared nurse is well qualified to practice in an ethical environment consistent with the ICN Code of Ethics for Nurses in all advanced practice roles, including those of educator, administrator, and researcher.

■ Table 8-3   ICN's Code of Ethics for Nurses

1. Nurses and People
   - The nurse's primary professional responsibility is to people requiring nursing care.
   - In providing care, the nurse promotes an environment in which the human rights, values, customs and spiritual beliefs of the individual, the family and the community are respected.
   - The nurse ensures that the individual receives sufficient information on which to base consent for care and related treatment.
   - The nurse holds in confidence personal information and uses judgment in sharing this information.
   - The nurse shares with society the responsibility for initiating and supporting action to meet the health and social needs of the public, particularly those of vulnerable populations.
   - The nurse also shares the responsibility to sustain and protect the natural environment from depletion, pollution, degradation and destruction.

2. Nurses and Practice
   - The nurse carries personal responsibility and accountability for nursing practice, and for maintaining competence by continual learning.
   - The nurse maintains a standard of personal health such that the ability to provide care is not compromised.
   - The nurse uses judgment regarding individual competence when accepting and delegating responsibility.
   - The nurse at all times maintains standards of personal conduct which reflect well on the profession and enhance public confidence.
   - The nurse, in providing care, ensures that use of technology and scientific advances are compatible with the safety, dignity and rights of people.

3. Nurses and the Profession
   - The nurse assumes the major role in determining and implementing acceptable standards of clinical nursing practice, management, research and education.
   - The nurse is active in developing a core of research-based professional knowledge.
   - The nurse, acting through the professional organization, participates in creating and maintaining safe, equitable social and economic working conditions in nursing.

4. The Nurse and Co-Workers
   - The nurse sustains a co-operative relationship with co-workers in nursing and other fields.
   - The nurse takes appropriate action to safeguard individuals, families and communities when their health is endangered by a co-worker or any other person.

Source: International Council of Nurses. (2006). *The ICN code of ethics for nurses.* Geneva, Switzerland: Author. Reprinted with permission.

Ethical Issues and Current Debates Relevant to the DNP

There are many issues relevant to health care today (Table 8-4). Those issues are local (practice) issues, national issues, and international issues, the latter primarily related to the problems of third world countries and their health-care systems. It is of utmost importance that advanced practice nurses be knowledgeable about these issues and able to articulate their ethical dimensions. The case studies presented here are by no means inclusive and do not reflect the personal biases of the authors. The goal for this section is to stimulate reflection, thought, and the development of ethical competency in the people who read it.

As part of the development of ethical competency, nurses must identify the ethical dimensions of current issues, practice analyzing ethical dilemmas, and explore potential interventions and solutions. The following examples are intended to precipitate reflection, discussion, and individual or group debate.

Local Ethical Issue: Refusal to Provide Care Based on Personal Beliefs

Abortion is now and has always been a divisive issue for society and can be especially challenging for nurses. The general consensus is that one either supports the right of women to choose abortion or one does not. Neither side seems to be able to find much middle ground. If a patient who had an abortion procedure and then experienced postprocedure complications were transferred to another hospital unit or clinic and assigned to a nurse whose religious beliefs were against abortion, would this nurse have the ethical right to refuse care to this patient? Is this a religious, moral, or ethical issue? If the nurse exchanged this patient assignment with a colleague who was not against abortion, would this still be considered an issue, and would it be considered an ethical one?

A second issue related to a belief system judgment could be one in which a liver transplant was performed on a man who was incarcerated for a felony conviction, and the advanced practice nurse on the transplant service who would provide postoperative care had an issue regarding organ allocation to an individual who had committed a heinous act against society. Again, would this nurse be within his or her right to refuse care to this patient if the nurse provided another qualified nurse to accept this patient? Is this an ethical or moral issue, and is this nurse within his or her right to refuse to care for this

■ Table 8-4 Ethical Issues and Current Debates Relevant to the DNP

Level	Issue
Intraprofessional	Safety of healthcare delivery Aging nursing population Shortage of nursing faculty Succession Impaired providers Maintenance of competence in a rapidly changing environment
National	Access to health care Economics of health care Stem cell research Abortion debate Privacy issues and advanced technology End-of-life issues Human cloning Discrimination and racism in health care Cultural issues Assisted suicide Reparations DNPs providing primary care ABCC primary care certification Disaster preparedness Organ transplantation (international aspects) Genetics and genomics
International	Genocide Worldwide oppression of women and minorities Genital mutilation Famine and disease Clean water Basic sanitation Spread of pandemic disease (e.g., HIV) Access to basic medical care
DNP	Faculty shortage Additional cost of education Titling issues Practice issues Parity between providers Impact on nursing research Time lag from discovery of new knowledge to dissemination

patient? What does the law of your state say about this issue? What does the ANA Code of Ethics say about these situations? How would you use these documents to guide your decisions?

National Ethical Issue: Genetic Testing

Recently there has been a proliferation of testing modalities for genetic markers of disease. One example is the BRACA gene for breast or ovarian cancer. Use of these tests has the potential to save many lives through monitoring and preventive surgery. However, they have also created the ethical dilemma of privacy concerns and the identification of genetic tendencies that will affect individuals' ability to get health insurance (ANA Code of Ethics Principle 3). Consider the ethical dimensions of genetic testing in conception and pregnancy. What is our ethical obligation to the couple who both test positive for sickle cell disease, cystic fibrosis, or Tay-Sachs disease? Should we counsel them to avoid having children or advise testing in utero? When considering all of these ethical aspects, should we even encourage testing? How do we respect the patient's or family's autonomy when they choose courses of action that are inconsistent with our own moral framework and beliefs? The ethical tension in this situation arises from the two apparently conflicting principles of patient autonomy versus the welfare of others (the ethical principle of justice). This issue has aspects of distributive justice as well: Is it ethical to bring children into the world who have numerous known medical issues that will consume enormous resources while others wait for care or cannot get insurance?

International Ethical Issue: Genocide

Genocide is an atrocity committed against an entire nation or group of people. The United Nations General Assembly adopted the Convention on the Prevention and Punishment of the Crime of Genocide in 1948 (Schabas, 2008), which defines genocide as follows:

> In the present Convention, genocide means any of the following acts committed with intent to destroy, in whole or in part, a national, ethnical, racial or religious group, as such:
>
> (a) Killing members of the group;
> (b) Causing serious bodily or mental harm to members of the group;
> (c) Deliberately inflicting on the group conditions of life calculated to bring about its physical destruction in whole or in part;

(d) Imposing measures intended to prevent births within the group;

(e) Forcibly transferring children of the group to another group. (Office of the United Nations High Commissioner for Human Rights, 2007)

The international group Genocide Watch has posted "Genocide Alerts" for eight countries: Sudan, Ethiopia, Burundi, Kenya, Myanmar, Uzbekistan, Chad, and Zimbabwe (Genocide Watch, 2009). We know of these situations through the news services that bring the issue into our homes daily. What is our ethical obligation as nurses to intervene, and how is that done? Provision 8 of the ANA's Code of Ethics clearly states that we have an ethical obligation to the world. People have the right to self-determination and respect, even if they are of different cultural, ethnic, or religious backgrounds (Hamric & Delgado, 2009). Is genocide a violation of the ethical principle of autonomy? Why or why not? Although the ANA's position statement on ethics and human rights (ANA, 1994) does not specifically identify international human rights as a focus, is action to eliminate genocide an extension of the ethical position the ANA has articulated? Is it an extension of the ICN's Code of Ethics? What group is best suited for international intervention?

Ethical Issues Surrounding the DNP Degree

Not long after the first utterance of the phrase "Doctor of Nursing Practice," a vigorous debate began within nursing and related fields about many aspects of this clinical doctorate. The pros and cons of the degree itself and the impact it will have as a requirement for entry into advanced practice have generated many articles and editorials in nursing journals and newspapers. The debate continues today and ranges from issues of the overall nursing shortage to the titling debate. Many of the issues raised have elements of ethical dilemmas. One article by Silva and Ludwick (2006) asked the question "Is the doctor of nursing practice ethical?"

This section examines some of the ethical issues that have been raised in regard to the DNP degree itself, the wisdom of requiring a clinical doctorate for entry into practice, and ethical issues for particular specialties within nursing. This is an evolving topic and deserves some reading, thought, reflection, and discussion by students, DNP faculty, and practicing DNPs.

Factors that contribute to the evolving nature of this ethics debate include the increasing complexity of care, the leadership roles that DNPs may take in health care and management, and business opportunities for the DNP. There will also be different practice settings and levels of practice open to the

DNP-prepared advanced practice nurse, and competency in several aspects of ethics is necessary. In addition to traditional clinical bioethics, the DNP must be competent in the areas of business, research, and legal ethics (Pierce & Smith, 2008). Pierce and Smith have proposed a framework for curricula that address all arenas of ethics that the DNP may need to enter. What we present in this section is a list of topics to spark vigorous but respectful debate in the nursing community about ethical aspects of the DNP degree as a requirement for entry into advanced nursing practice or expanded nursing roles.

COST

Cost is one of the issues frequently discussed as relevant to the proposed requirement of the clinical doctorate for nursing to enter into advanced practice. As we move from master's degree programs for preparation of advanced practice nurses into the DNP framework, the length of the programs will increase from a minimum of 24 months to a minimum of 36 months. An increase in the length of an educational program implies an increase in the cost of that education, which is borne by the student, the institution, and society.

Recent studies have demonstrated that care delivered by advanced practice nurses is comparable to that delivered by physician general practitioners (Dierick-van Daele, Metsemakers, Derckx, Spreeuwenberg, & Vrijhoef, 2009; Horrocks, Anderson, & Salisbury, 2002; Mundinger et al., 2000). Presently nurse practitioners are educated at the master's-degree level in the United States. If the quality of advanced practice nursing at the master's level is comparable to that delivered by primary care physicians, is it ethical to demand a program that increases the cost of educating these nurses? In the face of a shortage of nurses, is it ethical to demand that nurses who are preparing to enter advanced practice roles study for an additional year before they reenter the nursing workforce in an expanded capacity? Is the added benefit to society from nurses who are competent in the eight essentials as described by the AACN (2006) worth the added cost for this education? Are we doing harm to the population by requiring this additional education? Are we ensuring greater access to health care or merely delaying the entry into practice of providers we know are safe and efficacious? What is the greater good?

TITLING

The issue of titling has generated more comment than any other issue regarding the DNP. In April of 2008, the *Minneapolis Star-Tribune* ran an article highlighting several graduates of the University of Minnesota School of Nursing's first DNP program (Yee, 2008). Fourteen of the 32 comments posted concerned the title "Doctor" in some manner, including this one:

> What is in a word?
>
> It is interesting that the discussion is focused on the use of the title doctor. A doctorate simply means that the person who earned it is prepared at the highest level of that profession. Physicians are prepared at the highest level of medical practice. The DNP is prepared at the highest level of nursing practice. Nurses and physicians are licensed independently of each other. Both the MD and the DNP have earned the right to call themselves "doctor". Perhaps the confusion would be lessened if we identified ourselves as physicians or nurses or pharmacists or chiropractors or physical therapists or audiologists whose title is doctor. In the coming healthcare crisis, it will take all professionals in the healing arts to work together to provide solutions to the problems we face as a nation in making top notch care available to all of our people. Our energy might be better spent thinking about solutions instead of quibbling over titles.
>
> Posted by kwhitecrna April 27 @ 3:12 PM

In this blog, comments from the public reflect concerns that nurses will represent themselves as physicians. In turn, this reflects inadequate understanding of the difference between nursing practice and medical practice. Nevertheless, because nursing holds a high degree of public trust, ethical concerns raised by the public must be addressed by the profession and by individual nurses. Nurses should not misrepresent themselves as physicians, but they should use such opportunities to inform the patient population about the practice of nursing at the doctoral level.

The American Medical Association initially expressed considerable opposition to the use of the term *doctor* by practitioners who are not physicians (American College of Nurse Practitioners [ACNP], 2006). Not only were there concerns about use of the title "Doctor" in the clinical setting but also about encroachment of other professionals into the scope of practice of medicine. After some debate and compromise, the American Medical Association House of Delegates revised the language in the resolution to simply state that professionals in the healthcare setting should clearly identify themselves and their qualifications and degrees attained. This approach is similar to what other professional organizations recommend (ACNP, 2006). At the same time, the AMA also supports state legislation that would make it a felony crime to misrepresent oneself as a physician (ACNP, 2006).

The clinical doctorate is granted in recognition of the highest level of practice. It is not the exclusive property of physicians. There are doctors of pharmacy, doctors of chiropractic, doctors of physical therapy, doctors of audiology, doctors of psychology, doctors of naturopathy, doctors of optometry, and doctors of public health, as well as other emerging clinical doctorates. No single profession owns the title "Doctor," but it is important to note that none of the nonphysician specialties wants to use the title "physician." A degree is not a role; it is an academic credential. It is appropriate for DNP graduates to use the title of "Doctor" to introduce themselves in their role as advanced practice nurses. The emphasis must be on clarification of roles. Nursing and medicine are different roles that both recognize the attainment of the highest level of practice through the granting of a doctoral degree. Seven national nursing organizations met at the Nurse Practitioner Roundtable in June of 2008 and constructed a unified statement on certification and titling (Nurse Practitioner Roundtable, 2008). The statement from this body is that "Recognition of the title 'Doctor' for doctorally prepared nurse practitioners facilitates parity within the health care system."

Is it ethical for DNP-prepared nurses to use the title "Doctor" in the clinical setting, knowing that it may generate some confusion in the patient population? Is it ethical for one group of professionals to claim the title of "Doctor" when the degree is simply a degree? Who gets to decide who may call themselves a doctor? Does the use of the academic title "Doctor" facilitate parity among providers within the healthcare system?

THE DNP EXAMINATION

In 2008, the Council for Advancement of Comprehensive Care (CACC) and the National Board of Medical Examiners (NBME) met and developed a comprehensive examination for DNP graduates (American Board of Comprehensive Care [ABCC], 2008). The intent of the exam is to assess the knowledge and skills of the DNP, primarily as related to the advanced practice nurse in primary care settings. The exam is similar to the U.S. Medical Licensing Examination Step 3.

The use of the DNP examination has generated much debate within the nursing profession and within the medical profession. In 2009, the first examination was given and had a pass rate of about 50% (ABCC, 2009). These DNPs will have the additional credential of Diplomat in Comprehensive Care granted by the American Board of Comprehensive Care. In March of 2009, the American Association of Colleges of Nursing responded to questions and concerns with a statement about the examination (AACN, 2009a). The statement refers to the unified statement on credentialing and titling crafted by the seven national nursing organizations: all APRNs are credentialed through the use of national certification examinations administered by *nursing* certification bodies that address the skills and knowledge necessary for that specialty practice (APRN Consensus Work Group, 2008). These national examinations are then used by state boards of nursing to grant the authority to practice as an APRN (AACN, 2009a).

The American Medical Association has taken a stance objecting to the use of this examination and accused national nursing organizations of misrepresenting the examination (Sorrell, 2009). In this same article, Mary Mundinger, DPH, RN, Dean of Columbia University School of Nursing, is quoted as saying, "If nurses can show that they can pass the same test at the same level of competency, there's no rational argument for reimbursing them at a lower rate or giving them less authority in caring for patients" (Sorrell, 2009). Does this examination add to the confusion over the roles and qualifications of healthcare providers? Does it facilitate parity between healthcare providers? Will the use of this examination improve the ability of nurse practitioners to provide care to patients in primary care settings? Does it ensure a higher quality of care provided by nurse practitioners in this clinical setting? Do we really need this examination in the face of evidence that APN primary care is equivalent to that of general practitioners?

IMPACT ON NURSING RESEARCH

Will the DNP decrease the number of nurses entering existing PhD programs and potentially decrease the amount of nursing research? Meleis and Dracup (2005) posit that the development of the DNP course of study will inhibit the development of nurse scientists and potentially decrease research into the very evidence upon which the advanced practice nurse depends to deliver effective care. According to the AACN website, the number of nursing students in doctoral programs increased by 20.9% between 2007 and 2008 (AACN, 2009b). The enrollment increase was almost exclusively in DNP programs. For research-based doctoral programs, the growth in enrollment was 0.1%, indicating flat enrollment numbers.

Meleis and Dracup also point out that in many universities, membership in the faculty senate is reserved for tenured professors who hold a PhD. This would exclude the DNP faculty member from participation in the decisions and policies of that university. They predict creation of a "second class" citizen within the professorial ranks of the schools of nursing, with one class able to participate fully in the life and policies of the university and one class prohibited from doing so (Meleis & Dracup, 2005). Are we creating a two-tiered faculty? Is this ethical?

Is it ethical to potentially draw candidates away from research-focused programs into clinical doctoral programs and potentially impede the progress of nursing science development? Does the introduction of DNP-prepared faculty threaten the hard-won place of nursing in academia? Is there a middle ground, a clear pathway to collaboration between PhD-prepared nurses who develop new knowledge and DNP-prepared nurses who implement the new knowledge into clinical practice? Is clinical research strictly the domain of the PhD, or can the DNP conduct clinical research, thus addressing the need for clinical evidence of the efficacy of nursing interventions?

Conclusions

As of this writing, there are 93 DNP programs accepting students, and it is largely a given that advanced practice nurses will be educated within the DNP framework. We are moving full steam ahead on a major change in the education of advanced practice nurses based on recommendations, theories, and expert opinions. What is lacking is the evidence that DNP graduates will be better advocates, be better collaborators, or will incorporate more evidence-based guidelines into their practice than master's-prepared APNs. We are conducting a grand experiment in nursing education based on current thought. Is it ethical to move forward without the benefit of evidence that DNP practitioners have more skills than their master's-prepared colleagues do? Should we slow the pace of change to gain some evidence of the efficacy of the DNP programs, or does the crisis in American health care demand that we move forward now?

References

American Association of Colleges of Nursing. (2006). *The essentials of doctoral education for advanced practice nursing.* Retrieved from http://www.aacn.nche.edu/DNP/pdf/Essentials.pdf

American Association of Colleges of Nursing. (2009a). *AACN update on the new comprehensive care certification exam.* Retrieved from http://www.aacn.nche.edu/DNP/pdf/CCExamStatement.pdf

American Association of Colleges of Nursing. (2009b). *Despite surge in interest in nursing careers, new AACN data confirm that too few nurses are entering the healthcare workforce.* Retrieved from http://www.aacn.nche.edu/Media/NewsReleases/2009/workforcedata.html

American Board of Comprehensive Care. (2008, March 10). *CACC and NBME announce certification exams for Doctor of Nursing Practice graduates.* Retrieved from http://www.abcc.dnpcert.org /pressrelease.shtml

American Board of Comprehensive Care. (2009, January 29). *Fifty percent of candidates pass first certification exam in comprehensive care for doctors of nursing practice.* Retrieved from http://www.abcc.dnpcert.org/pressrelease2009.shtml

American College of Nurse Practitioners. (2006). *AMA meeting summary 6/2006.* Retrieved from http://www.acnpweb.org/i4a/pages/Index.cfm?pageID=3723

American Nurses Association. (n.d.). *Florence Nightingale pledge.* Retrieved from http://www .nursingworld.org/FunctionalMenuCategories/AboutANA/WhereWeComeFrom_1 /FlorenceNightingalePledge.aspx

American Nurses Association. (1994). *Position statement background information (Members only): Ethics and human rights.* Retrieved from http://www.nursingworld.org/position/ethics/ethics.aspx

American Nurses Association. (2001). *Code of ethics for nurses with interpretive statements.* Washington, DC: Author.

American Nurses Association. (2004). *Scope and standards of nursing practice.* Washington, DC: Author.

APRN Consensus Work Group and the National Council of State Boards of Nursing APRN Advisory Committee. (2008). *Consensus model for APRN regulation: Licensure, accreditation, certification and education.* Retrieved from http://www.aacn.nche.edu/Education /pdf/APRNReport.pdf

Beauchamp, T., & Childress, J. (2001). *Principles of biomedical ethics.* New York: Oxford University Press.

Centers for Disease Control and Prevention. (2009). *The Tuskegee timeline.* Retrieved from http://www.cdc.gov/tuskegee/timeline.htm

Dierick-van Daele, A., Metsemakers, J., Derckx, E., Spreeuwenberg, C., & Vrijhoef, H. (2008). Nurse practitioners substituting for general practitioners: Randomized controlled trial. *Journal of Advanced Nursing, 65*(2), 391–401.

Genocide Watch. (2009). *News monitors, current alerts.* Retrieved from http://www.genocide watch.org/resources.newsmonitors.html

Hamric, A., & Delgado, S. (2009). Ethical decision making. In A. Hamric, J. Spross, & C. Hanson (Eds.), *Advanced practice nursing: An integrative approach* (4th ed., pp. 315–346). St. Louis, MO: Saunders.

Horrocks, S., Anderson, E., & Salisbury, C. (2002). Systematic review of whether nurse practitioners working in primary care can provide equivalent care to doctors. *British Medical Journal, 324,* 819–823.

International Council of Nurses. (2006). *The ICN code of ethics for nurses.* Geneva, Switzerland: Author.

Meleis, A., & Dracup, K. (2005). The case against the DNP: History, timing, substance and marginalization. *Online Journal of Issues in Nursing, 10*(3). Retrieved from http://www.nursingworld.org/MainmenuCategories/ANAMarketplace/ANAPeriodicals/OJIN/Tableof Contents/Vol·ıme102005/No3/Sept05/tpc28_216026.aspx

Mitscherlich, A., & Mielke, F. (1947). The Nuremberg Code. In *Doctors of infamy: The story of the Nazi medical crimes.* New York: Schuman, 1949: xxiii–xxv.

Mundinger, M., Kane, R., Lenz, E., Totten, A. M., Tsai, W. Y., Cleary, P. D., et al. (2000). Primary care outcomes in patients treated by nurse practitioners or physicians: A randomized trial. *JAMA, 28*(1), 59–68.

National Commission for the Protection of Human Subjects of Biomedical and Behavioral Research. (1979). *Ethical principles and guidelines for the protection of human subjects of research.* Retrieved from http://www.hhs.gov/ohrp/humansubjects/guidance/belmont.htm

Nurse Practitioner Roundtable. (2008, June). *Nurse practitioner DNP education, certification and titling: A unified statement.* Washington, DC: Author.

Nurses top honesty list . . . again. (2009). *Nursing Economics.* Retrieved from http://www .accessmylibrary.com/coms2/summary_0286-36905697_ITM

Office of the United Nations High Commissioner for Human Rights. (2007). *Convention on the prevention and punishment of the crime of genocide.* Retrieved from http://www2.ohchp.english/law/genocide.htm

Pantilat, S. (2008). *Beneficence vs nonmaleficence.* Retrieved from http://missinglink.ucsf.edu/lm /ethics/Content%20Pages/fast_fact_bene_nonmal.htm

Pierce, A., & Smith, J. (2008). The ethics curriculum for Doctor of Nursing Practice programs. *Journal of Professional Nursing, 24*(5), 270–274.

Schabas, W. (2008). Introduction, Convention on the Prevention and Punishment of the Crime of Genocide. Retrieved from http://untreaty.un.org/cod/avl/ha/cppcg/cppcg.html

Silva, M., & Ludwick, R. (2006). Is the Doctor of Nursing Practice ethical? *Online Journal of Issues in Nursing, 11*(2).

Sorrell, A. (2009, June 8). Medicine decries nurse doctorate exam as being equal to physician testing. *AMA News.* Retrieved from http://www.ama-assn.org/amednews/2009 /06/08/prl10608.htm

White, G. (2001). The code of ethics for nurses. *AJN, 101*(10).

Yee, C. M. (2008, April 28). A doctor and a nurse—all in one package. *Minneapolis Star-Tribune.* Retrieved from http://www.startribune.com/business/18292444.html

Application of the Elements of the ICN Code of Ethics for Nurses

Element of the Code 1: Nurses and People

Practitioners and Managers	Educators and Researchers	National Nurses' Associations
Provide care that respects human rights and is sensitive to the values, customs and beliefs of all people.	In curriculum include references to human rights, equity, justice, solidarity as the basis for access to care.	Develop position statements and guidelines that support human rights and ethical standards.
Provide continuing education in ethical issues.	Provide teaching and learning opportunities for ethical issues and decision making.	Lobby for involvement of nurses in ethics review committees.
Provide sufficient information to permit informed consent and the right to choose or refuse treatment.	Provide teaching/learning opportunities related to informed consent.	Provide guidelines and continuing education relevant to informed consent.
Use recording and information management systems that ensure confidentiality.	Introduce into curriculums concepts of privacy and confidentiality.	Incorporate issues of confidentiality and privacy into a national code of ethics for nurses.
Develop and monitor environmental safety in the workplace.	Sensitize students to the importance of social action in current concerns.	Advocate for safe and healthy environment.

Element of the Code 2: Nurses and Practice

Practitioners and Managers	Educators and Researchers	National Nurses' Associations
Establish standards of care and a work setting that promotes safety and quality care.	Provide teaching/learning opportunities that foster lifelong learning and competence for practice.	Provide access to continuing education through journals, conferences, distance education etc.
Establish systems for professional appraisal, continuous education and systematic renewal of licensure to practice.	Conduct and disseminate research that shows links between continual education opportunities and quality care standards.	Lobby to ensure continuing education opportunities and quality care standards.

(continues)

Element of the Code 2: Nurses and Practice

Practitioners and Managers	Educators and Researchers	National Nurses' Associations
Monitor and promote the personal health of nursing staff in relation to their competence to practice.	Promote the importance of personal health and illustrate its relation to other values.	Promote healthy lifestyles for nursing professionals. Lobby for healthy workplaces and services for nurses.

Element of the Code 3: Nurses and the Profession

Practitioners and Managers	Educators and Researchers	National Nurses' Associations
Set standards for nursing practice, research, education and management.	Provide teaching/learning opportunities in setting standards for nursing practice, research, education and management.	Collaborate with others to set standards for nursing education, practice, research and management.
Foster workplace support of conduct, dissemination and utilization of research related to nursing and health.	Conduct, disseminate and utilize research to advance the nursing profession.	Develop position statements, guidelines and standards related to nursing research.
Promote participation in national nurses' associations so as to create favorable conditions for nurses.	Sensitize learners to the importance of professional nurses associations.	Lobby for fair social and economic working conditions in nursing. Develop position statements and guidelines in workplace issues.

Element of the Code 4: Nurses and Co-workers

Practitioners and Managers	Educators and Researchers	National Nurses' Associations
Create awareness of specific and overlapping functions and the potential for interdisciplinary tensions.	Develop understanding of the roles of other workers.	Stimulate co-operation with other related disciplines.

Element of the Code 4: Nurses and Co-workers

Practitioners and Managers	Educators and Researchers	National Nurses' Associations
Develop workplace systems that support common professional ethical values and behavior.	Communicate nursing ethics to other professions.	Develop awareness of ethical issues of other professions.
Develop mechanisms to safeguard the individual, family or community when their care is endangered by health care personnel.	Instill in learners the need to safeguard the individual, family or community when care is endangered by health care personnel.	Provide guidelines, position statements and discussion for a related to safeguarding people when their care is endangered by health care personnel.

Source: International Council of Nurses. (2006). *The ICN code of ethics for nurses.* Geneva, Switzerland: Author. Reprinted with permission from International Council of Nurses.

PART II

DOCTOR OF NURSING PRACTICE ROLES

CHAPTER 9

Traditional Advanced Practice Roles for the DNP

Clinical Nurse Specialist
Mary E. Zaccagnini and Germaine M. Edinger

I have an almost complete disregard of precedent, and a faith in the possibility of something better. It irritates me to be told how things have always been done. I defy the tyranny of precedent. I go for anything new that might improve the past.
—CLARA BARTON

It is apparent that these are tumultuous times in health care. Currently the United States is experiencing a flood of problems associated with health care and healthcare delivery systems. According to a Census Bureau report (2009), the numbers of Americans without insurance rose to 46.3 million in 2008, and healthcare premiums have grown faster than inflation. The United States allocates more of its economy to health care than any other developed country (Kaiser Family Foundation, 2009). The Centers for Medicare and Medicaid Services (CMS) report that the United States will spend over $2.5 trillion on health care in 2009, which equates to approximately 20.3% of the gross domestic product. According to the Institute of Medicine report *Crossing the Quality Chasm* (2001, p. 1), "The American healthcare delivery system is in need of fundamental change." The report additionally states that "in its current form, habits, and environment, American health care is incapable of providing the public with the quality health care it expects and deserves."

The Doctor of Nursing (DNP) degree is currently evolving into the terminal degree for advanced practice nursing and as such is lauded as the preparation nurses need to face the new complexities of patient care, healthcare delivery, and additional local and national healthcare concerns. According to the American Association of Colleges of Nursing (AACN, 2008), although the new degree will not alter the scope of practice of advanced practice nurses (APNs), transitioning to the DNP will better prepare them for the "growing complexity of health care." Because the clinical nurse specialist (CNS) is educated as a systems thinker and a practitioner who is primarily answerable for challenges and changes at the population, disease, or organizational level, the CNS is at the forefront of complex emerging issues in health care and at the cusp of shaping reform.

The clinical nurse specialist is a registered nurse functioning in an advanced role. The American Nurses Association (ANA) outlines the scope of practice for all nurses and the expectations of the professional roles within which all nurses must practice. It defines the role of the CNS as follows:

> CNSs are registered nurses who have graduate level nursing preparation at the master's or doctoral level as a CNS. They are clinical experts in evidence-based nursing practice within a specialty area, treating and managing the health concerns of patients and populations. CNSs practice autonomously and integrate knowledge of disease and medical treatments into the assessment, diagnosis, and treatment of patients' illnesses. In many jurisdictions, CNSs, as direct care providers, perform comprehensive health assessments, develop differential diagnoses, and may have prescriptive authority. CNSs serve as patient advocates, consultants, and researchers in various settings. (ANA, 2004)

The National Association of Clinical Nurse Specialists (NACNS) articulates CNS practice competencies, educational guidelines, and credentialing requirements. This organization describes the essence of CNS practice as clinical nursing expertise in diagnosis and treatment to prevent, remediate, or alleviate illness and promote health, with a defined specialty (NACNS, 2004). A type of health problem, a specific setting or unit, a disease, or a population can define the specialty. Currently, over 72,000 advanced practice nurses are prepared and credentialed to practice as CNSs (ANA, 2009).

History

Florence Nightingale has often been identified as the founder of modern nursing practice. She identified concepts that are the basis of contemporary CNS practices, including

> (1) differentiating nursing and medicine, with nursing focusing on illness/suffering and medicine focusing on disease, (2) easing suffering and preventing disease from nondisease factors were nursing responsibilities,

(4) using scientific approach to ground nursing practice, (5) identifying nurses' competency as critical to quality of care, and (6) influencing the health care system was nursing's responsibility. (NACNS, 2004)

The beginnings of specialized nursing practice began with a psychiatric nursing program in 1880 at McLean Hospital in Massachusetts (Critchley, 1985). There was more formal attentiveness to this role circa the 1940s, when it was ascertained that many soldiers returning from World War II were burdened with mental illness (Hamric, 1996). This was most probably post-traumatic stress syndrome, which had not been defined at this time. This diagnosed illness was originally treated with electroshock therapy, which required the assistance of nurses with specialized training.

Dr. Hildegard Peplau is considered the "founding mother" of CNS practice (NACNS, 2009). She was a psychiatric nurse and professor who described the CNS as an advanced practice nurse having expertise in the nursing care of complex patients. She established the first master's program at Rutgers University in 1954. This program in psychiatric nursing was considered the first CNS program and made more evident the link between academia and specialization.

The 1960s brought a time when CNS practice took its modern form. In 1965, Dr. Peplau "contended that development of areas of specialization is preceded by three social forces: (1) an increase in specialty-related information; (2) new technological advances; and (3) a response to public need and interest" (Hamric, 1996, p. 15). These could be correlated to current issues in health care and the call for the further evolution of advanced practice specialized nurses.

The need for and growth of psychiatric CNS programs was instrumental in defining and developing the CNS role. Psychiatric CNSs continued to proliferate during the 1970s, and the specialties of critical care and oncology emerged (Keeling, 2009). It was not until the mid-1970s that the American Nurses Association officially recognized the CNS role and title. Initially, ANA defined the CNS as an expert practitioner and a change agent; at the same time, it included a master's degree as a requirement for CNS practice.

CNS expansion continued in the 1980s as researchers studied outcomes related to CNS practice. CNS practice began to include the practice of nursing staff development and organizational aspects of nursing care. In the 1990s, CNS roles were challenged due to changes in the healthcare landscape regarding financial reimbursement in organizations and the rise in the need for primary care practitioners. A major step in the specialty occurred in 1995 when the professional organization, the National Association of Clinical Nurse Specialists, was established. In the same period, Medicare reimbursement was expanded to include direct payment to CNSs.

Historically, CNS practice was described by subroles of skills and activities. These included expert practitioner, educator, researcher, change agent, administrator, and consultant. In recent years, CNS practice has been described conceptually by integration of these subroles across the three spheres of influence: the patient/client sphere, the nurses/nursing sphere; and the system/organizational sphere. Direct care (the patient/client sphere) is the inner core of CNS practice.

Educational Preparation

CNS practice has expanded exponentially into over 40 specialties. The master's degree has always been an entry-level requirement for CNS practice. Only since the 1990s have the foundational specialty competencies been defined. Educational preparation may vary; however, it is desirable that the foundational graduate education prepare the CNS as a proficient advanced practice nurse regardless of venue. It would then be the intent that specialization education be subsequent to the core graduate tutelage. The curriculum dedicated to the expert portion should included a minimum of 500 hours of supervised clinical experience, and a CNS in the same or similar specialization should provide the supervision. The clinical hours would ensure that the practitioner met the criteria for certification.

Certification

The purposes of certification are to validate knowledge and competency for CNS entry into practice and to meet emerging regulatory trends (NACNS, 2007). Required certification is defined by individual states and may require one or both of the following: Clinical Nurse Specialist certification and specialty certification. The predominant trend is to require certification as a validation of attainment of initial advanced practice competencies and of recognition and authority to practice (NACNS, 2005). This may also be a factor in the application process for credentialing and prescriptive authority. Currently, the American Nurses Credentialing Center (ANCC) offers the certification exams listed in Table 9-1.

■ Table 9-1   American Nurses Credentialing Center Certification Examinations for Clinical Nurse Specialists

Clinical Nurse Specialists
Adult Health
Adult Psychiatric & Mental Health
Child/Adolescent Psychiatric & Mental Health
CNS Core Examination
Diabetes Management—Advanced
Gerontological
Home Health
Pediatric
Public/Community Health

Other Advanced-Level Examinations
Diabetes Management—Advanced
Forensic Nurse—Advanced Practice
Nurse Executive—Advanced
Public Health Nursing

In addition to the AANC certification process, many professional organizations offer examinations in specialty areas. However, some specialty areas do not offer a certification process or examination, and therefore a certification option may not be feasible in all practice areas. Unfortunately, many states now require a certification in order to practice in a specialty area as an advanced practice nurse. ANCC has attempted to satisfy this need by providing a CNS core exam.

Core Competencies

The core competencies for the CNS practice were developed by the National Association of Clinical Nurse Specialists and are applicable to all specialty areas. These competencies provide the foundation for practice and are written to reflect the three spheres of influence, with the patient/client sphere envisioned as the largest area of practice. There is an expectation that the competencies are then actualized within the specialty practice. These competencies include educational requirements and outcomes.

The core competencies were developed from evidence-based best practices, evidence from literature, and expert opinion. They were validated by a national study in 2005 and by Baldwin, Clark, Fulton, and Mayo (2009), who further validated and defined the entry-level core competencies' use in practice, their importance, and the potential gaps between competency and practice. The competencies were placed under the scrutiny of more than 30 national organizations, which were invited to provide critique and review (Baldwin, Lyon, Clark, Fulton, & Dayhoff, 2007), and they were presented to the organizations' membership for response.

Most recently, NACNS wrote a set of CNS core competencies for the Doctor of Nursing Practice. As with the original core competencies, they encompassed the three spheres of influence. The subject matter of these competencies is much broader and far-reaching. In the client sphere, the competencies speak to advanced clinical judgment and include pharmacologic interventions and prescribing. The nursing sphere dictates leadership and healthcare team processes that may affect both fiscal and clinical outcomes. Finally, the organizational/system sphere of influence includes areas such as organizational and system theory, and care that is evidence based, cost effective, and ethical. Again, in the evolution of the competencies, public scrutiny and feedback were solicited. Although this was not an endorsement of the DNP degree, it acknowledged that this degree was more than likely the terminal degree in the future of advanced practice nursing.

The Role and Scope of Practice

According to Hamric, Spross, and Hanson (2009), the role of the CNS has been dynamic and has moved from a listing and definition of roles (expert practitioner, educator, researcher, change agent, administer, and consultant) to the impact and influence CNSs have on their clients and environment. This delineation of influences was intended to diminish role ambiguity and "to distinguish CNSs from other APNs" (NACNS, 1998).

CNS role genesis is specialization, and the client sphere is at its core. Direct clinical practice is at the heart of care, as with all APNs, although the CNS will most likely be found in the inpatient setting. Direct care is not only the mainstay of practice but also directs and influences all spheres and outcomes. The CNS, in this sphere, will most probably oversee care for his or her population or area of practice and directly manage those clients whose needs are multifaceted, complicated, challenging, or unique. Direct care refers to CNS activities and responsibilities that occur within the patient–nurse interface (Sparacino & Cartwright, 2009). The goal of CNS patient care is to decrease or prevent symptoms and suffering and improve the functioning of the individual patient or population. Outcomes related to this role could include direct reduction in costs for the institution as well as improved quality of care. Studies have reinforced the realization that CNS involvement in patient care has consistently improved outcomes. The amount of direct care practice, however, varies from institution to institution and CNS to CNS. The direct care practice role may be overemphasized or underemphasized depending on the institution's needs and the availability of other expert resources.

In the nurse/nursing sphere of influence, the CNS affects practice through the integration of evidence-based interventions into nursing care. This includes the leadership and expert coaching the CNS provides for nursing, and the education furnished regarding the current science of practice and technology. CNSs also develop and provide nursing education in order to improve practice and assist the institution in meeting goals of safety and quality. In addition, it is generally incumbent upon the CNS to assist with the key indicators of magnet status accreditation.

In the organizational/system sphere, CNSs are skilled at "assessing organizational processes, including interdepartmental relationships/functioning, professional climate, multi-disciplinary collaboration, external relationships and regulations, and health policy to identify facilitators and barriers to effective patient care" (McKinley, 2007). In this context, CNSs work within the culture and mission of the institution and are in alignment with the organizational goals. CNSs lead multidisciplinary teams in developing new and inventive programs that improve care and are fiscally responsible. Given the complexity of health care and the need for expert clinical practice change agents, the practice doctorate enhances the CNS's effectiveness in the nurse/nursing practice and organization/system sphere.

The Future of CNS Practice

Regulatory Challenges

As with all APNs, the CNS is confronted with legislative and regulatory challenges that can restrict practice and withhold care. CNSs do not currently hold prescriptive authority in all states even though they are recognized as advanced practice nurses. This is beginning to change, and it is hoped the issue will be resolved so that CNSs can practice within their scope as APNs. It is important that all CNS curricula contain the content necessary for prescriptive practice so that CNSs will be prepared even if their specific state does not currently allow this provision of care.

Currently APN groups, which include CNSs, are debating with regulatory agencies in many areas regarding the supervision verbiage that is contained in many state boards of nursing's standards of practice. There is consensus that all APNs, including CNSs, should have autonomy in practice and not be required to have physician supervision or formalized collaborative practice agreements.

Titling issues specific to the CNS also exist. There is significant inconsistency in various state boards of nursing regarding the recognition of the title of Clinical Nurse Specialist. This includes the criteria necessary for attainment and use of the title. For example, in the state of Minnesota, a nurse may not use the title Clinical Nurse Specialist unless the nurse has graduated from a Clinical Nurse Specialist program within a college or university and the nurse has obtained a Board of Nursing–accepted national accreditation as a CNS. NACNS (2004) has stated and advocates that the CNS title should be protected in the statute of all boards of nursing.

The Future Role of the CNS and the DNP Degree

Patients, health care professionals, and policy makers are becoming all too painfully aware of the shortcomings of our current care delivery systems and the importance of finding better approaches to meeting the health care needs of all Americans.
—WILLIAM C. RICHARDSON

According to the National Association of Clinical Nurse Specialists, CNSs can meet the need to "[i]ncrease the effectiveness of transitioning care from hospital to home and prevent readmissions; improve the quality and safety of care and reduce health care costs; educate, train and increase the nursing workforce needed for an improved health system; increase access to community-based care; increase the availability of effective care for those with chronic illness; and improve access to wellness and preventative care" (NACNS, 2009). This assertion reflects many of the changes needed to help reform the current healthcare system. For example, according to a 2007 Milken Institute report, "people with chronic health conditions cost the United States more than $1 trillion a year. This figure could jump to nearly $6 trillion by 2050 unless the provision of preventive health services substantially improves" (Bedroussian & DeVol, 2007). At the heart of APN practice is preventive care, and APN-led chronic care clinics developed in order to better manage chronic illness and prevent hospital readmissions are a current and imminent trend. The CNS is skilled in symptom management and has commonly acquired program management skills within the foundation of education and practice. This affords the CNS the proficiency necessary to ensure positive outcomes related to the chronic care process or clinic. As a DNP graduate, the CNS would possess additional expertise in issues such as policy and economics, which would undoubtedly improve the prospect for the success of such ventures.

Studies have shown that those elders who received care from gerontological CNSs had fewer readmissions and fewer rehospitalization days (NACNS, 2009). A study demonstrated a decrease in costs and complications when CNSs used evidence-based guidelines to reduce pain and to reduce the incidence of pulmonary complications in the intensive care unit setting (NACNS, 2009). Several studies laud the success of the CNS as a practitioner who currently addresses healthcare needs and who will be an indispensable leader in healthcare reform in the future.

According to Hathaway, Jacob, Stegbauer, Thompson, and Graff (2006), "Graduates of DNP programs are already practicing up market and making important contributions. Their course-work and practical experiences acquired through doctoral study help prepare them for this phase of practice. For example, the study of policy and economics enables DNP graduates to knowledgeably and effectively represent the interests of nursing before regulatory agencies and legislative bodies. Epidemiology and advanced evidence-based practice courses help position DNP graduates for leadership in the burgeoning quality improvement movement." The CNS is currently knowledgeable in many of these matters, and the additional DNP degree will reinforce and strengthen those skills.

The CNS will continue to have extensive involvement in many healthcare settings. "The CNS is uniquely prepared to be the transprofessional collaborator, change agent, evidence-based practice integrator, and patient/client outcomes driver who will ensure safety and quality outcomes for patients now and into the future" (Goudreau et al., 2007).

Nurse Practitioner
Gwendolyn Short

> Transforming health care delivery recognizes the critical need for clinicians to design, evaluate, and continuously improve the context within which care is delivered ... Nurses prepared at the doctoral level with a blend of clinical, organizational, economic and leadership skills are most likely to be able to critique nursing and other clinical scientific findings and design programs of care delivery that are locally acceptable, economically feasible, and which significantly impact health care outcomes. (American Association of Colleges of Nursing [AACN], 2004, p. 3)

These words in the American Association of Colleges of Nursing's 2004 *Position Paper on the Practice Doctorate in Nursing* describe the need, rationale, and timeliness for the creation and development of the Doctor of Nursing Practice degree. Included in the AACN position paper is the recommendation that by 2015 the DNP become the terminal degree for nursing practice.

From its inception, demand for the DNP has been strong. The first DNP program began at the University of Kentucky in the fall of 2001, with a cohort of 13 students. Several other schools had similar programs or were in the process of developing them, including the University of Tennessee and Columbia University (AACN, 2004). Interest quickly proliferated around the country, and within 8 years, 91 schools of nursing were accepting students into their newly developed DNP programs, and another 50 schools were planning such a program (AACN, 2009).

Economics, technology, and politics have all affected and challenged the evolution of nursing education and practice. Important factors surrounding the development of the DNP are those that affect society at large: the rising costs of health care, the increasing complexity of disease care and healthcare delivery, the decline in the number of medical doctors entering primary care, and the integration of technology into patient care. The Institute of Medicine's (IOM) 1999 groundbreaking report, *To Err Is Human: Building a Safer Health System,* argued for the need to improve patient safety as well as the overall quality of healthcare organizations and systems (IOM, 1999). Subsequent work by the IOM (2001, 2003a, 2003b) provided additional direction on how to make these improvements and addressed the roles of specific groups of healthcare workers, including nurses. The IOM (2003a) proposed development of core competencies for all health professionals in the 21st century. These competencies will allow the health professional to provide patient-centered care, work in interdisciplinary teams, employ evidence-based practice, apply quality improvement, and utilize informatics.

The IOM competencies provide a supportive framework and share some common themes with the eight essentials of doctoral education for advanced nursing practice as developed and proposed by the American Academy of Colleges of Nursing (AACN, 2006). Both emphasize the goal of providing evidence-based, patient-centered health care to populations within systems of care that support collaboration between the different health disciplines.

Birth of a Movement

The first nurse practitioners began their education in 1965 at the University of Colorado as part of a demonstration project to determine whether nurses, working in an expanded role, could provide well-child care in community-based settings (Komnenich, 2005). Development of this program was the result of a collaborative effort by Loretta Ford, pioneer of the nurse practitioner movement, and pediatrician Henry K. Silver in direct response to an existing physician shortage as well as to the recognition among nursing leaders of a need to prepare graduate nurses for clinical specialization (Komnenich, 2005). The role of the graduate nurse practitioner (NP) was fully grounded in nursing, with a focus on well-child care, health promotion, and disease prevention, preparing the NP to "assess autonomously, innovate, and work collaboratively with families and physicians" (p. 29) to provide health care. These graduates were certified in the area of pediatrics and assumed the title of Pediatric Nurse Practitioner.

Nurses soon began to request educational preparation in the care of populations other than pediatrics, spawning the development of nurse practitioners who focused on other groups, including adults, the family, and women. Nurse practitioners currently comprise by far the largest group of advanced practice nurses—147,295 (Pearson, 2009). Close to 6,000 new NPs are graduated each year at over 325 colleges and universities within the United States (ANA, 2009).

Educational Requirements and Specialty Areas

Early nurse practitioner graduates received certificates as proof of their successful program completion, awarded jointly by the American Nurses Association and the American Academy of Pediatrics. Schools of nursing soon began to offer master's degree programs, and by the early 1970s, these programs began to outnumber those granting certificates (Bullough, 1995). By 1990, 90% of nurse practitioner programs were either master's degree programs or post-master's degree programs (Pulcini & Wagner, 2001).

A significant driving force for the development of the DNP is the amount of education required to earn a master's in a nurse practitioner program, which has increased over the years to 45 to 50 semester credits. The average number of credit hours required to earn a master's degree in almost any other specialty is 30 semester credits (Chase & Pruitt, 2006). Even at the level of 45 to 50 credits, many leaders in NP education have voiced their concern that increased complexity in the healthcare environment continues to drive the need for additional content in the educational curricula for nurse practitioners.

Areas of focus within the master's program determine the type of specialty area the graduate will enter, the most common being family, adult, pediatrics, gerontology, psychiatry, women's health, and acute care. The newly graduated student then takes a certification exam within the specialty area, administered by an accredited certification body, and on passing this exam can become eligible for state licensure.

Certification, Licensure, and Credentialing

Certification, licensure, and credentialing comprise the often complicated regulatory process that governs nursing, with the goal of maintaining standards of practice to protect the public and patients.

Certification is the process used by national professional nursing organizations to recognize advanced practice (ANA, 2004). Certification requires graduation from an accredited program and successful completion of a certification examination recognized nationally by the advanced practice specialty's professional organization (ANA, 2004). Forty-four of the 51 states and Washington, D.C., require some type of certification for APN practice (Pearson, 2009). Certification of the nurse practitioner currently occurs following graduation from the master's program. As schools adopt the DNP and drop their master's-level curricula, completion of the DNP will be required prior to certification. Some schools, however, are choosing to continue a master's-level program of study while adding the DNP; for students in these programs, certification would continue to occur following completion of the master's course of study.

Licensure is the process whereby a state agency grants authority to an individual to practice as a nurse practitioner. For nurse practitioners, licensing is granted following completion of an accredited educational program and passing of a national exam. The nurse practitioner is first licensed as a registered nurse, and in some states must then obtain an additional license to practice as a nurse practitioner (ANA, 2004; Hanson, 2009).

Credentialing is an additional step, required by a state regulatory agency or local institution, to ensure that an individual can provide all the documentation necessary to practice in a professional capacity, with a given title. The credentialing process for nurse practitioners not only assures the public that the individual meets professional practice standards (Hanson, 2009) but also is required before the NP can be reimbursed for services rendered. Certification and licensure are just two components of the credentialing process.

Accreditation

There is no uniform model of regulation of nurse practitioners across states, and currently each state independently determines the NP's scope of practice, recognized roles, criteria for entry into advanced practice, and certification examinations accepted for entry-level competence assessment. This lack of standardization has restricted the mobility of nurse practitioners and has created a barrier to health care for patients (APRN Joint Dialogue Group, 2008). In an attempt to help standardize the regulatory process, representatives from a number of nursing organizations organized a working group to develop a plan for the licensure, accreditation, certification, and education of advanced practice nurses. The outcome of this process—the Consensus Model for APRN Regulation, or the APRN Regulatory Model—addresses the licensure, accreditation, certification, and education of the four categories of advanced practice registered nurses: nurse anesthetists, nurse midwives, clinical nurse specialists, and nurse practitioners. Recommendations are included to clarify and improve the regulatory processes for each group (APRN Joint Dialogue Group, 2008).

Scope of Practice

Scope of practice describes the limits and boundaries of those practice activities within which nurses in the various advanced practice nursing specialties may legally practice (Hanson, 2009). Each advanced practice nursing specialty has its own scope of practice, based on its professional purpose and educational foundation. Furthermore, scope of practice differs from state to state and is based on state law described in the nurse practice acts and rules and regulations for advanced practice nurses (Hanson, 2009; Pearson, 2009).

Nurse practitioners have traditionally focused on health and wellness in a community-based primary care setting, their practice characterized by autonomy in clinical decision making, systematic collection of data through history taking, appropriate diagnosing and treatment, illness and injury prevention, patient advocacy, health counseling, and patient education (ANA, 2004; Komnenich, 2005). According to the American Academy of Nurse Practitioners (2007), NPs are "licensed independent practitioners who practice in ambulatory, acute, and long term care as primary and/or specialty care providers. According to their practice specialty, NPs deliver nursing and medical services to individuals, families, and groups."

The scope of practice for NPs has changed over time in response to the demands of the healthcare system and the natural evolution of the nursing profession. Scope of practice for nurse practitioners—and all advanced practice nurses—is an area of NP practice debated in many state legislatures. Through legislation, nurse practitioners strive to ensure an environment in which they can practice to the limit of their skills, while others (frequently physicians) attempt to limit and place restraints on their practice activities (Safriet, 2002).

The DNP is not intended to increase the nurse practitioner's level of clinical expertise, but rather to increase the NP's organizational, economic, and leadership skills (Chism, 2009). Although the master's degree has proven to be adequate preparation for a practitioner to function in an advanced nursing capacity, the healthcare environment is increasing in its complexity, requiring additional skills on the part of healthcare workers to improve the delivery of healthcare services. The DNP offers additional preparation to enable nurses to improve these services, especially in the areas of organizational leadership, project development and implementation, and quality improvement, all within the context of providing population-based health care. The DNP-prepared nurse practitioner should be poised to assume a substantial role in an era of healthcare reform.

Role of the DNP Nurse Practitioner

The nurse practitioner has much to add to the national discussion of health-care delivery and reform, and may very well become a key component of solutions to the challenges of improving and sustaining an effective and efficient health delivery system. The nurse practitioner who has obtained a DNP, with its additional focus on providing health care within complex systems, will have an even greater impact on the improvement of patient care delivery and patient outcomes. Indeed, the first three essentials of doctoral education for advanced nursing practice specifically deal with systems improvement based on scientific evidence:

1. Scientific underpinnings for practice
2. Organizational and systems leadership for quality improvement and systems thinking
3. Clinical scholarship and analytical methods for evidence-based practice (AACN, 2006)

The doctorate of nursing practice is a degree, and not a role (AACN, 2004). The role of the advanced practice nurse with the DNP degree will continue to reflect the specialty practice of the master's-prepared advanced practice nurse, as nurse anesthetist, nurse midwife, clinical nurse specialist, or nurse practitioner. The DNP-prepared nurse practitioner will continue to provide health care through assessment, diagnosis, and treatment of the complex responses of individuals, families, or communities to actual or potential health problems, prevention of illness and injury, maintenance of wellness, and provision of comfort (ANA, 2004).

With additional education at the doctoral level, the nurse practitioner will be better prepared to navigate, and to help their patients navigate, the increased complexity of the healthcare environment. DNP curricula focus on organizational leadership, project development and implementation, quality improvement, and the use of evidence-based health care through use of existing research. Addition of these skills to the nurse practitioner's existing skill set of providing patient-centered care, patient advocacy, and service coordination will ensure an even more competent nurse practitioner, and improved patient outcomes.

Certified Registered Nurse Anesthetist
Garrett J. Peterson

History

The first professional group to provide anesthesia services to surgical patients in the United States were nurses (Figure 9-1). In the late 1800s, nurse anesthesia became the first recognized clinical nursing specialty (Bankert, 1989). Surgeons were frustrated over the morbidity and mortality rates of their surgical patients and felt that it was associated with the administration of anesthesia (Bankert, 1989).

The initial methods of anesthesia delivery to surgical patients were dangerous because they involved either a handkerchief soaked in chloroform and held over the patient's nose and mouth or an ether-soaked sponge held over the nose and mouth of the patient (Bankert, 1989). These techniques

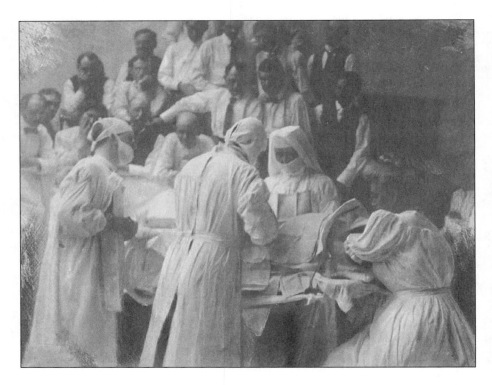

■ Figure 9-1   Nurse Anesthetist Alice McGaw Administers Anesthesia During Surgery at St. Mary's Hospital, Rochester, Minnesota, Circa 1910

Source: American Association of Nurse Anesthetists. Reproduced with permission.

allowed for minimal air inhalation by the patient, leading to death by suffocation. Surgeons therefore viewed nurses as practitioners with the ability to provide undivided attention to patients during administration of anesthesia. This resulted in nurses emerging as pioneers in anesthesia administration, providing anesthesia for all surgical specialties.

First Known Anesthetic Documentation by Nurses

Virginia S. Thatcher researched the history of nurse anesthetists and discovered that significant contributions to the profession of nurse anesthesia were made by the religious nursing sisters. The code of canon law required detailed documentation of each individual nun, which revealed that these nursing nuns were involved in anesthesia administration (Bankert, 1989). In 1877, a Catholic nun named Sister Mary Bernard (Figure 9-2) provided anesthesia administration at St. Vincent's Hospital in Erie, Pennsylvania. Her anesthetic documentation became the first known documentation of a nurse administering an anesthetic (Bankert, 1989).

In a textbook written by Isabel Adams Hampton Robb in 1893, *Nursing: Its Principles and Practices for Hospital and Private Use*, an entire chapter was titled "The Administration of Anesthetics." Robb explained that "A nurse is often called upon in private practice to administer an anaesthetic" (Robb, 1893). The

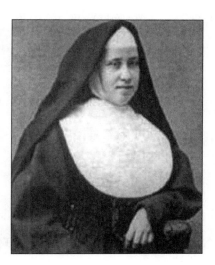

■ Figure 9-2   Sister Mary Bernard

Source: American Association of Nurse Anesthetists. Reproduced with permission.

Third Order of the Hospital Sisters of St. Francis established St. John's Hospital in Springfield, Illinois, which provided a place where the sisters were instructed in the administration of anesthesia by surgeons. Additional hospitals were built for employees of the Missouri Pacific Railroad, which were also managed by the Sisters of St. Francis, allowing the sisters to serve as the hospitals' anesthetists.

The Sisters of St. Francis traveled north from Illinois to Rochester, Minnesota, establishing St. Mary's Hospital in 1889, which was operated by Dr. William Worrell Mayo. Eventually, the hospital would become the Mayo Clinic. The hospital became a center point for interested health professionals to learn the techniques of the surgeons. The visitors were also privileged to observe the superior administration of anesthesia by nurse anesthetist Alice McGaw (Figure 9-3) and the other nurse anesthetists at St. Mary's Hospital. Dr. Mayo bestowed upon McGaw the title of "mother of anesthesia" for her many achievements, including mastery of the "open-drop" technique of anesthesia using ether and chloroform and her subsequent publication of her findings (Bankert, 1989).

Hundreds of nurses and physicians from around the world traveled to St. Mary's Hospital to observe Alice McGaw and Dr. Mayo and learn their techniques of anesthesia administration. McGaw documented the anesthesia practice outcomes at St. Mary's and published them in several medical journals between 1899 and 1906. In 1906, McGaw published an article in the medical journal *Surgery, Gynecology and Obstetrics,* "A Review of over

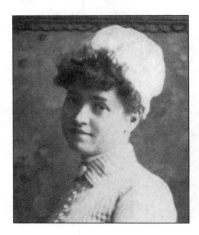

■ Figure 9-3 Alice McGaw

Source: American Association of Nurse Anesthetists. Reproduced with permission.

14,000 Surgical Anesthetics." She noted that during all of those anesthetic procedures, not one death was attributed to the anesthetic, an outstanding record for the time.

Sharing the Skill of Anesthesia Administration

Surgeon Dr. George Crile, known for his research in the treatment of surgical shock, followed the Mayo's model of training nurses in the administration of anesthesia. Dr. Crile chose a nurse, Agatha Cobourg Hodgins (Figures 9-4 and 9-5), to become his special anesthetist. Dr. Crile taught Miss Hodgins extensively about anesthesia administration, using laboratory animals to become familiar with the symptoms of impending death and to learn how to recognize and treat these symptoms before leading to death. Dr. Crile reported at the Southern Surgical and Gynecological Association that Miss Hodgins had administered thousands of anesthetics without an anesthetic death.

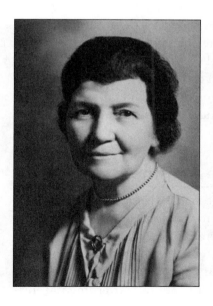

■ Figure 9-4   Agatha Hodgins

Source: American Association of Nurse Anesthetists. Reproduced with permission.

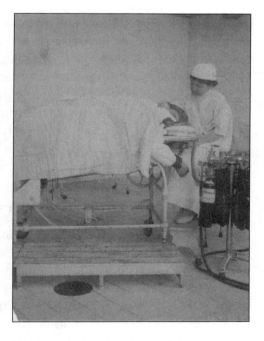

■ Figure 9-5   Agatha Hodgins Administers Anesthesia to a Patient, Circa 1914

Source: American Association of Nurse Anesthetists. Reproduced with permission.

Dr. Crile and Agatha Hodgins traveled together to France in 1914 and became instrumental in the creation of hospitals that provided care for the sick and wounded soldiers. It was during this visit that Hodgins had the opportunity to teach nurses and physicians in the art of anesthesia administration.

Nurse Anesthetists in World War I and Beyond

Nurse anesthetists have been the primary anesthesia providers to the U.S. military forces since World War I and in some instances the only anesthesia provider. During World War I, hospital administrator Gustaf W. Olson urged that Sophie Gran Winton, a graduate nurse from Swedish Hospital in Minneapolis, Minnesota, be trained as a nurse anesthetist. After administration of more than 10 thousand cases without a fatality, she joined the Army Nursing Corps in 1918 and traveled to Chateau-Thierry, France, to serve in Mobile Hospital No. 1. She received the French Croix de Guerre medal, along with six overseas service bars and honors for her anesthesia service (Bankert, 1989).

"Nurse anesthetists have been held as prisoners of war, suffered combat wounds during wartime service, and have lost their lives serving their country" (AANA, 2009a). The United States and foreign governments have recognized the efforts put forth by nurse anesthetists in caring for wounded military men and women and have honored them for their outstanding service (AANA, 2009a). The involvement of certified registered nurse anesthetists (CRNAs) in anesthesia administration during times of war increased the demand for CRNAs, resulting in an increased number of nurse anesthesia educational programs.

American Association of Nurse Anesthetists

In 1931, nurse anesthetist Agatha Hodgins became the founder of the American Association of Nurse Anesthetists, the first professional organization for nurse anesthetists. It currently represents more than 40,000 certified registered nurse anesthetists and student registered nurse anesthetists nationwide. "The AANA promulgates education, and practice standards and guidelines and affords consultation to both private and governmental entities regarding nurse anesthetists and their practice" (reprinted from the AANA website, www.aana.com, with permission from the American Association of Nurse Anesthetists, [© 2009]).

Nurse Anesthesia Education Programs

In 1909, nurse anesthetist Agnes McGee (Figure 9-6) established the first known school of nurse anesthesia at St. Vincent's Hospital in Portland, Oregon. The curriculum was six months long and included didactic instruction in anatomy and physiology, pharmacology, and the administration of the common anesthetic agents. Following the success of Agnes McGee's program, approximately 19 additional nurse anesthesia schools were opened between 1912 and 1920. All of these programs consisted of postgraduate training for nurses in the specialty of anesthesia delivery. A few of these programs included the Mayo Clinic, John Hopkins Hospital, Barnes Hospital, New York Post-Graduate Hospital, Presbyterian Hospital in Chicago, Charity Hospital in New Orleans, and Grace Hospital in Detroit.

Currently in the United States, 109 nurse anesthesia educational programs exist, all affiliated with or operated by academic institutions. Each program awards a degree of either master's or doctorate level, depending on the institution. The programs range from 24 to 36 months in length, determined

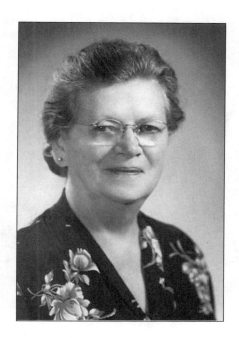

■ Figure 9-6   Agnes McGee

Source: American Association of Nurse Anesthetists. Reproduced with permission.

by the academic requirements of the individual institution. The total number of nurses enrolled in the current nurse anesthesia programs throughout the United States is more than 4,200 graduate students. These graduate nurse anesthesia programs provide the scientific underpinnings of anesthesia practice, including an average of 1,694 hours of clinical anesthesia administration to prepare highly competent nurse anesthesia graduates (Figure 9-7).

The future of nurse anesthesia education will require educational institutions to award only a clinical doctorate degree to those seeking a nurse anesthesia education. The AACN introduced the Doctor of Nursing Practice in 2004 and published this statement regarding the DNP: "In many institutions, advanced practice registered nurses (APRNs), including Nurse Practitioners, Clinical Nurse Specialists, Certified Nurse Midwives, and Certified Nurse Anesthetists, are prepared in master's-degree programs that often carry a credit load equivalent to doctoral degrees in the other health professions." The AACN's position statement calls for educating all APRNs and

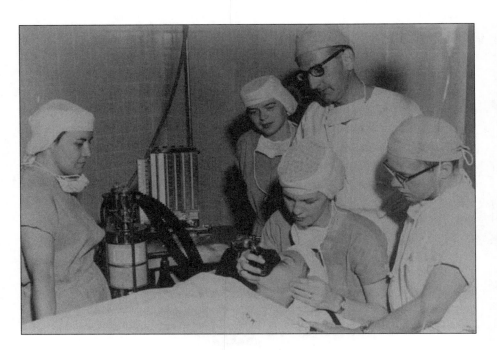

■ Figure 9-7   Nurse Anesthesia Students Learning How to Administer Inhalation Anesthesia at Easton Hospital, Circa 1964

Source: American Association of Nurse Anesthetists. Reproduced with permission.

nurses through doctoral education. The organization's decision to move the level of preparation for advanced practice nursing from the master's degree to the doctoral level is suggested to be in place by 2015.

The DNP is a natural progression in CRNA education, which began with the six-month course at St. Vincent's Hospital in Portland, Oregon, moved to the certificate level and then the bachelor's level, and then to all programs being required to award a master's degree. The DNP continues this advancement in CRNA education. CRNA education is already a two- to three-year postbaccalaureate program. At the completion of law school, a Juris Doctor is awarded as a recognition of the advanced level of education. The DNP will recognize the advanced level of education involved in CRNA training.

What does the DNP do for nurse anesthetists? The DNP will recognize the continuing advancement of the quality and depth of CRNA education. The DNP recognizes the tremendous responsibility of the CRNA, who literally makes life-and-death decisions and takes lifesaving measures with every anesthetic administered. Many early anesthesia programs were considered apprenticeships. Modern CRNA training programs require extensive didactic instruction, clinical training, and research. This level of academic progress will now result in a DNP. This recognition gives additional credibility to a time-honored advancing profession.

The educational requirements for nurse anesthetists have substantially evolved throughout the 20th century. During most of the 1980s and 1990s, the AANA and the Council on Accreditation evaluated whether there was a need for nurse anesthesia education to move to the practice-oriented doctoral level. After the 2004 release of the AACN's *Position Statement on the Practice Doctorate in Nursing*, the 2005 AANA president, Brian Thorson, appointed a task force (the DTF) to develop options related to the doctoral preparation of nurse anesthetists. The DTF presented its final report to the AANA board of directors in April 2007. In June 2007, the AANA board of directors unanimously adopted the position statement in support for the requirement of doctoral education for entry into nurse anesthesia practice by 2025.

Accreditation of Educational Programs: Council on Accreditation

In 1952, the American Association of Nurse Anesthetists created an accreditation body for nurse anesthesia educational programs in the United States. In 1975, a major revision to the accreditation criteria by the U.S. Office of Education triggered the transfer of the accreditation body from the AANA to a self-governing multidisciplinary body under the AANA's business structure. The newly formed accreditation body became the Council on Accreditation of Nurse Anesthesia Educational Programs/Schools (COA). The Council on Accreditation sets the standards and policies that must be followed by all nurse anesthesia educational programs located in institutions offering a post-master's certificate or a master's- or doctoral-level nurse anesthesia degree. The standards address administrative policies and procedures, institutional support, curriculum and instruction, faculty, evaluation, and ethics. Each year the council reviews the standards and presents revisions if warranted (AANA, 2009b).

The council consists of a 12-member assembly who represent the following groups: nurse anesthesia educators and practitioners, nurse anesthesia students, healthcare administrators, university representatives, and the public. The goal of accreditation is to advance the quality of nurse anesthesia education and provide competent practitioners to healthcare consumers and employers (AANA, 2009b).

The U.S. Department of Education and the Council for Higher Education Accreditation recognize the COA as an accrediting agency for the nurse anesthesia profession. Nurse anesthesia students must graduate from an accredited nurse anesthesia programs to become eligible to sit for the national certification exam.

Accreditation of nurse anesthesia programs occurs for established as well as new programs desiring accreditation. For a nurse anesthesia program to be accredited, it must be in compliance with each of the standards and policies set forth by the COA. Established programs are required to submit a self-evaluation of their program and welcome a review from the COA's team of reviewers. A summary of the visit is presented to the council for a decision as to the permission of continued accreditation and the time frame of the award, which can be up to ten years. Possible accreditation actions are as follows (AANA, 2009b):

- *Accreditation:* The program has successfully completed the accreditation process.
- *Probation:* The program has deficiencies that jeopardize the quality of nurse anesthesia education.
- *Revocation:* The program is noncompliant with the standards set forth by the council or there is evidence of a decrease in quality of the educational program.

Academic institutions seeking consideration for accreditation of a new nurse anesthesia program are required to submit a capability study and welcome an on-site evaluation. If the council deems the study and on-site evaluation have met the standards, accreditation will be awarded (AANA, 2009b). Each year, the Council on Accreditation publishes a list of current and newly added anesthesia programs to inform the public, other agencies, and prospective students.

Academic Curriculum Requirements

The Council on Accreditation has set forth curriculum requirements for the education of nurse anesthetists. The minimum requirements of a nurse anesthesia program provide the student with the clinical, scientific, and professional foundations to build a safe and sound clinical practice (Table 9-2).

Nurse anesthesia students spend many hours gaining clinical experience while being supervised by a nurse anesthetist, allowing them to learn and master the different anesthesia techniques. This intense clinical experience allows the student to apply the knowledge learned in the classroom directly to surgical patients. A 1998 survey of nurse anesthesia program directors revealed that the nurse anesthesia programs provide an average of 1,595

■ Table 9-2 Coursework and Minimal Contact Hours Required by the Council on Accreditation of Nurse Anesthesia Educational Programs

Coursework	Minimal Contact Hours
Pharmacology of anesthetic agents and adjuvant drugs, including concepts in chemistry and biochemistry	105
Anatomy, physiology, and pathophysiology	135
Professional aspects of nurse anesthesia practice	45
Basic and advanced principles of anesthesia practice, including physics, equipment, technology, and pain management	105
Research	30
Clinical correlation conferences	45

Source: American Association of Nurse Anesthetists. (2009). *Qualifications and capabilities of the certified registered nurse anesthetist.* Retrieved from http://www.aana.com/qualifications.aspx. Modified with permission.

hours of experience in the clinical area (AANA, 2009c). Nurse anesthesia students are given the opportunity to gain experience with anesthesia administration with patients of all ages in need of medical, surgical, pediatric, dental, and obstetrical surgeries and procedures (Figure 9-8).

Certification and Recertification of Nurse Anesthetists

The National Board on Certification and Recertification of Nurse Anesthetists (NBCRNA) is a governing body consisting of two councils: the Council on Certification of Nurse Anesthetists (CCNA) and the Council on Recertification of Nurse Anesthetists.

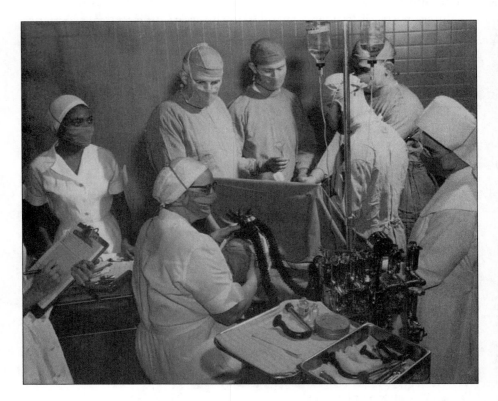

■ Figure 9-8   Nurse Anesthesia Students Administering Anesthesia at St. Mary of Nazareth Hospital, Date Unknown

Source: American Association of Nurse Anesthetists. Reproduced with permission.

Council on Certification of Nurse Anesthetists

The mission statement of the CCNA states, "The Council on Certification of Nurse Anesthetists (CCNA) is charged with protecting and serving the public by assuring that individuals who are credentialed have met predetermined qualifications or standards for providing nurse anesthesia services" (AANA, 2009d).

In 1945, the American Association of Nurse Anesthetists introduced a certification exam that was administered by the Credentials Committee of the AANA. All nurse anesthesia graduates from around the country were required to sit for the examination to obtain certification. The Councils for Certification and Recertification of nurse anesthetists were established in 1975, with the CCNA taking over responsibility for the certification exam. The CCNA resides under the structure of the NBCRNA and is responsible for the certification of registered nurse anesthetists who have fulfilled the educational requirement for the practice of nurse anesthesia. The CCNA membership appoints ten representatives as part of the governing body composed of seven CRNAs (three practitioners and four educators), two anesthesiologists, and one public member.

The CCNA oversees the credentialing requirements of examination and certification to assure the public that those certified in nurse anesthesia have met the qualifications for providing nurse anesthesia care. Table 9-3 lists the four primary goals of the CCNA.

The National Commission for Certifying Agencies (NCCA), a division of the National Organization for Competency Assurance (NOCA), is an

---

■ Table 9-3   Primary Goals of the Council on Certification of Nurse Anesthetists

---

1. Formulate and adopt requirements for eligibility for admission to the certification examination and for certification of registered nurse anesthetists.
2. Formulate, adopt and administer the certification examination to those registered nurse anesthetists who have met all requirements for examination and have been found eligible by the CCNA.
3. Evaluate candidates' performance on the certification examination.
4. Grant initial certification to those candidates who pass the certification examination and fulfill all other requirements for certification.

Source: American Association of Nurse Anesthetists. (2009). *Council on Certification of Nurse Anesthetists (CCNA) overview.* Retrieved from http://www.aana.com/Credentialing.aspx?id=138. Reprinted with permission.

accreditation body that sets standards that must be met by organizations which offer certification programs. The CCNA was awarded accreditation from the NCCA in 1980 and has maintained this accreditation to date. Accreditation from the NCCA signifies that the CCNA certification program has demonstrated compliance with the NCCA's Standards for the Accreditation of Certification Programs.

Recertification of Nurse Anesthetists

The Council on Recertification of Nurse Anesthetists is a self-governing body responsible for the recertification of nurse anesthetists. The council's purposes are to "(1) recertify qualified CRNAs on a biennial basis; (2) formulate, adopt and continuously evaluate the criteria for recertification of CRNAs; (3) formulate, adopt and continuously evaluate the criteria for approval of continuing education (CE) activities; (4) develop and maintain appellate mechanisms for CRNAs who have been denied recertification; and (5) develop and maintain a mechanism for the investigation and final resolution of charges or other allegations against CRNAs who are currently recertified" (reprinted from the AANA website, www.aana.com, with permission from the American Association of Nurse Anesthetists, [© 2009]).

Biennially, every nurse anesthetist must engage in the recertification process. The council's goal of recertification is to maintain high levels of knowledge, skill, and professionalism among CRNAs and to promote high-quality anesthesia care for patients.

Scope and Standards of Practice for Nurse Anesthetists

In 1974, the AANA created a set of standards to guide the practice of nurse anesthetists according to their amount of experience, state regulations, and the policy at the employed institution. The CRNA's scope of practice provides the responsibilities that must be maintained during the practice of anesthesia performed in collaboration with other healthcare providers.

Anesthesia care delivered by CRNAs consists of four general categories:

- Preanesthetic preparation and evaluation
- Anesthesia induction, maintenance, and emergence
- Postanesthesia care
- Perianesthetic and clinical support function

A nurse earning certification as a nurse anesthetist holds the qualifications to provide the functions of the CRNA's scope of practice shown in Table 9-4.

■ Table 9-4   Scope of Practice for Certified Registered Nurse Anesthetists

1. Performing and documenting a preanesthetic assessment and evaluation of the patient, including requesting consultations and diagnostic studies; selecting, obtaining, ordering, or administering preanesthetic medications and fluids; and obtaining informed consent for anesthesia
2. Developing and implementing an anesthetic plan
3. Selecting and initiating the planned anesthetic technique, which may include general, regional, and local anesthesia and intravenous sedation
4. Selecting, obtaining, or administering the anesthetics, adjuvant drugs, accessory drugs, and fluids necessary to manage the anesthetic, to maintain the patient's physiologic homeostasis, and to correct abnormal responses to the anesthesia or surgery
5. Selecting, applying, or inserting appropriate noninvasive and invasive monitoring modalities for collecting and interpreting patient physiological data
6. Managing a patient's airway and pulmonary status using endotracheal intubation, mechanical ventilation, pharmacological support, respiratory therapy, or extubation
7. Managing emergence and recovery from anesthesia by selecting, obtaining, ordering, or administering medications, fluids, or ventilatory support in order to maintain homeostasis, to provide relief from pain and anesthesia side effects, or to prevent or manage complications
8. Releasing or discharging patients from a postanesthesia care area, and providing postanesthesia follow-up evaluation and care related to anesthesia side effects or complications
9. Ordering, initiating, or modifying pain relief therapy through the utilization of drugs, regional anesthetic techniques, or other accepted pain relief modalities, including labor epidural analgesia
10. Responding to emergency situations by providing airway management, administration of emergency fluids or drugs, or using basic or advanced cardiac life support techniques
11. Additional nurse anesthesia responsibilities that are within the expertise of the individual CRNA, including administrative and management, quality assessment, education, research, committee assignments, and interdepartmental liaison efforts

Source: American Association of Nurse Anesthetists. (2007). *Scope and standards for nurse anesthesia practice,* pp. 1–2. Park Ridge, IL: Author. Modified with permission.

Standards for Nurse Anesthesia Practice

The standards of nurse anesthesia practice are designed to guide the practice of a nurse anesthetist. The intention of the standards is to

1. Assist the profession in evaluating the quality of care provided by its practitioners.
2. Provide a common base for practitioners to use in their development of a quality practice.
3. Assist the public in understanding what to expect from the practitioner.
4. Support and preserve the basic rights of the patient. (AACN, 2007, p. 3)

Each standard applies to all anesthetizing locations. Table 9-5 outlines the standards that are intended to encourage the nurse anesthetist to provide the highest quality of patient care.

Clinical Practice Outside the Operating Room

A majority of nurse anesthetists provide anesthesia in the operating room, but there is also opportunity for CRNAs to administer anesthesia outside the operating room. Anesthesia services have expanded to areas such as cardiac catheterization labs, MRI units, and lithotripsy suites. Anesthetists are also contacted by referrals outside the anesthesia department to provide consultation for respiratory concerns including intubation, to participate in emergency situations such as cardiopulmonary resuscitation, and to manage blood, fluid, electrolyte, and acid–base balance.

CRNAs also perform administrative activities for the department of anesthesia. The overall function of an anesthesia department depends on services provided by the directors and managers of the anesthesia division to ensure the efficiency and quality of the provided anesthesia services. Functions include but are not limited to continuing education, financial management, personnel and resource management, quality assurance, and risk management.

CRNA Scholarship

Nurse anesthetists participate on healthcare centers' committees and are involved as educators for both professional and nonprofessional staff. CRNAs serve on committees within their state and governmental agencies, including the state boards of nursing and the U.S. Food and Drug Administration. Nurse anesthetists are also directly involved in professional and standard-

■ Table 9-5   Standards for Nurse Anesthesia Practice

Standard I	Perform a thorough and complete preanesthesia assessment.
Standard II	Obtain informed consent for the planned anesthetic.
Standard III	Formulate a patient-specific plan for anesthesia care.
Standard IV	Implement and adjust the anesthesia care plan based on the patient's physiologic response.
Standard V	Monitor the patient's physiologic condition as appropriate for the type of anesthesia and specific patient needs. 1. Monitor ventilation continuously. 2. Monitor oxygenation continuously. 3. Monitor cardiovascular status continuously. 4. Monitor body temperature continuously. 5. Monitor neuromuscular function and status. 6. Monitor and assess the patient positioning.
Standard VI	Document pertinent information on the patient's medical record completely, accurately, and in a timely manner.
Standard VII	Transfer the responsibility for care of the patient to other qualified providers in a manner that assures continuity of care and patient safety.
Standard VIII	Adhere to appropriate safety precautions, as established within the institution, to minimize the risks of fire, explosion, electrical shock, and equipment malfunction. Document on the patient's medical record that the anesthesia machine and equipment were checked.
Standard IX	Take precautions to minimize the risk of infarction to the patient, the CRNA, and other health care providers.
Standard X	Assess anesthesia care to assure its quality and contribution to positive patient outcomes.
Standard XI	Respect and maintain the basic rights of patients.

Source: American Association of Nurse Anesthetists. (2007). *Scope and standards for nurse anesthesia practice*, pp. 4–6. Park Ridge, IL: Author. Modified with permission.

setting organizations such as the National Fire Protection Association and the American Society for Testing and Materials.

Research is a fundamental component of anesthetic administration. Nurse anesthetists have served in multiple roles related to research as early as the beginning of the 20th century. Nurse anesthetists' involvement in research has included roles as principle investigators, consultative and collaborator positions, and users of the research findings. Nurse anesthesia programs include research as part of the standard curriculum, providing the graduate student with the basic skills necessary for conducting research. The AANA Foundation promotes nurse anesthetists' involvement with research, focusing on the quality of anesthesia care and outcome-based research. Funding for research by CRNAs and nurse anesthesia students has been provided by private and governmental grants and by the AANA Education and Research Foundation. Students and CRNAs are given the opportunity to present and disseminate their research findings at the AANA's annual meeting.

Nurse anesthetists have been involved in authoring or contributing to anesthesia textbooks and clinical, educational, and research topics published in peer-reviewed journals. Some of these professional publications include the *AANA Journal, CRNA: The Clinical Forum for Nurse Anesthetists, Nurse Anesthesia, Anesthesiology, Anesthesia and Analgesia, Journal of the American Society of Regional Anesthesia, Journal of the American Medical Association, Nursing Research,* and *Hospitals and Nursing Forum.*

The needs of the healthcare environment are in constant change. The Doctor of Nursing Practice degree will provide nurse anesthetists with an education that is comparable to other practice-focused professional degrees such as the Doctor of Pharmacy, the Doctor of Physical Therapy, and the Doctor of Occupational Therapy. Research conducted by Linda Aiken in 2003 revealed that in hospitals with higher proportions of nurses educated at the baccalaureate level or higher, surgical patients experienced lower mortality and failure-to-rescue rates. (Aiken, 2003). This shows a clear link between higher levels of nursing education and better patient outcomes. The DNP degree will prepare tomorrow's nurse anesthetists at the highest education level and will provide them with the capability to transform healthcare delivery by designing, evaluating, and continuously improving the framework within which care is delivered. Also, CRNAs educated within a doctoral framework will have the capability to influence local and national health care by demonstrating effective leadership and political advocacy.

Nurse Midwife
Deborah Ringdahl

Nurse midwives represent a vital part of advanced practice nursing, with a long history of patient advocacy, leadership, service to underserved populations, development of new models of healthcare delivery, and commitment to the provision of high-quality health care for women and families. In many important ways, nurse midwives have broken ground for all advanced practice nurses, leading the way in APN outcome-based research, the development of educational programs, and access to healthcare systems through legislative reform. From the time nurse midwifery was first introduced into this country in 1925 to the present, the midwifery profession has demonstrated many of the attributes that are now associated with the doctorally prepared nurse practitioner. Awareness and understanding of a larger practice context is required for the midwifery profession to remain strong and viable. The formal integration of midwifery clinical practice skills with a DNP education will serve to further strengthen the midwifery profession and ultimately improve the health of women and families. This section provides an overview of midwifery practice, followed by a discussion of the role of the DNP-prepared midwife.

Midwifery Practice

As an organized profession, nurse midwives have worked hard to define who they are, maintain high standards of education and practice, and interact with other professional organizations. The professional documents of the American College of Nurse-Midwives (ACNM) define the standards of midwifery practice (ACNM, 2003a) and also serve to educate the public about the roles and responsibilities of the nurse midwife. The *Philosophy of the American College of Nurse-Midwives* affirms the entitlement of basic human rights in health care and the value of the midwifery model of health care, which includes supporting normalcy in women's lifecycle events (ACNM, 2004a). The majority of practicing midwives in this country are certified nurse midwives (CNMs), individuals "educated in the two disciplines of nursing and midwifery, who possess evidence of certification according to the requirements of ACNM" (ACNM, 2004b). In 1994 the ACNM approved adding a non-nurse midwifery option to its educational programs, resulting in the addition of the title certified midwife (CM), "an individual educated in the discipline of midwifery, who possesses evidence of certification according to the requirements of ACNM" (ACNM, 2004b). The decision to include non-nurses in ACNM-accredited education programs and the certification process was made in order to set uniform standards for midwifery education and practice, leading to the development of direct-entry educational programs. Not surprisingly, developing one midwifery standard for nurses and non-nurses has presented many challenges, including consumer awareness, institutional credentialing, legislative practice regulations, and policy development. Legal recognition of midwifery practice exists primarily through nursing boards, requiring licensure in nursing as a prerequisite to practice.

Midwives have made significant progress toward gaining legitimacy within the healthcare system, even though their numbers are small (11,546 CNMs/CMs) and they have encountered legislative and institutional barriers to practice. Certified nurse midwifery practice is legal in all 50 states, and CMs can practice in New Jersey, New York, and Rhode Island. Medicaid reimbursement for CNM/CM care is mandatory in all states, and 33 states mandate private insurance reimbursement for nurse midwifery services. CNMs have prescription-writing authority in all 50 states, and CMs have prescription-writing authority in New York and Rhode Island (ACNM, 2009a).

Many important professional issues affect access to clients and the financial viability of CNM/CM practice, among them being direct access; liability insurance; reimbursement, including Medicare and Medicaid; antitrust laws; and midwifery admitting privileges. These issues require development of legislative and policy strategies. The ACNM has provided leadership by developing resources on the politics and business of midwifery practice, as well as allocating more resources for legislative work.

Midwives work primarily in hospitals, and the number of women choosing midwives as their birth attendants continues to increase. In 2006, 10.8% of all vaginal births were attended by CNMs in the United States, which represents more than a doubling of the 1990 rate (Declercq, 2009). Of these CNM/CM-attended births, 97% occurred in hospitals, 2% occurred in freestanding birth centers, and 1% occurred in homes. More than 60% of CNMs/CMs list physician practices or hospitals/medical centers as their principal employers. Midwives also provide primary care: 90% of visits to CNMs/CMs are for primary, preventive care, including annual exams and reproductive health visits (ACNM, 2009a).

There are currently 38 midwifery accredited educational programs in the United States, mostly housed in nursing schools as graduate programs. Nineteen of these programs offer a DNP option, mostly after masters' programs (ACNM, 2009a). The majority (80%) of CNMs have a master's degree, and 5%

hold a doctoral degree. For the remainder of this section, the term *midwife* will be reserved for the CNM, as CMs are not currently eligible for DNP educational programs.

History

Midwives have moved from serving as home birth attendants within their communities during the 1800s and 1900s to an organized group of healthcare professionals who now meet the primary healthcare needs of women in a variety of healthcare settings. These changes have been influenced by social trends and the shifting healthcare landscape. Understanding the history of midwifery in this country provides perspective on two of the recurring themes that accompany midwifery practice: recognition of midwifery as a legitimate profession and access by midwives to the healthcare system. It is particularly noteworthy that a vital connection was made between the practice of midwifery and the nursing profession when midwifery was formally introduced into this country. Although there is ongoing debate about whether midwifery practice requires a nursing background, it is clear that midwifery's connection to nursing has been instrumental in establishing professional legitimacy in midwifery practice (Burst, 2005).

The informal origins of midwifery practice in the United States can be traced to the immigrant midwives who arrived during the late 1800s and early 1900s and the African American midwives who provided care to women in the South. At the beginning of the 20th century, 50% of births occurred at home with a midwife (Dawley, 2003). During this same time period, studies revealed alarmingly high infant and maternal mortality rates, resulting in a chain of events that dramatically affected midwifery practice. Health officials were concerned that midwives did not have adequate education or training, and several strategies were developed to resolve this "midwife problem," including training public health nurses to provide maternity care (Varney, Kriebs, & Gegor, 2004). The Sheppard-Towner Act was passed in 1921 and funded through 1929, providing training of midwives by public health nurses. During this same time, medical schools started to include obstetrics in their curricula; obstetrics became a medical specialty in 1930, and birth began moving out of the home into the hospital (Varney, Kriebs, & Gegor, 2004).

Mary Breckinridge introduced the nurse midwifery model of care to the United States when she brought British-trained nurse midwives to rural Kentucky in 1925. The Frontier Nursing Service (FNS) was a carefully crafted program that used nurse midwives as birth attendants and provided a comprehensive scope of healthcare services, yielding dramatic improvements in both maternal and infant mortality rates, lower than the national rates from 1931 to 1950 (Varney, Kriebs, & Gegor, 2004). These outcomes were particularly significant given that most births occurred in homes with primitive living conditions, and further advanced the credibility of nurse midwives as competent healthcare providers.

The first educational nurse midwife program opened in 1931, and by the end of the 1950s there were seven nurse midwifery educational programs nationwide. Practice opportunities remained limited until the 1970s, with the majority of nurse midwifery practices providing care to low-income women who lived in underserved areas of the country. Many events occurred during the 1960s and 1970s that led to greater acceptance of the nurse midwifery model of care and extended nurse midwifery care into the middle-class population. Social movements promoting more autonomy for women, federally funded projects using nurse midwives, a 1971 joint statement between the nurse midwife and obstetrician/gynecologist professions, the need for more birth attendants to provide care to the baby boomer generation, the inclusion of family planning and gynecologic care in clinical competencies, and the demonstration of the safety and efficacy of nurse midwives all converged to create a more favorable climate for the proliferation of nurse midwifery educational programs and clinical practice opportunities (Varney, Kriebs, & Gegor, 2004).

Midwifery history is rich with examples of leadership "in the areas of clinical excellence, educational strategies, business savvy, and policy development" (Ament, 2006, p. 328), contributing to increased access to the healthcare system. By the 1980s, nurse midwives were practicing in a wide range of settings, providing a wide range of services and providing care to all classes of women. Physicians became aware that nurse midwives were now competing for their middle- and upper-class clients, and some efforts were made to restrict midwifery practice (Varney, Kriebs, & Gegor, 2004). Nonetheless, midwifery education and practice experienced more growth in the 1990s, in part as a response to managed care and the focus on providing high quality and cost-effective care.

Professional Organization

The American College of Nurse-Midwives, incorporated in 1955, provides a foundation for the growth and development of nurse midwifery education and practice. The mission of the ACNM is to "promote the health and well-being of women and infants within their families and communities through the development and support of the profession of midwifery as practiced by certified nurse-midwives (CNMs) and certified midwives (CMs)" (ACNM, 2003b). The ACNM has developed position statements, political and legislative resources, and executive staff positions that reflect a strong commitment to professional involvement in local, state, and national politics. At the national level, the ACNM provides leadership through the board of directors, divisions, and committees that work to address clinical practice issues, health policy, and educational standards. The ACNM conducts research, accredits midwifery education programs, administers and promotes continuing education programs, establishes clinical practice standards, and creates liaisons with state and federal agencies and members of Congress.

The International Confederation of Midwives (ICM) confers membership to ACNM members, promoting professional relationships with midwives throughout the world. The ACNM website (acnm.org or midwife.org) has become a particularly useful vehicle for keeping its membership up to date with current issues affecting nurse midwifery practice.

Education and Certification

The education of midwives is central to professional credibility and viability. Midwifery education has undergone many changes since the first program was introduced in 1931. Requirement of a baccalaureate degree upon entrance or completion of the program was initiated in 1996, and in 2006 the ACNM issued a position statement requiring a graduate degree by 2010 for entry into midwifery practice (ACNM, 2009d). Although the ACNM supports a graduate degree, it does not require the Doctor of Nursing Practice degree for entry into midwifery practice (ACNM, 2009e). "At the present time, evidence points to the fact that current education requirements produce safe, knowledgeable, competent midwives. Because data are lacking regarding the potential impact of the proposed Doctor of Nursing Practice on the cost of education to both the institution and the student, on the applicant pool, and the health care system, the Directors of Midwifery Education (DOME) endorse a statement affirming support for multiple routes of midwifery education based on the ACNM Core Competencies, and does not endorse a mandatory requirement for the clinical doctorate for entry into practice" (Avery & Howe, 2007, p. 14).

The ACNM Accreditation Commission for Midwifery Education (ACME) sets standards for the educational programs. All programs accredited by ACME provide curricula as defined by ACNM's *Core Competencies for Basic Midwifery Practice* (ACNM, 2008). *The Knowledge, Skills, and Behaviors Prerequisite to Midwifery Clinical Coursework* (ACME, 2005) was developed for direct-entry (CM) midwifery programs, ensuring that all graduates emerge with the foundational knowledge that nursing education provided for nurse midwife graduates. All accredited educational programs have required affiliation with a university, college, or other institution of higher learning accredited by a U.S. Department of Education–recognized accrediting agency since 1996 (ACNM, 2009c).

CNM and CM candidates must sit for the national certification exam (NCE), which was first offered in 1971 by the ACNM. The ACNM Certification Council became the certifying body in 1991, changing its name to the American Midwifery Certification Board in 2005. Since 1995, all candidates passing the NCE have received an eight-year time-limited certificate, with two options for renewal through the Certificate Maintenance Program. All other CNMs/CMs are expected to demonstrate continuing competency through continuing competency assessment (Slattery, 1999, 2006).

Scope of Practice

Midwifery practice has changed over time, reflecting the need for expanding the scope of practice beyond pregnancy and childbirth. Midwifery practice now includes providing reproductive and primary health care to women from menarche to menopause. The ACNM's position statement *Definition of Midwifery Practice* (2004d) outlines the parameters of clinical practice:

> Midwifery practice as conducted by Certified Nurse-Midwives (CNMs) and Certified Midwives (CMs) is the independent management of women's health care, focusing particularly on common primary care issues, family planning and gynecologic needs of women, pregnancy, childbirth, the postpartum period and the care of the newborn. The CNM and CM practice within a health care system that provides for consultation, collaborative management or referral as indicated by the health status of the client. CNMs and CMs practice in accord with the Standards for the Practice of Midwifery, as defined by the American College of Nurse-Midwives. (p. 1)

The *Core Competencies for Basic Midwifery Practice* (ACNM, 2008) provides the practice and educational template for CNMs and CMs and applies to all midwifery settings, including hospitals, ambulatory care settings, birth centers, and home. These competencies were first developed in 1978 in order to provide a set of uniform standards for clinical practice and nurse midwifery education and have been revised five times, illustrating the evolving nature of midwifery practice. Some of the major points of revision have been delineation of the role of midwifes in collaborative management; expansion of the components of midwifery care outside the maternity cycle; description of professional responsibilities; identification of the hallmarks of midwifery; inclusion of primary care; and addition of business competencies (Avery, 2005). The changes made to this document provide evidence of the professional growth of midwifery practice, the changing healthcare environment, and the need for expanding the scope of practice beyond maternity care and the development of nonclinical skills. The AACN's *Essentials of Doctoral Education for Advanced Nursing Practice* (AACN, 2006) and the National Organization of Nurse Practitioner Faculties' *Practice Doctorate Nurse Practitioner Entry Level Competencies* (2006) are reflected in several of the nonclinical components of the core competencies, such as leadership, business, research, and policy development (Table 9-6).

■ Table 9-6   Congruency of ACNM Core Competencies for Basic Midwifery Practice with DNP Competencies

ACNM Core Competencies for Basic Midwifery Practice	*Essentials of Doctoral Education for Advanced Nursing Practice:* American Association of Colleges of Nursing (AACN)	DNP Entry-Level Competencies: National Organization of Nurse Practitioner Faculties (NONPF)
Incorporation of scientific evidence into clinical practice	Scientific underpinnings for practice	Scientific foundation
Participation in evaluation, peer review, other activities that ensure and validate quality practice, understanding of bioethics related to women, newborns, families	Organizational and systems leadership for quality improvement and systems thinking	Quality, ethics
Ability to evaluate, apply, interpret, and collaborate in research	Clinical scholarship and analytical methods for evidence-based practice	Practice inquiry

(continues)

■ Table 9-6   Congruency of ACNM Core Competencies for Basic Midwifery Practice with DNP Competencies (CONTINUED)

ACNM Core Competencies for Basic Midwifery Practice	Essentials of Doctoral Education for Advanced Nursing Practice: American Association of Colleges of Nursing (AACN)	DNP Entry-Level Competencies: National Organization of Nurse Practitioner Faculties (NONPF)
Standards for Practice of Midwifery (VI): accessible and complete documentation	Information systems/ technology and patient care technology for the improvement and trans- formation of health care	Technology and information literacy
Support of legislation and policy initiatives which promote quality healthcare, knowledge of issues and trends in health- care policy and systems	Healthcare policy for advocacy in health care	Policy
Development of leadership skills, collaboration with other members of the healthcare team	Interprofessional collaboration for improving patient and population health outcomes	Leadership
Health promotion, disease prevention, and health edu- cation, cultural competence, promotion of a public health perspective, care to vulnerable populations	Clinical prevention and population health for improving the nation's health	Health delivery system
Midwifery management process, fundamentals, primary care, childbearing family, knowledge of legal basis for practice, knowledge of licensure, clinical privileges, credentialing	Advanced nursing practice	Independent practice

Sources: American College of Nurse-Midwives (ACNM). (2008). *Core competencies for basic midwifery practice.* Retrieved from http://www.midwife.org/siteFiles/descriptive/Core_Competencies_6_07.pdf; ACNM. (2003). *Standards for the practice of midwifery.* Silver Spring, MD: Author; American Association of Colleges of Nursing. (2006). *The essentials of doctoral education for advanced nursing practice.* Washington, DC: Author; and National Organization of Nurse Practitioner Faculties. (2006). *Practice doctorate nurse practitioner entry-level competencies.* Retrieved from http://nonpf.org/NONPF2005/CoreCompsFINAL06.pdf.

Federal and state laws, institutional regulations, and practice guidelines also play a role in determining scope of practice. Federal and state laws affect scope of practice primarily through federal regulations and state regulatory boards, such as boards of medicine or nursing. Institutional regulations, typically hospital bylaws, can restrict scope of practice by preventing midwives from obtaining hospital or admitting privileges. "Practice guidelines define the legal basis for a clinician's practice, describe parameters or scope of practice, and describe situations in which a physician should be consulted" (Slager, 2004, p. 38). Supervisory language in practice guidelines is strongly discouraged, because it implies a dependent relationship with the physician consultant rather than supporting independent clinical decision making within a defined scope of practice. It is generally recommended that practice guidelines not be overly proscriptive and leave room for clinical judgment and the experience level of the midwife. Practice guidelines are typically updated on a yearly basis to include new research and professional standards.

The DNP-Prepared Midwife

The DNP-prepared midwife learns knowledge and skills that further support autonomy, leadership, and the role of change agent in an increasingly complex healthcare system. Advancing knowledge of leadership, educational and change theories, health policy, economics, and epidemiology add depth and breadth to midwifery education and practice. As change agents, midwives need to develop skills that promote evidence-based practice, evaluation of clinical practice, integration of nursing theory into practice, and effective use of information systems to document outcomes. Educational programs leading to the master's degree for midwives include some of this content in their coursework, but the primary focus is the development of clinical competencies, leaving little time for in-depth study of less clinically based practice competencies.

Table 9-6 provides an overview of the congruency between the ACNM's *Core Competencies for Basic Midwifery Practice* (ACNM, 2008) and the DNP competencies developed by the American Association of Colleges of Nursing (AACN) and the National Organization of Nurse Practitioner Faculties (NONPF). Within the ACNM core competencies, the majority of the DNP competencies are found in the "Hallmarks of Midwifery" and "Professional Responsibilities" (ACNM, 2008). These ACNM core competencies are incorporated into all CNM and CM educational programs, and must be present in the curriculum for programs to achieve accreditation. DNP course content that addresses healthcare economics, policy, evidence-based practice, leadership and change theories, and program evaluation will further develop these midwifery core competencies. "Although the focus of the practice doctorate is not on basic research, the potential exists for the development of much needed evaluation and systems research in the practice and business of midwifery" (Avery & Howe, 2007, p. 17).

Midwives have provided leadership in many healthcare arenas, from safeguarding normal pregnancy and childbirth to advocating for high-quality, affordable, and accessible health care for all women. DNP-prepared midwives should retain strong leadership in their primary area of expertise, namely, providing high-quality health care to women. Midwives have long advocated for the healthcare needs of all women by building alliances with other professional organizations, using public health and business strategies, creating new models of health care, developing international programs, and remaining committed to the normalcy of women's lifecycle events. DNP-prepared midwives can further advance women's health by assuming leadership in the following areas: development of maternal–child health public policy; development of quality measures and data collection tools that promote maternal–child health; creation of a healthcare model that safeguards the normalcy of women's lifecycle events and promotes cultural competency; development of standards for midwifery that promote safe motherhood; development of programs that teach healthcare business acumen; and active engagement in healthcare reform. These areas are discussed in more detail in the following sections.

Maternal–Child Health Public Policy

The roots of midwifery practice lie in providing care to disadvantaged and vulnerable women and children. Research on the socioeconomic component of health status has informed the public health perspective and provided a better understanding of how poverty directly and indirectly affects health. The Healthy People Initiative provides a framework for addressing health disparities, examining both healthcare access and healthcare delivery. The midwife's expert clinical skills and experience in working effectively with vulnerable populations provide a strong foundation for improving maternal–child health outcomes and achieving the public health goals outlined in this initiative (Jesse & Blue, 2004). The DNP-prepared midwife can further advance the public policy agenda for maternal–child health by integrating epidemiologic and evidence-based research into the development of community health programs and engaging in legislative work that informs public policy.

Quality Measures and Data Collection

Midwives have achieved recognition as healthcare providers who provide high-quality care. The first midwifery service in this country maintained careful records that demonstrated improved outcomes with nurse midwifery care; a statistical analysis of the first 30 years of Frontier Nursing Service practice (1925–1954) estimated that national adoption of their processes would prevent 60,000 perinatal deaths every year (Metropolitan Life Insurance Company, 1960). Since then, there have been numerous studies that document highly favorable outcomes in births attended by nurse midwives (ACNM, 2005).

The value of accurate record keeping cannot be underestimated: midwifery statistics lead to both recognition of high standards of care and credibility within the healthcare system. Data collection should be integrated into every clinical practice, selecting quality measures that reflect the high standard of care that is provided. Intrapartal (1996) and antepartal (1999) data sets have been developed by the ACNM that provide a template for midwifery data collection. The ACNM recently initiated a benchmarking project aimed at collecting data from midwifery practices across the country, and three years of data on best practices have been collected to date. The DNP-prepared midwife has the knowledge and resources to further develop quality management skills, including development of clinically relevant data sets, consolidation and organization of data through information technology, and developing partnerships with other organizations invested in providing high-quality care.

Safeguarding the Normalcy of Women's Lifecycle Events

Midwives have maintained a philosophy of birth as normal, and incorporated this model of health care into a variety of healthcare settings. According to Barger (2005), "The midwifery model of care emanates from the belief that pregnancy, birth, and menopause are normal processes of life and that it is, therefore, part of the role of the midwife to help protect the normalcy of these events from a culture or society that might believe otherwise" (p. 88).

Safeguarding the normalcy of birth is no small feat in the current climate of rising cesarean sections, representing 31.8% of all births in 2007 (Hamilton, Martin, & Ventura, 2009). The ACNM supports the normalcy of birth by using research to demonstrate the safety of out-of-hospital births, developing position statements supporting nonintervention in normal processes, and supporting evidence-based research as the gold standard in providing health care. The DNP-prepared midwife can move this agenda further forward by maintaining currency with clinical research and educating consumers, healthcare providers, and policy makers about the risks associated with intervening unnecessarily in normal processes.

Cultural Competency

A long history of providing health care to women who are uninsured, immigrant, adolescent, and ethnically, racially, and socioeconomically diverse (Declercq, Williams, Koontz, Paine, Streit, & McClosky, 2001) has given midwives many avenues for cultivating cultural competency. According to Varney, Kriebs, and Gegor (2004), "Midwives must be at the forefront in the implementation of cultural competence training programs, which are now considered key interventions in reducing the health care disparities that disproportionately affect women of color" (p. 56). Although there is no specific DNP competency addressing cultural competency (see Table 9-6), development of effective healthcare policy requires cultural understanding and research on health outcomes among different cultural groups. The DNP-prepared midwife has a more comprehensive understanding of health policy and epidemiologic trends, contributing to a wider application of cultural competency, including clinical practice, research, and policy development.

Midwifery Standards and Safe Motherhood

Midwives exist in all cultures and countries, and although educational backgrounds may differ, all midwives are part of the global community. Midwives carry the international torch for safe motherhood, playing a central role in "global efforts to make pregnancy and birth safe throughout the world and promote the health and well-being of girls and women wherever they reside" (Varney, Kriebs, & Gegor, 2004, p. 60). The ACNM has a long history of active involvement in the International Confederation of Midwives, as well as developing international programs to support safe motherhood. The ACNM Department of Global Outreach has undertaken projects to support the education of traditional birth attendants (TBAs) and the development of *The Lifesaving Skills Manual for Midwives* (Varney, Kriebs, & Gegor, 2004). In 1997 the ACNM spearheaded a Safe Motherhood Initiative, leading to partnership with other professional organizations in developing priorities for improving maternity care in the United States. More recently, the ACNM formed the Ad Hoc Committee on Disaster Preparedness, providing leadership in managing the needs of mothers and infants during disasters (ACNM, 2009f; Al Gasseer, Dresden, Keeney, & Warren, 2004).

As a birth attendant, the midwife assumes a unique position among advanced practice nurses in the care of women during labor and birth, demonstrating commitment and leadership in preserving the health of mothers and babies. The word *vivant*, or *let them live*, takes center stage on the ACNM seal, representing midwives' "unremitting dedication to safeguarding and promoting the health and wellbeing of family life, particularly the mother and infant" (Varney, Kriebs, & Gegor, 2004, p. 22). Evidence-based practice needs to be recognized as an international standard and applied to improving maternal and child outcomes in all countries (Miller, Sloan, Winikoff, Langer, & Fikree, 2003). In addition to improving maternal outcomes by providing excellent clinical care, the DNP-prepared midwife has access to knowledge and resources that will activate leadership in health policy, education, and program evaluation.

Healthcare Business Acumen

Most healthcare providers do not learn business skills in conjunction with their healthcare education. Midwives learned about the business aspects of clinical practice as a survival strategy. Viability meant learning the nuts and bolts of marketing and financial management, as well as developing skills to influence legislative and institutional barriers to practice. Educational programs responded by adding more professional issues into their curricula, and the ACNM developed guidelines for starting a practice and resources on marketing and managed care. The Nurse-Midwifery Service Director's Network (SDN) published editions of *An Administrative Manual for Midwifery* in 1994, 1996, and 2005 (Slager), focusing on the administrative and business aspects of midwifery practice. The Midwifery Business Institute has sponsored annual conferences since 1996, and the ACNM publishes handbooks on specific aspects of business practice, such as billing and coding.

According to Joan Slager, author of *Business Concepts for Healthcare Providers* (2004), "[Business] ignorance has resulted in inadequate compensation, inappropriate restriction, and unfair representation of the non-physician provider" (p. ix). Although each nursing specialty may have some unique business needs, the business knowledge and resources culled through the experience of midwives can serve as a template for all advanced practice nurses. This template, combined with coursework in health economics, informatics, and policy, will generate advanced practice nurses with healthcare business acumen.

Healthcare Reform

The unique role that midwives play in healthcare reform needs to be framed within the context of quality and cost-effectiveness. The concepts of high-quality and cost-effective care are embedded in midwifery philosophy, making the midwifery model of care useful as a healthcare exemplar. The Pew Health Professions Committee convened a task force in 1998 that concluded that "the midwifery model of care should be incorporated into the health care system in order to make it available to all women and their families" (Paine, Dower, & O'Neil, 1999). A 2008 Cochrane review by Hatem, Sandall, Devane, Soltani, and Gates showed that midwifery care is associated with many positive outcomes, including shorter hospital stays and increased probability of vaginal birth. The overuse of costly interventions and underuse of evidence-based care were recently outlined in *Evidence-Based Maternity Care*, emphasizing the need to use a low-intervention model of maternity care (Sakala & Corry, 2008). Additionally, the midwifery model of care places a strong emphasis on health promotion and disease prevention, positioning midwives as effective primary care providers (Shah & King, 2006).

The ACNM issued a set of seven key principles for healthcare reform that highlights the need for improved access to women's healthcare services, including primary, gynecologic, family planning, and maternity care, and the urgency of removing barriers to midwifery practice in these vital areas of health care (ACNM, 2009b). According to Melissa Avery, president of the ACNM, "Let us make the voice of midwifery heard by uniting toward one goal—improving health care access, quality, and value for women and their families" (2009, p. 3). The ACNM Government Affairs Committee assists in the development of a federal legislative and regulatory agenda that advocates for healthcare reform in women's health services, professional liability, third-party reimbursement, and access to midwifery care.

The DNP-prepared midwife is prepared to assume leadership in advocating for healthcare reform that provides accessible, high-quality, and cost-effective care for all citizens, integrating information from leadership and change theory, health policy, the economics of health care, evidence-based practice, and epidemiology. Successful development and implementation of healthcare reform requires the expertise of healthcare providers who understand the complexity of our healthcare system and have the necessary skills to develop solutions.

Conclusion

Midwives are an innovative and tenacious lot, functioning as leaders and change agents within our healthcare system. In spite of many barriers to practice, midwives have persisted in making inroads into mainstream health care. The vision of the early nurse midwife leaders, development of a strong professional organization, and strategic educational and practice changes have greatly contributed to professional recognition and access to the healthcare system. It is also clear that visibility and viability in the healthcare system require cultivation of business acumen and legislative engagement. In addition to maintaining high clinical practice standards, gaining recognition and access to the healthcare system requires an understanding of business, politics, data collection, public health, and quality improvement. Successful completion of a doctorate in nursing practice prepares graduates to provide leadership in the clinical practice arena.

The DNP-prepared midwife is especially well suited to assume leadership roles in the clinical arena. She or he will enter the healthcare system with additional knowledge and skills that will strengthen her or his capacity to interact effectively with the healthcare system. Strong clinical expertise in maternal–child health combined with an understanding of healthcare economics and policy will increase the effectiveness of midwives as they practice within an increasingly complex healthcare system. Utilization of information systems, program evaluation, and evidence-based research will enhance clinical practice and serve to reinforce the merits of the midwifery model of care. The DNP-prepared midwife will have new tools for promoting high-quality care for women and children, adding value to the role of the midwife as a woman's healthcare provider.

References

Accreditation Commission for Midwifery Education. (2005). *The knowledge, skills, and behaviors prerequisite to midwifery clinical coursework*. Silver Spring, MD: Author.

Aiken, L. H. (2003). Educational levels of hospital nurses and surgical patient mortality. *Journal of the American Medical Association, 290,* 1617–1623.

Al Gasseer, N., Dresden, E., Keeney, G., & Warren, N. (2004). Status of women and infants in complex humanitarian emergencies. *Journal of Midwifery and Women's Health, 49*(4 Suppl. 1), 7–13.

Ament, L. (2006). *Professional issues in midwifery*. Sudbury, MA: Jones and Bartlett.

American Academy of Nurse Practitioners. (2007). *Scope of practice for nurse practitioners*. Retrieved from http://aanp.org/NR/rdonlyres/59523729-0179-466A-A7FB-BDEE68160E8E/0/NPCurriculum.pdf#search="scope of practice"

American Association of Colleges of Nursing. (n.d.). *The doctor of nursing practice*. Retrieved from http://www.aacn.nche.edu/Media/FactSheets/dnp.htm

American Association of Colleges of Nursing. (2004). *Position statement on the practice doctorate in nursing*. Retrieved from http://www.aacn.nche.edu/DNP/pdf/DNP.pdf

American Association of Colleges of Nursing. (2006). *The essentials of doctoral education for advanced nursing practice*. Washington, DC: Author.

American Association of Colleges of Nursing. (2008). *Doctor of nursing practice (DNP) talking points*. Retrieved from http://www.aacn.nche.edu/DNP/talkingpoints.htm

American Association of Colleges of Nursing. (2009). *Doctor of nursing practice programs*. Retrieved from http://www.aacn.nche.edu/dnp/DNPProgramList.htm

American Association of Nurse Anesthetists. (2007). *Scope and standards for nurse anesthesia practice*. Park Ridge, IL: Author.

American Association of Nurse Anesthetists. (2009a). *History of nurse anesthesia practice*. Retrieved from http://www.aana.com/crnahistory.aspx

American Association of Nurse Anesthetists. (2009b). *Council on Accreditation of Nurse Anesthesia Educational Programs: Overview*. Retrieved from http://www.aana.com/councilaccreditation.aspx

American Association of Nurse Anesthetists. (2009c). *Qualifications and capabilities of the certified registered nurse anesthetist*. Retrieved from http://www.aana.com/qualifications.aspx

American Association of Nurse Anesthetists. (2009d). *Council on Certification of Nurse Anesthetists (CCNA) overview*. Retrieved from http://www.aana.com/Credentialing.aspx?id=138

American College of Nurse-Midwives. (2003a). *Standards for the practice of midwifery*. Silver Spring, MD: Author.

American College of Nurse-Midwives. (2003b). *ACNM mission statement*. Silver Spring, MD: Author.

American College of Nurse-Midwives. (2004a). *Philosophy of the American College of Nurse-Midwives*. Silver Spring, MD: Author.

American College of Nurse-Midwives. (2004b). *Position statement: Definition of midwifery practice, certified nurse-midwife, and certified midwife*. Silver Spring, MD: Author.

American College of Nurse-Midwives. (2005). *QuickInfo: Quality and effectiveness of nurse-midwifery practice.* Silver Spring, MD: Author.

American College of Nurse-Midwives. (2008). *Core competencies for basic midwifery practice.* Retrieved from http://www.midwife.org/siteFiles/descriptive/Core_Competencies_6_07.pdf

American College of Nurse-Midwives. (2009a). *Essential facts about midwives.* Silver Spring, MD: Author.

American College of Nurse-Midwives. (2009b). *Health care reform: Seven key principles.* Silver Spring, MD: Author.

American College of Nurse-Midwives. (2009c). *Position statement: Midwifery education.* Silver Spring, MD: Author.

American College of Nurse-Midwives. (2009d). *Position statement: Mandatory degree requirements for entry into midwifery practice.* Silver Spring, MD: Author.

American College of Nurse-Midwives. (2009e). *Position statement: Midwifery education and the doctor of nursing practice (DNP).* Silver Spring, MD: Author.

American College of Nurse-Midwives. (2009f). *ACNM Ad Hoc Committee on Disaster Preparedness.* Retrieved from http://www.midwife.org/disaster_preparedness.cfm

American Nurses Association. (2004). *Nursing: Scope and standards of practice* (4th ed.). Silver Spring, MD: Author.

American Nurses Association. (2009). *More about RNs and advanced practice RNs.* Retrieved from http://www.nursingworld.org/EspeciallyForYou/StudentNurses/RNsAPNs.aspx

APRN Joint Dialogue Group. (2008). *Consensus model for APRN regulation: Licensure, accreditation, certification and education.* Retrieved from http://www.aacn.nche.edu/Education/pdf/APRNReport.pdf

Avery, M. (2005). The history and evolution of the core competencies for basic midwifery practice. *Journal of Midwifery and Women's Health, 50*(2), 102–107.

Avery, M. (2009). Speak out for health care reform. *Quickening, 40*(1), 3.

Avery, M., & Howe, C. (2007). The DNP and entry into midwifery practice: an analysis. *Journal of Midwifery and Women's Health, 52*(1), 14–22.

Baldwin, K. M., Clark, A. P., Fulton, J., & Mayo, A. (2009). National validation of the NACNS clinical nurse specialist core competencies. *Journal of Nursing Scholarship, 41*(2), 193–201.

Baldwin, K. M., Lyon, B. L., Clark, A. P., Fulton, J., & Dayhoff, N. (2007). Developing clinical nurse specialist practice competencies. *Clinical Nurse Specialist, 21*(6), 297–302.

Bankert, M. (1989). *Watchful care: A history of America's nurse anesthetists.* New York: Continuum Publishing Group.

Barger, M. (2005). Midwifery practice: Where have we been and where are we going? *Journal of Midwifery and Women's Health, 50*(2), 87–90.

Bedroussian, A., & DeVol, R. (2007). *An unhealthy America: The economic burden of chronic disease.* Santa Monica, CA: The Milken Institute.

Bullough, B. (1995). Professionalization of nurse practitioners. *Annual Review of Nursing Research, 13*, 239–265.

Burst, H.V. (2005) The history of nurse-midwifery education. *Journal of Midwifery and Women's Health, 50*(2), 129–137.

Centers for Medicare and Medicaid Services. (2009). *National healthcare data projected.* Retrieved from http://www.cms.hhs.gov

Chase, S. K., & Pruitt, R. H. (2006). The practice doctorate: Innovation or disruption? *Journal of Nursing Education, 45*(5), 155–161.

Chism, L. (2009, January 12). Understanding the DNP. *Advance for Nurse Practitioners.* Retrieved from http://nurse-practitioners.advanceweb.com/Editorial/Content/Editorial.aspx?CC=191812

Critchley, D. L. (1985). Evolution of the role. In D. L. Critchley & J. T. Maurin (Eds.), *The clinical specialist in psychiatric mental health nursing* (pp. 5–22). New York: John Wiley & Sons.

Dawley, K. (2003). Origins of nurse-midwifery in the United States and its expansion in the 1940s. *Journal of Midwifery and Women's Health, 48*(2), 86–95.

Declercq, E. (2009). Births attended by certified nurse-midwives in the United States reach an all-time high: Trends from1989 to 2006. *Journal of Midwifery and Women's Health, 54*(3), 263–265.

Declercq, E. R., Williams, D. R., Koontz, A. M., Paine, L. L., Streit, E. L., & McClosky, L. (2001). Serving women in need: Nurse-midwifery practice in the United States. *Journal of Midwifery and Women's Health, 46*(1), 11–16.

Goudreau, K. A., Clark, A., Lyon, B., Rust, J. E., Baldwin, K., Fulton, J., et al. (2007, July). *A vision of the future for clinical nurse specialists.* Harrisburg, PA: National Association of Clinical Nurse Specialists.

Hamilton, B., Martin, J., & Ventura, S. (2009). Births: Preliminary data for 2007. *National Vital Statistics Reports, Volume 57, Number 12,* 1–23.

Hamric, A. B. (1996). A definition of advanced nursing practice. In A. B. Hamric, J. A. Spross, & C. M. Hanson (Eds.), *Advanced nursing practice: An integrative approach.* Philadelphia: Saunders.

Hamric, A. B., Spross, J. A., & Hanson, C. M. (Eds.). (2009). *Advanced practice nursing: An integrative approach* (4th ed.). St. Louis, MO: Saunders Elsevier.

Hanson, C. M. (2009). Understanding regulatory, legal, and credentialing requirements. In A. B. Hamric, J. A. Spross, & C. M. Hanson. *Advanced practice nursing: An integrative approach* (4th ed.). St. Louis, MO: Saunders Elsevier.

Hatem, M., Sandall, J., Devane, D., Hora Soltani, H., & Gates, S. (2008). Midwife-led versus other models of care for childbearing women. *Cochrane Database of Systematic Reviews,* Issue 4.

Hathaway, D., Jacob, S., Stegbauer, C., Thompson, C., & Graff, C. (2006). The practice doctorate: Perspectives of early adopters. *Journal of Nursing Education, 45*(12), 487–496.

Institute of Medicine. (1999). *To err is human: Building a safer health system.* Washington, DC: National Academy Press.

Institute of Medicine. (2001). *Crossing the quality chasm: A new health system for the 21st century.* Washington, DC: National Academies Press.

Institute of Medicine. (2003a). *Health professions education: A bridge to quality.* Washington, DC: National Academies Press.

Institute of Medicine. (2003b). *Keeping patients safe: Transforming the work environment of nurses.* Washington, DC: National Academies Press.

Jesse, D., & Blue, C. (2004). Mary Breckinridge meets Healthy People 2010: A teaching strategy for visioning and building healthy communities. *Journal of Midwifery and Women's Health, 49*(2), 126.

Kaiser Family Foundation. (2009). Trends in health care costs and spending. Retrieved from http//www.kff.org

Keeling, A. W. (2009). A brief history of advanced practice nursing in the United States. In A. B. Hamric, J. A. Spross, & C. H. Hanson (Eds.), *Advanced practice nursing: An integrative approach* (4th ed., pp. 3–32). St. Louis, MO: Saunders Elsevier.

Komnenich, P. (2005). The evolution of advanced practice in nursing. In J. M. Stanley (Ed.), *Advanced practice nursing: Emphasizing common roles.* Philadelphia: F. A. Davis.

McKinley, M. G. (2007). *Acute and critical care clinical nurse specialists: Synergy for best practices.* Wheeling, MO: Saunders Elsevier.

Metropolitan Life Insurance Company. (1960). Summary of the ten thousand confinement records of the Frontier Nursing Service. *Bulletin of the American College of Nurse Midwifery, 5,* 1–9.

Miller, S., Sloan, N. L., Winikoff, B., Langer, A., & Fikree, F. F. (2003). Where is the "e" in MCH? The need for an evidence-based approach in safe motherhood. *Journal of Midwifery and Women's Health, 48*(1), 10–18.

National Association of Clinical Nurse Specialists. (1998). *Statement on clinical nurse specialist practice and education.* Glenview, IL: Author.

National Association of Clinical Nurse Specialists. (2004). *Statement on clinical nurse specialist practice and education.* Harrisburg, PA: Author.

National Association of Clinical Nurse Specialists. (2005). *White paper on the nursing practice doctorate.* Retrieved from http://www.nacns.org/LinkClick.aspx?fileticket=xHLMMg MYJ98%3D&tabid=138

National Association of Clinical Nurse Specialists. (2007). *Vision of the future for clinical nurse specialists.* Retrieved http://www.nacns.org/LinkClick.aspx?fileticket=7AX5Ga5RbTg%3D&tabid=117

National Association of Clinical Nurse Specialists. (2009). *Clinical nurse specialist meeting the new demands of a reformed health care system.* Retrieved from http://www.nacns.org /LinkClick.aspx?fileticket=7AX5Ga5RbTg%3d&tabid=117

National Organization of Nurse Practitioner Faculties. (2006). *Practice doctorate nurse practitioner entry-level competencies.* Retrieved from http://nonpf.org/NONPF2005/CoreCompsFINAL06.pdf

Nurse-Midwifery Service Director's Network. (1994). *An administrative manual for nurse-midwifery services.* Dubuque, IA: Kendall/Hunt.

Nurse-Midwifery Service Director's Network. (1996). *An administrative manual for nurse-midwifery services* (2nd ed.). Dubuque, IA: Kendall/Hunt.

Paine, L., Dower, C., & O'Neil, E. (1999). Midwifery in the 21st century: Recommendations from the Pew Health Professions Commission/UCSF Center for the Health Professions 1998 Taskforce on Midwifery. *Journal of Midwifery and Women's Health, 44*(4), 341–348.

Pearson, L. (2009). A national overview of nurse practitioner legislation and healthcare issues. *American Journal of Nurse Practitioners, 13*(2), 9.

Pulcini, J., & Wagner, M. (2001). *Perspectives on education and practice issues for nurse practitioners and advanced practice nursing.* Retrieved from http://66.219.50.180/NR/rdonlyres

/eghts6f2qqae5hmknha7shtrws46y4m2yh3e34yak3h325ltfuwszkfgu46pa3tj3jttj4ciail4g
izkzvg47kyesna/pulciniarticle0305.pdf

Robb, I. (1893). *Nursing: Its Principles and Practice for Hospital and Private Use.* Philadelphia: W.B. Saunders.

Safriet, B. (2002). Closing the gap between can and may in health care providers' scopes of practice: A primer for policymakers. *Yale Journal of Regulation, 19,* 301–334.

Sakala, C., & Corry, M. (2008). *Evidence based maternity care: What it is and what it can achieve.* New York: Milbank Memorial Fund.

Shah, M., & King, T. (2006). Primary health care by midwives: Comprehensive and competent health services for women. *Journal of Midwifery and Women's Health, 51*(3), 139–140.

Slager, J. (2004). *Business concepts for healthcare providers.* Sudbury, MA: Jones and Bartlett.

Slager, J. (Ed.). (2005). *An administrative manual for nurse-midwifery services* (3rd ed.). Greenwood Village, CO: Midwifery Business Network.

Slattery, L. (1999, 2006). *CCA vs. CMP: Do you know the difference?* Retrieved from http://www.midwife.org/cca_cmp.cfm

Sparacino, P. S., & Cartwright, C. (2009). In A. B. Hamric, J. A. Spross, & C. H. Hanson (Eds.), *The clinical nurse specialist* (4th ed., pp. 349–379). St. Louis, MO: Saunders.

U.S. Census Bureau. (2009). *Income, poverty and health insurance coverage in the United States: 2008.* Retrieved from http://www.census.gov/prod/2009pubs/p60-236.pdf

Varney, H., Kriebs, J., & Gegor, C. (2004). *Varney's midwifery* (4th ed.). Sudbury, MA: Jones and Bartlett.

CHAPTER 10

Emerging Roles for the DNP

Nurse Educator
Michelle Riley

Advances in the body of nursing knowledge promote educational development of professional nurses beyond entry-level practice to meet the increasing healthcare needs of society. Research to increase the body of nursing knowledge is important to improving the nation's health. There is also a significant need for advanced practice nurses (APNs) with clinical knowledge and skills to facilitate collaborative practice and leadership in the profession. Professional nurses require highly developed skill sets for continuous quality improvement in diverse systems and healthcare settings where APNs work (Heller, Oros, & Durney-Crowley, n.d.).

Nurses with a practice doctorate who have advanced their education in clinical practice and leadership can use specialized skills and clinical judgment to perform roles in complex healthcare systems (American Association of Colleges of Nursing [AACN], 2006). The Doctor of Nursing Practice (DNP) degree is a doctoral degree that is different from a research doctorate, but no less important (Steefel, 2005, as cited in Stein, 2008). According to Stein (2008), the Doctor of Philosophy (PhD) focuses on theoretical developments leading to an advanced body of knowledge in nursing, whereas the DNP is more practice based. Furthermore, the PhD is the benchmark against which other forms of doctoral education are measured (Ellis, 2007).

According to the National League for Nursing (NLN), educator roles in nursing require preparation of leaders in higher education (NLN, 2007). Furthermore, "Educators who are not educated in pedagogy, evaluation, and educational theory will not be in a position to engage meaningfully in nursing education research or make evidence-based contributions to reform" (p. 2).

Strong proponents of the DNP understand the impact clinical expertise and education can have on client outcomes (AACN, 2008). Even though curricula may differ from state to state, educational programs that prepare doctoral-level clinicians offer courses in leadership and research translation (Fain, Asselin, & McCurry, 2008). In addition, doctorally prepared clinical experts can complete additional courses to acquire knowledge needed for academic positions (Long, 2006).

This section explores how DNP graduates, as expert clinicians, can use skills gained in their educational programs to perform effectively in the role of nurse educators in practice and academic settings. The section also explores the expanded role of the DNP nurse educator and suggests methods for seeking practice and leadership opportunities in a variety of settings.

DNP Nurse Educator Roles and Responsibilities

Practice Settings

Nurses with advanced education at the doctoral level can perform their roles at the bedside, at the table of college boards, or in community settings. In each of these scenarios and settings, a DNP graduate can perform the practice of nursing effectively. According to Riley, "The DNP will be the new standard for advancing practice nursing education" (2009, p. 12).

The clinical practice doctorate prepares nurses with advanced education to do research, apply new knowledge in practice, and educate nursing students (Stein, 2008). According to Ellis (2007), applying the knowledge nurses gain to clinical practice is at the heart of the clinical doctorate. This may explain why more clinicians are interested in pursuing this type of doctorate over the more traditional PhD.

Furthermore, graduates of DNP programs can seek leadership roles in settings that allow for enhancement, restructuring, and improvements in the quality of health services delivery (National Organization of Nurse Practitioner Faculties [NONPF], 2005). Clinically proficient, doctorally prepared nurses are needed as a result of increased demands for health professionals who are skilled in providing complex clinical care. Practice responsibilities in the clinical setting for DNPs may include overseeing medical centers, home care, and hospice services, as well as nursing education (Stein, 2008).

Academic Settings

Practice-focused doctorates allow practitioners to use clinical expertise at an advanced level in a variety of educational settings. Advanced practice nurses who are doctorally prepared and teach in baccalaureate and higher-degree programs can help to transform the education of nurses who will be practicing at the highest level of practice (Douglas, 2005). Developments in healthcare education and the demand for increasing the educational requirements in master's-level education have extended the credit requirements beyond conventional credits at the master's level, which has helped to increase interest in the practice doctorate (Douglas, 2005).

DNP graduates practicing in complex systems and organizational levels are called on to help define potential problems and to develop interventions to address these problems. Therefore, DNPs must be competent in identifying and developing interventions to facilitate healthcare delivery across multifaceted systems. DNP programs prepare expert clinicians who not only identify and implement systems changes, but also who facilitate the expert clinical teaching needed for the communities and health systems they service: clients, students, families, communities, and expert colleagues (NONPF, 2005). Even though not all institutions offering the DNP are prepared to place faculty in tenure-track positions, students in bachelor, master, and doctoral programs will need access to faculty who are expert clinicians in various practice settings, which will increase the demand for DNP graduates (Yale Nursing, 2009). Furthermore, according to Loretta Ford, cofounder of the nurse practitioner role, since the DNP is the next appropriate step toward clinical excellence, it would seem that education programs would have "expectations for translational research, clinical teaching and institutional leadership" from DNPs (Ford, 2009).

Nurses with practice doctorates will have a voice in research and have a bigger stage on which to show how they can positively affect client outcomes (Riley, 2009). DNPs in today's complex systems must maintain expert levels of clinical competence in order to make a positive impact on such systems. DNP-prepared individuals who participate in scholarship can reach beyond traditional definitions of teaching and research (Boyer, 1990, 1996). According to Boyer's concepts of scholarship, DNP-prepared faculty members can bring new perspectives to original research and can explore how research is applied to problems. Holland (2005) also speaks to the tradition of scholarship and balancing this with discovery, interpretation, and application by those with a practice doctorate.

More and more academic institutions are reviewing policies related to research scholarship and are trying to expand the definition of scholarship to support the work of faculty who bring practice-based experience to academia. In addition, educators are needed in nursing schools to teach students how to perform their roles as advanced practice nurses upon graduation by helping them to fill vacancies in educator and advocacy roles related to health, nursing policy, and client care outcomes within political and health-care communities (Fain, Asselin, & McCurry, 2008).

Faculty members who have devoted their careers to research over practice cannot be expected to maintain the clinical competence needed to educate advanced practice students pursuing careers in clinical practice. Enrollment of students into PhD programs who want advanced clinical practice is controversial. Fitzpatrick (2003) postulates that "it is unethical to accept students into PhD programs that do not develop research careers" (p.9). Since the introduction of the practice doctorate as a terminal degree allowing for permanent faculty roles in colleges and universities, students pursuing clinical practice or clinical teaching at the advanced level can now pursue careers in academia (Long, 2006).

Society will need educators with different doctorates to educate expert practitioners of the future. Given the complexity of health care, it is clear that master's-level education will no longer be sufficient to educate future nurses. The practice doctorate in nursing is evolving, and faculty members with doctoral preparation will need to move toward formal education beyond the master's level (Pennsylvania State Board of Nursing, 2005).

Nurses in clinical practice prepared at the doctoral level can also hold faculty appointments in academic settings, provide clinical oversight, and participate in teaching roles (AACN, 2005). With more and more DNP students graduating, the number of clinically prepared faculty holding a practice doctorate will continue to increase. The National Academy of Sciences supports the development of a "nonresearch" clinical doctorate to train advanced-level practitioners who will serve as clinical faculty (Long, 2006). More colleges and universities that offer the PhD are now offering the DNP as the terminal degree for clinical expertise. These clinical experts holding faculty roles can choose to take coursework to facilitate their transition to the academic educator role and add teaching skills to their clinical skill set (National League for Nursing, 2007).

Role Expansion Strategies for DNPs from a Nurse Educator Perspective

Nurses with practice doctorates have clinical, organizational, economic, and leadership skills to positively affect client outcomes at the systems level. These healthcare leaders can also use their considerable practice expertise to make management and policy decisions in health care while educating the interdisciplinary healthcare team on issues affecting the health of diverse client populations (Fain, Asselin, & McCurry, 2008).

Individuals who obtain the DNP degree will continue to seek faculty roles to educate future DNPs as more clinical doctorate programs for nurses are developed. It is estimated that approximately 60 schools with DNP programs are now admitting students to these programs, and more DNP programs are being developed (AACN, 2008).

It is important to remember that DNP curricula are not designed to prepare nurses to become educators necessarily, any more than PhD programs. However, in states such as Florida and Texas, graduates of doctoral programs who want to work in academia will be able to receive additional education to prepare and support their clinical expertise (Green, Starck, & Long, 2006).

In order for DNPs to continue to expand their roles in academia and contribute to the body of nursing knowledge, socializing them to their faculty roles through mentoring programs should be considered. Given the varied roles of faculty, supporting faculty members throughout their time in academia facilitates development of teaching research as well as service skills (National League for Nursing, 2007). The orientation and mentoring provided to DNP graduates who will work in academia are also essential to developing their ability to conduct research, apply empirical knowledge in practice, and educate future students (Stein, 2008).

The knowledge that DNP graduates gain in nursing programs will allow them to transition into practice and leadership roles with more confidence and skills to perform effectively in their new roles. As clinical leaders with nursing leadership, business, and healthcare management skills, these experts can use their knowledge of financial and business concepts to effect change on a global level.

Conclusions and Future Directions

Several demands in health care have provided momentum for the DNP degree. These demands include the changing complexity of our country's healthcare environments and improvements in the care of clients in clinical settings where advanced levels of practice expertise are needed at the bedside (Sperhac & Clinton, 2004; Williams, 2006). Parity with other healthcare professionals is another reason for the positive momentum behind the call for the DNP to be the highest degree for experts dedicated to the clinical role (Williams, 2006; Sperhac & Clinton, 2004).

Each nurse who completes the DNP degree can use that knowledge in a different way based on the individual's area of clinical expertise. Many will continue to fill faculty roles as more DNP programs are developed. Programs that offer practice doctorates will need DNP nurse educators in academic settings to educate students across all levels of nursing education to ensure that clinically competent faculty are educating students. Nurses who educate students and no longer practice in clinical care lose the connection to clinical care and tend to use more theoretical than clinical knowledge to educate students (Williams, 2006).

Improving communications channels in terms of how DNPs can help in practice and academic settings through mentoring relationship with experienced academic faculty will continue to be important to the transition of DNPs to academia (National League for Nursing, 2007). This key component of faculty transition is essential for faculty who are clinically competent and desire to have a career in academia because it affords the profession and society an opportunity to have clinical experts at clinical sites and in the classroom (Williams, 2006).

With the new emphasis on practice doctorates such as the DNP, nurse experts will continue to focus their work within areas of specialization that may not necessarily include the process of teaching. Some nurses with practice doctorates will be assuming needed roles in health care to meet various practice expectations, and others will remain in clinical work to facilitate healthcare policy changes (Riley, 2009). While working in various settings with other healthcare personnel with the title of "Doctor," DNPs will need to continue educating the public on the role and responsibilities related to their title (Green, Starck, & Long, 2006). Practice issues related to certification and reimbursement will continue to be a concern for some DNPs as the need for this level of clinical knowledge and expertise results in better client outcomes. It is essential that experts in clinical practice, academia, and research collaborate to facilitate changes in complex systems that lead to healthier outcomes for all of society.

Nurse Administrator/Executive
Don R. Hirschman

Your goal is to become or be a better leader and administrator/executive. What steps should you take to prepare yourself for the challenges and responsibilities of this role? This section posits the Doctor of Nursing Practice, or DNP, as a major step toward your nursing leadership goal. Why go to the effort, expense, and commitment of earning a DNP? You have experience; the DNP is the education you need to help you reach your potential, become a better leader, and "Be all you can be," as the U.S. Army slogan says.

The University of California, San Francisco School of Nursing, defines nursing administration as "the specialty that integrates nursing science, business principles, organizational behavior, and resource management to prepare nurses to participate as full partners in managing and leading healthcare organizations." For our purposes, the term *nurse administrator/executive* will be used.

In the military, leaders are taught to balance the accomplishment of the mission with the welfare of the troops. The nurse administrator/executive must balance the welfare of patients and staff and the needs of the healthcare organization. Whatever the title, the nurse administrator/executive must not stray far from his or her role as patient advocate, because this is what distinguishes the role from the rest of the healthcare executive team, that is, the chief financial officer (CFO), chief executive officer (CEO), chief operating officer (COO), and the chief nursing officer (CNO). Of these important management team officers, only the nurse has ever had the primary role of patient advocate.

This section's goal is to answer some questions regarding the DNP. Is the DNP better prepared for the role of administrator/executive? If so, then in what ways? Several words are key to answering this question: *leadership* (University of Colorado, 2008; University of Tennessee, 2008; Wall, Novak, & Wilkerson, 2005), *parity* (i.e., similar to other professional doctorates) (Case Western Reserve University, 2008), *commensurate, credibility, management, increased complexity* (Fain, Asselin, & McCurry, 2008), and *policy* (Marion, Viens, O'Sullivan, Crabtree, Fontana, & Price, 2003).

Leadership

The DNP, as described by universities offering the degree, "educates students for leadership roles" (University of Tennessee, 2008). In addition to clinical and course work, the University of Tennessee requires a dissertation.

Graduates of their rival, the University of Kentucky, "will be expert in designing, implementing, managing and evaluating health care delivery systems and will be prepared to lead at the highest clinical and executive ranks." DNP program graduates from the University of Colorado at Denver "will be prepared as leaders who will design models of health care delivery, evaluate clinical outcomes, identify and manage health care needs of populations, and use technology and information to transform health care systems" (University of Colorado, 2008). Case Western Reserve (2009) states, "Nurses with a DNP can move to the absolute pinnacle of their field: those with practice doctorates are the most highly educated and qualified practitioners in their profession. These advanced practice nurses apply their education and expertise in leadership roles on the front lines of nursing, in clinical practice, teaching and research, and in health policy design and development."

Clearly, the stated intentions of DNP programs are to prepare nursing leaders. The programs cited are merely examples, because all programs cannot be mentioned in this text due to space limitations. As of December 2007, there were 45 programs offering the DNP, and at least 140 programs being considered (Partin, 2008).

The author's experience in the U.S. Army is relevant to this brief discussion of leadership. The Army defines leadership as "influencing, providing purpose, motivating and directing to accomplish the mission and improve an organization" (Department of the Army, 2004). The Army has been consistent in this definition since 1968 (Department of the Army, 1968). Although this section is specifically directed to nurse administrators/executives, the concept of leadership has many universal applications. The military has developed some great leaders. Nurse administrators/executives would be well advised to develop leadership skills by studying and learning from the captains of infantry as well as the captains of industry.

Parity

The Merriam-Webster Online Dictionary defines parity as "the quality or state of being equal or equivalent." Case Western Reserve University's Frances Payne Bolton School of Nursing (2009) describes its DNP program as "similar in concept [to] practice doctorates in other professions such as medicine (MD), law (JD) and dentistry (DDM)." Joyce Fitzpatrick of Case Western University further notes that the "practice doctorate allows both degree parity and additional strengthening of the educational program to assume full leadership roles in clinical practice, clinical teaching, and clinical action research" (Fitzpatrick, 2003). The entrance level of pharmacists is the PharmD. Psychologists earn a PhD. The professions of optometry, osteopathy, public health, physical therapy, audiology, chiropractic, and naturopathy all offer practice doctorates (Brown-Benedict, 2008), and the DNP offers parity with these professionals (Brown et al., 2006).

The Institute of Medicine (IOM) has suggested that all disciplines need to raise the bar in leadership training (IOM, 2003). The DNP degree is commensurate with more responsibility as a healthcare professional, and offers increased credibility to facilitate better management to meet the demands for delivery for modern health care and its increased complexity (Fain, 2008). The increased educational requirements of DNP-prepared nurses can improve the U.S. healthcare system.

Credibility and Personal Experience

Credibility is characterized by belief and trustworthiness. Knowledge, self-confidence, and reputation increase credibility. Does the DNP degree add to credibility? Jolley (2007) suggests the answer is yes. Clearly the title "Doctor" implies knowledge, academic achievement, scholarship, trust, and a list of other positives. The author's brother graduated from the University of Michigan Medical School in 1959. From then until 2002, whenever I heard "Dr. Hirschman," that always meant my brother. The first time I was introduced as "Dr. Hirschman" was as a speaker at the Ophthalmic Anesthesia Society. At that point the purpose of the sacrifice, expense, and efforts of the previous four years at Rush University became much clearer. A nursing doctorate paved the way for me to become part of a research team at Kansas University and the Department Veterans Affairs studying delayed cataract surgery and adverse effects on veterans. If funded, this study could reduce the time veterans wait to have sight-restoring cataract surgery through the Veterans Health Administration. The DNP will have opened the door to allow research to improve practice.

The percentages of DNP-prepared nurses are increasing, but this is still a very small group. DNPs, similar to those nurses who were motivated to earn master's degrees, are successful, productive nurses who have much to contribute. Nurses need to "be all we can be." Nurse want to be able to contribute at the highest levels of healthcare delivery. One of my fellow contributors is the administrator/president of Alterna-Care Home Health. No doubt there are many highly qualified, fine nurses working for this company, but the administrator/president is a DNP-prepared nurse.

The author's doctorate helped to secure an adjunct teaching appointment at Wichita State University. This enables teaching, motivating, and demonstration by example of what a Doctor of Nursing Practice is and can do. My doctorate has not been to my financial advantage, earned me more vacation, gained me promotions, or had any other material benefit. Through doctoral studies I researched a question that had interested me for eight years. The question I studied was whether it was safe to continue anticoagulant therapy for cataract surgery patients. The common practice was to discontinue anticoagulants such as warfarin and aspirin for days or weeks before cataract surgery. This put patients at risk for developing the serious conditions the drugs were being used to prevent. Anecdotally, patients were reported to be experiencing embolisms, strokes, and other life-threatening conditions as a result of the withdrawal of anticoagulation therapy. There were no published data to confirm this, however. The study I led collected data from ophthalmic ambulatory surgery centers retrospectively. Without changing any medications pre- or postoperatively, we studied and compared the peri- and postoperative complications of patients on anticoagulation in over 2,100 cases. There was no difference. We concluded that it was safe to continue anticoagulation therapy for cataract surgery patients (Hirschman & Morby, 2005). To some, this is just another study. To some patients, however, it may mean the difference between continuing important medications or having them interrupted and putting them at unnecessary risk. The DNP you earn may touch lives, most of whom you will never know. The leadership you provide may touch many lives as well.

Management

A traditional master of science in nursing (MSN) may emphasize leadership and management. Advanced registered nurse practitioner programs also may or may not have a management track. Some DNP programs combine a healthcare leadership track using a combined faculty of nursing and business (Hardy, DeBasio, Warmbrodt, Gartland, Bassett, & Tansey, 2004).

The DNP manager can employ the techniques of the great management masters for better effectiveness. Some of the great names in management that DNP managers should study and emulate are W. Edwards Deming and Peter F. Drucker.

W. Edwards Deming, PhD, Yale University

Deming has written several books on management, productivity, and quality. One may ask how nursing relates to research on how post–World War II Japanese factories advanced from rubble to economic powerhouses so quickly. The answer is that the principles of building quality into the product at every stage rather than simply checking the end product can be adapted to healthcare delivery as well. Instead of inspecting a car as it rolls off the assembly line, Deming's method teaches quality to the designers and production workers and urges inspection during the process rather than simply at the end (Deming, 1986; Walton, 1986, 1991). In the realm of healthcare delivery, instead of relying on incident reports or chart reviews to discover problems, the DNP manager would develop a positive atmosphere of quality at every step of patient care.

Deming formulated 14 points for management, one of which is to "drive out fear" (Deming, 1986). All too often, incident reports are used punitively. Most nurses have been required to complete one after a real or perceived mistake. The DNP nurse administrator/executive would do well to drive out fear from his or her team and replace it with a "new philosophy" of leadership (Deming, 1986). DNP students should study Deming's management method. Do not limit your vision of leadership to only medical or nursing authors. Executive leadership by nurses must not be limited to the examples of nursing leadership.

Peter F. Drucker, Doctor of Law, University of Frankfurt

Peter Drucker has authored at least nine books on management and nine others on economics. His work is widely studied in graduate schools of business and management. Evidence of his timelessness is that *The Practice of Management*, first published in 1954, is still in print. The DNP nurse administrator/executive has both the research and additional management training to face the increased expectations of staff and CEOs. The DNP administrator/executive is prepared to face the increased complexity of delivering modern health care.

Increased Complexity

Bob Dylan sang, "The times they are a-changin'." Nursing care is certainly becoming more complex (Draye, 2006). We have come a long way. The role of the nurse administrator/executive has come a long way as well. Nursing has come from the 1860s, when one sponge and one basin of water would be used to clean wounds on multiple patients, to the present use of disposables (Helmstadter, 2002). The nurse's role in leadership, management, and the boardroom has also evolved. The word "transformation" is often used to describe the changes (Draye, 2006). The DNP can help prepare nurses for the complex changes in clinical practice and leadership opportunities. Nurses could at one time aspire to be the "head nurse." Now complex healthcare delivery systems are led by doctorally prepared nurses. DNP nurses are trained to be community leaders and healthcare policy makers (Wall, Novak, & Wilkerson 2005). Health policy administration is a very timely subject. Congress is debating healthcare reform, and DNP nurses are well prepared to participate in that debate and form and implement policy (Acorn, Lamarche, & Edwards, 2009).

Experience dictates that doing well in a chosen field is one key to advancement to management. Salespersons are presumed to know how to train and motivate others to similar success. So too in nursing do exemplary nurses seek more knowledge and responsibility. A portion follow the clinical track, a portion the research track, and some gravitate to management and leadership. Master's-level nurses learn more to advance their clinical knowledge base and become nurse practitioners, clinical nurse specialists, certified registered nurse anesthetists, and certified nurse midwives. Those nurses who choose the management track may earn a master of business administration, or MBA. The curriculum for the clinical master's degrees may not offer enough training for strategic planning. This nurse may not be ready for collaboration with the highest levels of corporate management (Marion et al., 2003). The DNP is uniquely prepared in strategic planning, organizational development, and systems.

Whatever path to graduate nursing education a nurse chooses, he or she is likely to study the concept of evidence-based practice.

Evidence-Based Practice

An important hallmark of doctoral programs is the focus on evidence-based practice. The term *evidence-based practice* (EBP) is common now when discussing nursing practice. This concept is addressed elsewhere in this book and others. One very simple definition is that evidence-based practice examines all that we do to determine whether there is scientific evidence to support the practice. EBP means we do not do things just because we were taught to do so or because "we have always done it this way." It may well be that a common practice is a good one and should be continued, but not simply because "that's the way we always do it." One practical example of EBP suggests a zero-based method, in which one starts with a blank policy and procedure manual and only adds a procedure after there is sound evidence to support it. Is this report, meeting, or process based on scientific evidence? Envision the savings of time, paper, and energy this would create. EBP must be the gold standard in every aspect of leadership, management, and administration.

Conclusions

The DNP prepares nurses for more responsibility in delivering health care. Having a doctoral preparation enhances the career path of nurses, whatever their specialty. The educational process is a component of this enhancement. The DNP-educated nurse will contribute to higher-quality health care with greater confidence gained from knowledge. The doctoral degree will help nurses gain parity when working with other doctorally prepared professionals as well as the leaders of healthcare organizations. It is reasonable to expect that CEOs, CFOs, and others who often are not doctorally prepared will give more credence to those who are. The DNP confers increased credibility. There will often be an assumption that the DNP-prepared individual is more knowledgeable and more credible than the individual with a master's degree.

The ideas and plans of DNP-prepared nurses are more likely to be tested than dismissed. The DNP program provides leadership training and the management emphasis track that will give the DNP enhanced skills. For those interested in management, executive leadership, patient care, and in making healthcare policy, the DNP is for you! As this is being written, our national government leaders are pushing very hard for healthcare reform. Whatever policies emerge, the DNP-prepared nurse will have strategic leverage to be at the table to determine and implement national healthcare policies. If in doubt about earning a DNP, remember and be guided by what may be the most appropriate and generally motivating ad slogan in current history: "Be all that you can be!"

Nurse Entrepreneur
Deonne J. Brown Benedict

The nurse entrepreneur is at the forefront as a change leader. Innovative, creative, forward thinking, risk taking, visionary, strategic, emotionally intelligent, and persevering (Faugier, 2005; Kowal, 1988; Shirey, 2008; West, 2008) are all characteristics that have been ascribed to the nurse entrepreneur. "Entrepreneurship takes a lot of devotion and courage" (Grace Grymes Chapman, personal communication, July 10, 2009). "It requires compassion, passion for your specialty, and drive" to weather the unrelenting juggling act, frequent obstacles encountered, and multiple competencies required (Scharmaine Lawson-Baker, personal communication, July 21, 2009). "Entrepreneurs create something new, something different—*they change values*" (Drucker, 1985). What is less well known is that the ideal nurse entrepreneur also merges flexibility, patience, self-discipline, a customer service emphasis, and, in particular, planning and management expertise into his or her skill set (Castledine, 2006; Wilson, Averis, & Walsh, 2003). Strategic planning and process management tools are characteristics and competencies identified within the DNP.

Historically, nursing has often, but not always, been an employed occupation. The birth of nurse practitioners and advanced practice nursing in the 1960s set the stage for a new wave of innovative transformation in nursing, as nursing leaders such as Loretta Ford began to blaze new paths and take risks. Today, although exact figures on the numbers of nurse entrepreneurs are difficult to obtain, data from the U.S. Department of Health and Human Services (2004) indicate that 5.5% of RNs and 3% of nurse practitioners (NPs) are self-employed, a percentage that has been rising rapidly in recent years (Rollet & Lebo, 2007, 2008). Self-employed nurses report enhanced job satisfaction, especially in relation to empowerment for making a difference in the lives of the patients with whom they work (Wilson, Averis, & Walsh, 2003). Other benefits include autonomy, flexibility to work around personal and work schedules, control of quality improvements, improved patient satisfaction, and the ability to subspecialize (Caffrey, 2005; Elango, Hunter, & Winchell, 2007). Additionally, surveys of nurses have historically found that advanced practice nurses (APNs) who own their practice are more highly compensated than employed NPs (Rollet & Lebo, 2008).

At least as important as any one of the preceding factors is that nurse entrepreneurs provide services not within the dominant medical model or under the oversight of other professionals, but in an interprofessional context within a distinctly nursing framework. Dr. Gregory Lind, owner of Lake Serene Clinic, an all–nurse practitioner practice in Washington State, says entrepreneurs recognize opportunity and apply their assets to a niche. When he started out as an NP in the late 1970s, local physicians transferred all of their nursing home patients to his practice. Through nursing interventions such as reducing overmedication and promoting safety and function, he was later rewarded with the responsibility of involvement in the development of a hospital birthing center. After obtaining his doctorate and briefly teaching at the university, he realized there was a need for an independent primary care open-access nurse practitioner practice. His walk-in clinic now employs seven nurse practitioners, with standard full time being three 11-hour days weekly alternating with four 11-hour days (personal communication, July 10, 2009).

Entrepreneurship provides the medium for an engaged and creative nursing populace without the subservience, sexism, inaccurate fettered public image, and other "cultural impediments" (Faugier, 2005, p. 50) that have historically tripped up nursing. Nurse entrepreneurship reminds the public that we are "far more than assistants to MDs," says Grace Grymes Chapman, owner of West Seattle Community Clinic (personal communication, July 10, 2009). Entrepreneurship provides the necessary conditions for "liberating" nurses to fulfill their professional promise (Howkins & Thornton, 2003, p. 219), while advancing technology and the growth of medical and nursing knowledge and in many ways continuing to aid the metamorphosis of nursing itself (Faugier, 2005). When Scharmaine Lawson-Baker, DNP and nurse practitioner, was asked why entrepreneurship is important for nursing, she responded, "Many patients are searching for affordable health care, and nurse entrepreneurs offer the holistic care, the quality care they need" (personal communication, July 21, 2009).

Although only recently identified as such through the use of the term *social entrepreneur* (Bishop, 2006), a contemporary term used to describe individuals who "bring about catalytic changes . . . in the perception of . . . social issues" (Waddock & Post, 1991), nursing history is replete with examples of entrepreneurship. Lillian Wald, together with Mary Brewster, founded the Henry Street Settlement. Lillian coined the term "public health nursing," offering a new vision of a collaborative, problem-solving, community-based approach to social, economic, and mental health issues in addition to medical concerns (Abrams, 2008). Mary Breckenridge founded the Frontier

Nursing Service, which introduced the first nurse midwives to the United States, radically reducing pregnancy complications, maternal deaths, and stillborn rates in rural areas (Osborne & Dawley, 2005). Dorothea Dix became a champion for expanding appropriate, compassionate mental health care (Parry, 2006). In more recent times, there is Florence Wald, who changed the paradigm of care for the dying by introducing comprehensive hospice care services (Hoffmann, 2005), and others such as Loretta Ford, who founded the movement that became nurse practitioners (Houser & Player, 2004).

Nurse entrepreneurs pave new roads. They engage in novel healthcare delivery forms. Dr. Lawson-Baker pioneered comprehensive home visit services for elders, providing necessary health services in Louisiana after Hurricane Katrina when other healthcare providers left the state.

Nurse entrepreneurship changes public perceptions, as communities begin to better understand the capabilities of the profession. "NPs make decisions in concert with patients. As NPs become decision makers and not just decision-deliverers, clients see our worth and experience a different kind of care" (Gregory Lind, personal communication, July 22, 2009). Nurse entrepreneurs are found in legal consulting, care coordination services, camp nursing, continuing education provision, nursing staffing agencies, home care, stand-alone nurse anesthetist centers, adult day programs for elders, foot care services, energy work and complementary services, infection control, health writing, lactation consulting, medical coding, nursing informatics, nurse recruiting, occupational health, parish nursing, social programs for the uninsured, telehealth, telephone triage services, nursing marketing services, nursing research, wellness coaching, and vaccination services. They have private practices in psychiatric, family, and geriatric care, and subspecialty services as diverse as convenience care clinics, chronic disease home care, dermatologic services, integrative services, sexual assault services, palliative care, travel medicine, wound care, weight management, urgent care, urinary incontinence, and aesthetics (Bullock, 2009; Hardy, 2008; Kacel, 2008; Keyes, 2009; Marra, 2008; Moen, 2009; Pronsati, 2008; Rollet, 2008; Schiff, 2009; Smith, 2009; Veilleux, 2009).

Nurse entrepreneurship seems appropriately and inextricably linked to many of the DNP essentials (AACN, 2006). The second essential, organizational and systems leadership, identifies "practice management" (p. 10), specifically, the need to balance productivity, quality of care, and budgetary issues. The development and evaluation of alternate delivery approaches and leading healthcare initiatives rings familiar to the ear of the entrepreneur. Dr.

Lawson-Baker, owner of Advanced Clinical Consultants, a nurse practitioner house call service (personal interview, July 22, 2009), says the DNP promotes improved problem solving and education regarding the factors that promote successful change, but that additional content in business topics such as computer software, human resource management, billing, and accounting are needed because nurse entrepreneurs often still require seminars in these areas or experience learning through the school of hard knocks.

Clinical scholarship and evidence-based practice, the third essential, is also seen in the entrepreneur as she or he "designs and implements . . . [new] practice patterns and systems of care" (p. 12), using current research to improve healthcare outcomes for the population or populations she or he serves (AACN, 2006). Additionally, much entrepreneurship is being fueled by rapid gains in healthcare technologies (Essential IV) as entrepreneurs design or use existing technology to advance outcomes and assist consumers in understanding the vast amount of information available. At Charis Family Clinic, we use 100% electronic systems to coordinate care, bill claims, fax, strengthen patient education resources, and document visits, resulting in more space and time for the personalized human element of care.

Nurse entrepreneurs are advocates (Essential V) by nature. Often faced with barriers such as lack of reimbursement for nursing services and directly accountable to the clients they serve, they are often the nurses most involved in educating others about nursing and advocating for the advancement of the profession and the development of new policy. Dr. Lawson-Baker has been a regular visitor to lawmakers' offices in Washington, D.C., since 2006 to remove barriers to the care she and other NPs provide. The more entrepreneurs changing health care's landscape, the more nurses who will be calling for legislative change. Essential VI is often foundational for nurse entrepreneurs, as they lead interprofessional teams for the purpose of positive change and provide consultative services for individuals and other health entities (AACN, 2006). "Nurse entrepreneurs need to understand hiring, firing, employee rights," and team concepts, says Dr. Lawson-Baker. Finally, the competency of advanced practice has laid the groundwork for much recent entrepreneurial activity.

Will the DNP facilitate nurse entrepreneurship? The answer is yes and no. "All professions have a practice base at the doctoral level. I applaud nursing for setting this standard instead of arguing for decades. . . . A recent presidential panel on health care lamented that medicine has abandoned primary care. [Fortunately,] there is no trouble finding nurses who want to become advanced practice nurses," said Dr. Gregory Lind. "I couldn't be more excited for the public, for nursing, or for countless advanced practice nurses to follow." The DNP places additional tools in the entrepreneurial toolbox. "[The DNP] helped me to practically apply evidence-based practice and to understand factors in addressing change," says Dr. Lawson-Baker. "The DNP will give more nurses the courage to follow their dream and go out on their own," says Grace Grymes Chapman. However, the DNP is a vital but insufficient condition for promoting nurse entrepreneurship. "It is the person with the degree, not the degree itself," that makes the entrepreneur, says Dr. Lind (personal communication, July 10, 2009).

As information technology continues to transform the delivery of care, clients continue to seek out customized wellness information and disease intervention, and organizations and skilled professionals continue to limit their long-term commitment to each other, opportunities for nursing entrepreneurship will grow and novel healthcare ventures will continue to flourish (Wilson, 1998). "Nursing must support entrepreneurship because medicine has abandoned setting up solo practices for the comfort of being employed . . . a true role reversal" (Gregory Lind, personal communication, June 12, 2009). The DNP will continue to provide the context for an adept nursing profession empowered to do what it was envisioned to do and what it does uniquely well—to radically alter and to deliver optimal health care.

Biosketches of Successful Nurse Entrepreneurs

Grace Grymes Chapman, MSN, FNP
West Seattle Community Clinic, PLLC

Grace Grymes Chapman, an Advanced Registered Nurse Practitioner owns her own family practice clinic in West Seattle serving families of all ages with a focus on women and adolescents. She has been an active presence on the boards of state and local nurse practitioner organizations. Grace provides full spectrum healthcare to people of all ages in West Seattle and surrounding communities. Grace provides health care to medically insured and the uninsured and is contracted with Washington State Breast and Cervical Health Program, a state funded program aimed at women without insurance between the ages of 40–65. Grace is also contracted with the Vaccines for Children Program with the Public Health department, as well as the Washington State Take Charge Family Planning program.

Scharmaine Lawson-Baker, DNP, FNP-BC
Advanced Clinical Consultants, LLC, President/CEO
http://www.advancedclinicalconsultants.com
http://www.geriatricinitiatives.org

Scharmaine Lawson-Baker is the founder of Advanced Clinical Consultants. She is the Family Nurse Practitioner for the only NP-owned housecall practice in New Orleans, Louisiana established in 2004. Housecalls are made daily to elderly, disabled, and indigent patients who would otherwise not receive healthcare. In 2008, she founded Geriatric Initiatives, a non-profit organization formed to raise funding for medical supplies, diapers, pads, nutritional supplies, and other items not covered by Medicare or Medicaid. After being featured on CBS with Katie Couric, *Forbes* magazine, *Washington Post*, and countless other news sources, Dr. Lawson-Baker is a frequent speaker on health disparities and elder care issues. She has 19 years of experience as a Registered Nurse and Nurse Practitioner providing care in almost every specialty from Pediatrics to Level 1 trauma. She has also traveled on various mission trips caring for the underserved in Puerto Rico and Dominican Republic. In 2007, she received the Housecall Clinician of the Year award from the American Academy of Home Care Physicians and has recently received the 2008 NP Entrepreneur of the Year award from ADVANCE for Nurse Practitioners.

Gregory A. Lind, PhD, ARNP
Lake Serene Clinic, Practice Owner

Gregory Lind is a nurse entrepreneur pioneer. He has graduate degrees from the University of Missouri in Columbia and the University of Kansas in Kansas City. In the 1970's he worked with Missouri's School of Family and Community Medicine to start a NP role in a rural clinic. He later served for a short period of time as assistant director of a nurse practitioner program, but felt the pull towards reentering practice after Washington state changed the laws to allow independent NP practice with mandated insurance and prescriptive parity. In 1990, he founded Lake Serene Clinic, developing his vision of an all-NP urgent care practice that currently employs 7 NPs. He devised the clinic to be open every day 9 A.M.–8 P.M. and 11 A.M.–4 P.M. on holidays, allowing staff to work 3–11s one week and 4–11s the next week while also meeting a community need. His is still one of the oldest group FNP clinics owned and operated by a NP and has been featured in Advance for Nurse Practitioners.

Public and Community Health Practitioner
Kathleen Sgro

The Doctor of Nursing Practice graduate specializing in public and community health nursing is able to take the advanced practice nursing role to a new level. Being able to identify systems problems in the delivery of health care and the promotion of wellness in our communities requires advanced training in evaluation of research, evidence-based nursing, and measurable outcomes. The DNP graduate possesses these skills and is able to apply them to these settings in many ways. Being able to measure responses to disasters, pandemic flu, treatment of chronic illnesses, women, infant, and children health programs, and so on will contribute to better care of populations, promotion of health, and prevention of illness.

Historical Development of Community and Public Health Nursing

In essence, public health nursing *requires specific educational preparation, and* community health nursing *denotes a setting for the practice of nursing.*
—U.S. DEPARTMENT OF HEALTH AND HUMAN SERVICES, 1985

It is important for us to recognize the contribution of Lillian Wald to the profession of public health nursing. Lillian Wald was the originator of public health nursing and the founder of the Visiting Nurse Service in New York City. She focused her practice on caring for the poor on the Lower East Side. She established Henry House as a neighborhood program to provide care for those who were sick and at home. After the turn of the century, over 90% of the sick stayed home. The poor had no money to pay physicians, and hospitals were reserved for extreme cases and generally did little good. Wald's influence on public health was felt worldwide through her visits to England, Germany, Italy, Mexico, and the Soviet Union (Falk, 2006). Modern public health nursing services emerged from the work of Lillian Wald.

Today public health nurses "provide population-focused care. Assessment, planning and evaluation occur at the population level. The nursing process is used in the planning and delivery of care to individuals, families, groups, populations, and communities" (ANA, 2007). The focus of the public health nurse is on promoting, restoring, and maintaining the health of the population or community, which is quite a different practice from what occurs in a facility or clinic. As our society has become more complex, so has public health nursing. Broad capabilities in systems thinking are foundational to the understanding of population health. The DNP graduate possesses the skills to identify these populations and incorporate evidence-based practice in addressing healthcare promotion and disease prevention for patient populations. In contrast, community health nursing is "the identification of needs, along with protection and improvement of collective health, within a geographically defined area" (Rector, 2010). The American Association of Colleges of Nursing supports the practice of doctoral education for public health and community nursing with Essential VII of doctoral education.

The DNP program prepares the graduate to:

1. Analyze epidemiological, biostatistical, environmental, and other appropriate scientific data related to individual, aggregate, and population health.
2. Synthesize concepts, including psychosocial dimensions and cultural diversity, related to clinical prevention and population health in developing, implementing, and evaluating interventions to address health promotion/disease prevention efforts, improve health status/access patterns, and/or address gaps in care of individuals, aggregates, or populations.
3. Evaluate care delivery models and/or strategies using concepts related to community, environmental and occupational health, and cultural and socioeconomic dimensions of health. (AACN, 2006)

Please see Chapter 7 for additional discussion of AACN Essential VII.

Measuring Progress in Population Health

Assessment of progress in population health is measured differently from that of an individual person's health. Progress is measured through collection and analysis of large data sets and the development of population wellness goals. This data collection and goal development is facilitated through the U.S. Department of Health and Human Services (DHHS). These national goals are known as Healthy People 2010, which will soon be replaced by Healthy People 2020. An advisory committee is developing new goals for the nation's health in an attempt to set national objectives and provide benchmarks against which progress can be measured toward the new goals (DHHS, 2008). It is thought that such objectives and benchmarks will focus actions toward the overall goal of improving the nation's health (see Figures 10-1 and 10-2).

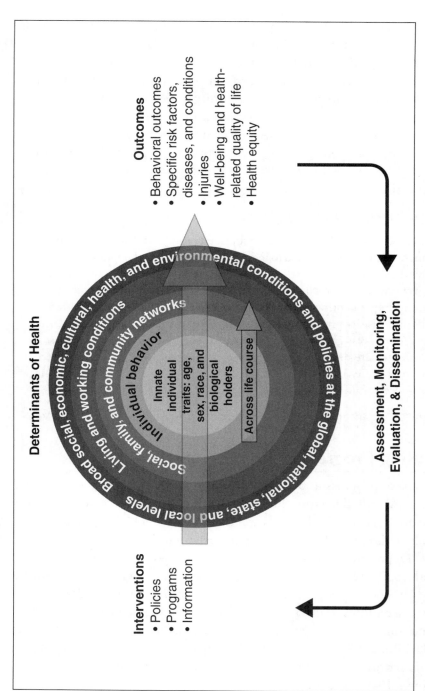

■ Figure 10-1   Action model to achieve Healthy People 2020's overarching goals.

Source: U.S. Department of Health and Human Services, Secretary's Advisory Committee on Health Promotion and Disease Prevention Objectives for 2020. (2008). *Phase I report: Recommendations for the framework and format of Healthy People 2020* (p. 8). Retrieved from http://www.healthypeople.gov/hp2020/advisory/PhaseI/PhaseI.pdf

---

Vision
A society in which all people live long, healthy lives.

Mission
To improve health through strengthening policy and practice,
Healthy People will:

- Identify nationwide health improvement priorities;

- Increase public awareness and understanding of the determinants of health, disease, and disability and the opportunities for progress;

- Provide measurable objectives and goals that can be used at the national, state, and local levels;

- Engage multiple sectors to take actions that are driven by the best available evidence and knowledge;

- Identify critical research and data collection needs.

■ Figure 10-2   Healthy People 2020 Vision and Mission Statement

Source: Secretary's Advisory Committee on National Health Promotion and Disease Prevention Objectives for 2020. (2008). *Phase I report: Recommendations for the framework and format of Healthy People 2020*, p. 5. Retrieved from http://www.healthypeople.gov/HP2020/advisory/PhaseI/PhaseI.pdf.

Organizational Aspects of Public and Community Health

The Quad Council on Public Health Nursing Organizations is a group of member organizations that includes the Association of State and Territorial Directors of Nursing (ASTDN), the American Nurses Association (ANA) Council on Nursing Practice and Economics, the Association of Community Health Nursing Educators (ACHNE), and the Section of Public Health Nursing of the American Public Health Association (APHA). The purpose of the Quad Council is to provide a forum for developing ideas about issues. It also identifies public health nurse experts to advocate for public health nursing on national and other committees (ACHNE, n.d.). The DNP graduate has the skills and competencies to participate in the dialogue and present the perspective of public health nursing to legislators (AACN, 2006).

Community Health

The DNP graduate who practices in the community health role must integrate these initiatives into the planning and treatment of patients within the community setting. There are many venues for community health nursing. Local county and city health departments, home health agencies, wellness programs, and government-sponsored community health programs are a few settings in which community and public health nurses focus on disease prevention and wellness promotion. The DNP's role in community health nursing is to maintain a knowledge base of the healthcare delivery system across the continuum of care and focus on evidence-based interventions when developing a comprehensive plan of care. The plan of care incorporates available community healthcare resources and established treatment guidelines in managing patients and clients. The DNP identifies illnesses that are being addressed through community health systems, develops interventions to improve the health of the patients and families who are part of the community, and assists them in managing acute and chronic illnesses within the community setting. The community health nurse integrates outcomes and cost-control measures in the development and provision of nursing interventions. The DNP graduate in community health "has and continues to demonstrate great promise in reshaping nursing practice and health care management" (Cohen & Cesta, 2001). As more complex nursing interventions are provided to patients in settings outside the hospital, the need for doctorally prepared community health nurses will increase.

Another aspect of community nursing that the DNP graduate is well suited for is the development of disease management protocols that include the integration of technology in the delivery of community health services. Remote monitoring and electronic healthcare records are changing the delivery of healthcare services for the better. According to the AACN's *Essentials of Doctoral Education*, the DNP graduate has competencies in technology and information systems (AACN, 2006). The DNP's skills also promote the analysis of systems for cost containment measures across the entire healthcare delivery system. Given the current financial climate, many local, state, and national legislatures are attempting to restructure the current system in the United States. The DNP is uniquely positioned to advocate for those who are unable to have a voice in the decision-making process. Vulnerable patient populations continue to need ongoing nursing care, and the DNP graduate has the skills to participate in policy formation to ensure that these patient populations have their needs addressed.

Community Healthcare Settings

County Health Departments

Disease prevention and control, emergency preparedness, maternal–child health, family health, clinic services, elder care, the homeless, and environmental health are all areas that government-operated health departments oversee. The DNP's expertise in identification of problems facing the community and development of evidence-based interventions contributes to continued preparedness in dealing with public health issues. County and city health departments vary in the number and types of services they offer. Some oversee the inspection and licensing of local restaurants. Many provide Medicare and Medicaid skilled home health services; women, infant, and children (WIC) programs; and wellness and prevention programs such as smoking cessation, disease management, and weight loss programs. The DNP graduate is well prepared to play a role as a member of the interdisciplinary team that plans and develops education programs that focus on disease prevention and health promotion.

The DNP graduate has a role in policy setting and in the tracking of illnesses in order to continue to improve the lives of these populations. Identification of gaps in services to populations lies with the advanced practice nurse. Ongoing reevaluation of the effectiveness of these programs will lead to improved care, and the DNP must develop tracking and intervention criteria and outcome measures. The public health DNP uses evidence-based practice and research to develop needed programs for populations in the community. Since September 11, 2001, the focus on disaster preparedness has required the advanced practice nurse to develop strategic plans to deal with potential disasters such as bioterrorism and to work as a team member with other community resources in developing comprehensive response plans.

PANDEMIC FLU AND TUBERCULOSIS PREVENTION

Local county health departments are also the main distributors of flu vaccines and healthcare worker protective equipment during pandemic flu episodes. They usually provide tuberculosis testing for the public, and many provide annual flu vaccine clinics for the general public. Identification of public health concerns and potential infections requires the skills of the DNP. Development of action plans and coordination of dissemination of vaccines to communities requires advanced skills in developing strategic plans in order to have positive outcomes. Being able to measure these outcomes is also the role of the DNP in controlling the spread of disease, educating the community, and promoting health.

DISASTER PREPAREDNESS

County and city health departments are a focal point in implementing community disaster responses. They work closely with area hospitals, the Red Cross, and law enforcement in providing services to the community during a disaster. The public health DNP's input is vital to the development of comprehensive disaster preparedness programs. Hurricane Katrina was a wake-up call to our country that more work on our national disaster preparedness is needed. Examining our past failures leads us toward improved systems for providing services to our communities during disasters. The DNP plays a significant role in development of policies and disaster preparedness plans, as well as educating the healthcare workforce on the proper response.

CLINICS

County and city health departments provide for health clinics and dental clinics for the uninsured as well as immunization programs for school-aged children. The public health nurse who works at a county health department wears many hats. County and city health departments are funded through local taxes and grants. The DNP has a major role in program development, cost controls, and adherence to grant requirements and other funding sources. Identification of patient populations and needs is important for the advanced practice nurse in order to prepare grant applications that will have an impact on the prevention of illnesses. Advanced practice nurses in government-sponsored health programs must develop methodologies for measuring the success of many programs. Treatment programs must be evidence based, with measurable outcomes, in order to provide a continuing evaluation of the effectiveness of programs.

Home Healthcare Settings

Community nursing is provided through several venues. One of these venues is home health services. Home health agencies are licensed by state departments of public health. The licensing acts cover skilled intermittent and part-time services. Some states require a certificate of need (CON) before a license is issued. These states attempt to control costs and manage services through the licensing process. Many states are beginning to develop standards and licensing requirements for private-duty skilled and nonskilled hourly home services. The state of Illinois recently amended its home health licensing act to include these levels of home care services. This policy change was achieved through the work of community health nurses and social workers in Illinois who requested oversight of the delivery of hourly home care to homebound patients in the state. Issues relating to unlicensed care were identified as a problem-prone area by community nurses. Through their efforts, the state now has oversight of the nursing care and home care services delivered to one of the most vulnerable patient populations, the homebound disabled and elderly. The advanced practice nurse can effect change through policy development and testifying before legislatures in order to meet the needs of the community.

MEDICAID AND MEDICARE ISSUES IN HOME HEALTH SERVICES

Skilled home health services are funded through the Medicare Part A benefit. Senior citizens aged 65 and older and disabled adults are covered under the Medicare home health benefit. When a patient is admitted to a home health agency, a plan of care is established by the community health nurse assigned to the patient and the patient's primary care physician. The community health nurse coordinates the care needed and develops a plan of care that may include other disciplines, such as therapy, social services, and home health aides for assistance with personal hygiene. Most home health agencies provide these services on an intermittent basis. Community health nurses and therapists make visits on a predetermined frequency. All services must be ordered by a medical doctor, doctor of osteopathy, or psychiatrist.

The DNP has a role as a program and treatment manager in a home health agency, as well as in identification of developing trends and gaps in services available to patient populations within the community. The advanced practice nurse is able to serve as a liaison to community healthcare nurses in directing disease management programs that will reduce hospitalization and emergency room usage for these patient populations. Evidence-based practice protocols need to be designed for home health nursing. The DNP has the expertise to identify best practices that will lead to management of chronic illnesses that produces improved outcomes.

DISEASE MANAGEMENT AND EVIDENCE-BASED PRACTICE IN HOME HEALTH

Development of disease management programs that are evidence based provides the DNP with a challenging role in the community setting. The Disease

Management Association of America (DMAA) has established the following criteria for disease management programs:

- Population identification process
- Evidence-based practice guidelines
- Collaborative practice models to include physician support
- Patient self-management education
- Process outcomes measurement evaluation and management
- Routine reporting/feedback loop (DMAA, 2009)

Disease management programs are beginning to show evidence of improved quality of life for patients with chronic illnesses. Further research needs to be done in this area, and the DNP has the necessary tools to evaluate the effectiveness of disease management programs.

HOME HOSPICE AND INPATIENT SERVICES

Hospice services provided to terminally ill patients and their families focus on symptom management, pain control, medical equipment, and emotional and pastoral care services as well as bereavement follow-up for survivors. Hospice programs are home health based and are reimbursed under Medicare Part A. Coordinating care and managing patient symptoms must be designed to meet the individual needs of each patient. The advanced practice nurse specializing in hospice and palliative care collaborates with other healthcare providers in management of pain and symptoms related to the terminal illness.

TECHNOLOGY

Home healthcare agencies are incorporating technology into their practice. Electronic clinical records and telehealth vital sign monitoring devices are being used to provide accurate and immediate health status information to the community health nurse. Daily vital sign monitors transmit information such as pulse, weight, blood pressure, pulse oxygen levels, temperature, blood glucose readings, and prothrombin times to the agency so that community health nurses or therapists are able to intervene when a patient's condition fluctuates. The goal is to intervene early and prevent an emergency room visit or inpatient admission. DNPs collaborate with physicians and other healthcare professionals to develop standardized treatment protocols for chronic diseases. In the community health setting, DNPs also collaborate with other community resources and develop programs that incorporate technology to bridge the gap in information that is shared across the healthcare continuum.

Evidence-Based Practice and Community Health

It is the role of the community health nurse to provide evidence-based clinical treatments. Home health agencies are developing disease management programs in order to prevent exacerbations of illnesses such as diabetes, congestive heart failure, and so forth, as well as implementing fall reduction programs. Outcome measurements provide nursing staff with measurable results to identify areas of success and areas needing improvement.

Case Study

In 2006, Alterna-Care Home Health Agency, located in Springfield, Illinois, completed a two-year project aimed at reducing emergency room visits and repeat hospitalizations among its diabetic and cardiac patient populations. Evidence-based treatments and a disease management model of care were implemented. After the two-year project, repeat hospitalizations and emergency room visits were significantly reduced in these patients. Evidence-based practice that provides interventions to reduce acute care services will add cost savings to the Medicare program. Disease management using specialized nursing and collaboration with physician specialists are two components of the program that led to improved outcomes. This was a DNP project that showed successful results. The DNP must develop these types of programs that are replicable to other patient populations. The disease management model of care is easily replicable to other diagnoses, which is important for a DNP project (Sgro, 2007). The DNP identifies areas that need improvement or unmet needs of patient populations and develops a plan to improve the outcomes for this population. There is continued work to be done in the disease management arena.

Future and Proposed Legislation

In 2008 several states were chosen to pilot a pay-for-performance (P4P) reimbursement methodology for home health agencies. Value-based purchasing for services provided to Medicare beneficiaries will be the focus of P4P. The DNP must have the ability to track patient outcomes and efficacy of treatment in order to survive in the P4P environment. At this writing, the proposal is for home health agencies to receive a bonus if their outcome measures are in the top 10% of the national average and a penalty if their outcome measures are in the bottom 10%. This is an example of the type of outcomes-based payment strategies being proposed on a national level as a result of cost overruns and concerns about the sustainability of current Medicare and Medicaid benefits.

The need for long-term-care home- and community-based services is straining the Medicare system. By 2050 one in four Americans will be 65 years or older, making up 18.5% of the U.S. population by 2025 (U.S. Census Bureau, 1990). The DNP will need to focus on cost-effective and evidence-based interventions to meet the needs of the senior population in the community.

The Independence at Home Act (S.1131) was introduced on May 21, 2009. This bill would allow Medicare to authorize chronic care coordination programs for Medicare beneficiaries with multiple chronic conditions under the traditional fee-for-service program. The goal is to help patients to remain in their homes with additional support, at a lower cost than institutional care. The DNP graduate is well prepared to track legislation in order to prepare for the provision of nursing care to the large volume of aging baby boomers. "Research is needed to address and evaluate the effectiveness of our current public health system," and the DNP will play a major role in this research, American Academy of Home Care Physicians (AAHCP, 2009).

Wellness Programs in the Community

Insurance- and Employer-Sponsored Programs

Insurance payers are focusing on preventive care programs. Health insurance companies provide wellness programs to their beneficiaries. Employers are also developing these programs in an effort to decrease the cost of care for chronic illnesses such as diabetes, asthma, congestive heart failure, obesity, and smoking-related illnesses. Insurance companies use advanced practice nurses who provide phone teaching through case management to enrollees of the insurance program. The DNP is able to provide evidence-based preventive care programs while monitoring the cost effectiveness of interventions. Measuring the outcomes of a wellness program provides feedback to the organization on the benefits of preventive programs.

Government-Sponsored Community Health Programs

Specialized Services for Children

Each state receives federal money for home care services to support families who are caring for children with multiple handicaps. Many children who need complex nursing care are managed at home. Family members are taught to provide this type of care with support from community nursing services.

These state grants use case managers to oversee and approve the care provided in the home. This vulnerable patient population needs ongoing evaluation by the advanced practice nurse to ensure the delivery of adequate community services in order for them to remain independent. Proper funding and policy making are the goal of the DNP.

Community Mental Health Services

Community-based case management systems for chronically mentally ill patients integrate the role of the case manager as a coordinator of community resources and as coordinator of care. Two models of community-based care to support the mentally ill have emerged. The assertive community treatment model and the intensive case management model both have a low patient-to-staff ratio, with services provided in the community rather than mental health centers. The assertive community model uses a team approach with nurses and physicians sharing the case load. The intensive case management model provides for a stronger relationship between the nurse and the patient (Cohen & Cesta, 2001). Further research is needed to measure the effectiveness of these programs.

Senior Community Care Programs

State-sponsored community care programs for senior citizens are similar to the services provided through the Department of Rehabilitative Services. The community care programs for seniors provide assistance with daily living. Clients must qualify financially to receive the services. A case coordination assessment is completed using a scoring system to determine the number of hours of assistance for which each applicant qualifies. The doctor of nursing practice must be aware of all the programs available in the community. The DNP needs to bring these services together to meet the needs of each individual.

Summary

The advanced practice nurse has numerous roles in public and community health nursing across the life span of individuals. Research into the efficacy of community programs is needed to provide the best evidence-based and cost-effective interventions. As the population ages, the provision of care in the home will become more common in an attempt to keep seniors in their own homes. Emerging technologies will provide much-needed improvements in communication and valuable outcome measurements. Implementing evidence-based care and using feedback and outcome measures to improve care provide direction for improvement of community-based healthcare services.

Healthcare issues such as pandemic flu outbreaks, natural disasters, and treatment of chronic illnesses require a global perspective. Nursing must be involved in policy making and the identification of trends and the needs of patient populations in the community. Advanced practice nurses are instrumental in developing programs, influencing policy, and providing research for evidence-based practice in community and public health nursing.

Integrative Practitioner
Joy Elwell and Kathryn Waud White

Integrative health care is growing as a choice for Americans. The National Institutes of Health reported that in 2005 38% of American adults and 12% of children use alternative or complementary therapies of some type ("Americans Continue," 2009). Integrative health care is just that: the integration of the best concepts of traditional medicine with the best concepts of alternative therapies (Center for Spirituality and Healing, 2008). The skills gained in the DNP program will enhance the advanced nurse practitioner in integrative therapy. Essential III states that the DNP program prepares advanced practice nurses to "[c]ritically appraise existing literature and other evidence to implement the best evidence for practice" (AACN, 2006). Essential VI speaks to interprofessional collaboration, which is truly an essential for the practice of this specialty that reaches across so many different healthcare fields (AACN, 2006). Essential VII describes clinical prevention and population health, all facilitated through integrative health care (AACN, 2006). The DNP-prepared integrative health practitioner will have much to offer patients.

To address the DNP-prepared advanced practice nurse as an integrative practitioner, it is essential to explore integrative health as a specialty within health care. Integrative health, also known as *holistic health*, is described as "treating the whole person, helping the person to bring the mental, emotional, physical, social, and spiritual dimensions of his or her being into greater harmony, using the basic principles and elements of holistic healing and, as much as possible, placing reliance on treatment modalities that foster the self regenerative and self reparatory processes of natural healing" (Otto & Knight, 1979, p. 3). Nursing's approach to wellness from a holistic perspective makes nursing and integrative health perfect partners for the advanced practice nurse.

Nurses as Integrative Practitioners

Historically, Florence Nightingale may be considered one of the first professional integrative health practitioners in nursing. Nightingale "was a mystic, visionary, healer, reformer, environmentalist, feminist, practitioner, scientist, politician and global citizen." (Dossey, Selanders, Beck, & Attewell, 2005). She looked beyond the era's traditional medical and surgical treatment of disease and injury to include nutrition and sanitation, lighting, and activity. She addressed the mind, body, and spirit connection that would pave the way for modern professional integrative practitioners.

Since Nightingale's death in 1910, professional nursing has evolved in numerous ways, including the development of advanced practice nursing roles. Numerous nursing pioneers have explored integrative modalities to assist clients in achieving optimum levels of wellness, alleviating suffering, and facilitating healing. Founded in 1980, the American Holistic Nurses Association (AHNA) focuses on holistic nursing as "all nursing practice that has healing the whole person as its goal" (AHNA, 1998, cited in AHNA, n.d.).

New York University established the first holistic nurse practitioner program; others have followed. Within the United States, certain states (e.g., New York) identify holistic health as a specialty (New York State Office of the Professions, n.d.). There are also holistic clinical nurse specialists. The American Nurses Association now recognizes holistic nursing as a specialty, and certification can be obtained through the American Holistic Nurses' Certification Corporation (AHNCC). The American Holistic Nurses Organization (AHNO) has also articulated standards of practice, core values, a certification curriculum, and requirements for endorsement of holistic nursing programs. A current listing of nursing programs that are endorsed by the AHNCC can be found at http://ahncc.org/home/endorsedschools.html.

Nurses can pursue educational programs for integrative or holistic modalities at all levels of post-licensure preparation; generally, there is no prescribed level of degree preparation for an integrative practice. Certain roles within the realm of integrative practitioners, such as chiropractors, acupuncturists, and massage therapists, are licensed and do have educational requirements. Nurses who pursue these roles must fulfill those requirements in addition to any nursing curriculum.

That nurses practice integratively is not a novel concept. Major nursing theorists incorporate holism into their theories. Dr. Jean Watson's theory of human caring is one example. She identifies caring beliefs and behaviors that benefit not only the client but the nurse as well.

Types of Integrative Healing Modalities

Integrative health care includes many healing modalities. There are five different approaches to care as organized by the National Center for Complementary and Alternative Care (NCCAM): whole medical systems, manipulative and body-based practices, mind–body medicine, biologically based practices,

■ Table 10-1   Websites for Further Information on Integrative Health

American Holistic Nurses' Certification Corporation
http://www.ahncc.org

Center for Spirituality and Healing at the University of Minnesota
http://www.csh.umn.edu

Life Science Foundation
http://lifesciencefoundation.org

National Center for Complementary and Alternative Medicine (NCCAM)
http://nccam.nih.gov/health/whatiscam

University of Michigan, Doctor of Nursing Practice Program
http://www.nursing.umn.edu/dnp/ProspectiveStudent/Specialties/Integrative_
Health_and_Healing/home.html

and energy medicine (NCCAM, 2007). The modalities described here are not intended to be an exhaustive list of every integrative healing modality known. Table 10-1 lists websites where further information can be found.

Whole Medical Systems

- *Homeopathy:* A medical discipline that facilitates healing through the administration of substances prescribed according to three principles: (1) like cures like, also known as the "law of similars"; (2) the more a remedy is diluted, the greater the potency; and (3) illness is specific to the individual. Homeopathy is based on the belief that symptoms are signs of the body's effort to get rid of disease; treatment is based on the whole person, rather than on the symptoms (NCCAM, 2009).
- *Osteopathic medicine:* A form of medicine focusing on the relationship between the structure of the body and its function, identifying that both structure and function are subject to a range of illnesses. In treating the client, osteopathic practitioners use various types of physical manipulation to stimulate the body's self-healing ability, as well as traditional allopathic medical modalities. Osteopathic physicians are licensed to diagnose, treat, and prescribe nationally.

Manipulative Modalities

- *Acupressure:* Pressure, by fingers and hands, over specific areas of the body, is used to alleviate pain and discomfort and to positively influence the function of internal organs and body systems. Various approaches are used to release tension and restore the natural flow of energy in the body.

- *Acupuncture:* Use of fine-gauged needles inserted into specific points on the body to stimulate or disperse the flow of energy. This ancient Oriental technique is used to alleviate pain or increase immunity by balancing energy flow. Massage, herbal medicine, and nutritional counseling are often used in conjunction with acupuncture.

- *Alexander technique:* This technique, developed by the Australian actor Frederick Matthias Alexander, involves learning a series of lessons in rebalancing the body through awareness, movement, and touch. As the student explores new ways of reorganizing neuromuscular function, the body is reintroduced to healthy posture and direct, efficient movement (Trivieri & Anderson, 2002).

- *AMMA therapy:* AMMA therapy is a form of Oriental massage that focuses on the balance and movement of energy within the body.

- *Applied kinesiology:* Originated by chiropractic physician George Goodheart Jr. in the 1960s, applied kinesiology incorporates the principles of a number of holistic therapies, "including chiropractic, osteopathic medicine and acupuncture, and involves manual manipulation of the spine, extremities, and cranial bones in performing its procedures" (Trivieri & Anderson, 2002, p. 71).

- *Aromatherapy:* Aromatherapy incorporates the use of essential oils extracted from plants and herbs to treat physical imbalances, as well as to achieve psychological and spiritual well-being. The oils are inhaled, applied externally, or ingested. According to Dr. Kurt Schnaubelt, "the chemical makeup of essential oils gives them a host of desirable pharmacological properties, ranging from antibacterial, antiviral, and antispasmodic, to uses as diuretics, vasodilators, and vasoconstrictors. Essential oils also act on the adrenals, ovaries, and thyroid, and can energize, pacify or detoxify, and facilitate the digestive process" (Trivieri & Anderson, 2002, p. 76).

- *Breema bodywork:* Breema bodywork incorporates simple, playful bodywork sequences along with stretch and movement exercises that help create greater flexibility, a relaxed body, a clear mind, and calm, supportive feelings. Developed by chiropractic physician Jon Schraiber, Breema bodywork is based on nine principles: body comfortable, no extra, firmness and gentleness, full participation, mutual support, no judgment, single moment/single activity, no hurry/no pause, and no force (Mann, 2009).

- *Chiropractic medicine:* A healthcare system emphasizing structural alignment of the spine. Adjustments involve the manipulation of the spine and joints to reestablish and maintain normal nervous system functioning. Some chiropractors employ additional therapies, such as massage, nutrition, and specialized kinesiology.
- *Cranial osteopathy:* Gentle and almost imperceptible manipulation of the skull to reestablish its natural configuration and movement. Such correction can have a positive influence on disorders manifested throughout the body.
- *Craniosacral therapy:* Diagnosis and treatment of imbalances in the craniosacral system. Subtle adjustments are made to the system through light touch and gentle manipulations.
- *Dance therapy:* Dance therapy is a modality in which dance and music combine to allow the body, mind, soul, and spirit to be refreshed and uplifted and to experience the freedom that natural bodily movement allows.
- *Feldenkrais method:* The Feldenkrais method is a method of instruction, through movement and gentle manipulation, to enhance self-image and restore mobility. Students are taught to notice how they are using their bodies and how to improve their posture and move more freely.
- *Jin shin jyutsu:* This is a bodywork technique that balances body energy as it travels along specific pathways. Specific combinations of healing points are held with the fingertips to restore balance and harmony.
- *Lymphatic therapy:* Lymphatic therapy is a vigorous form of massage that helps the body release toxins stored in the lymphatic system— excellent for the immune system and rebuilding the body.
- *Massage:* Massage involves the use of strokes and pressure on the body to dispel tension, increase circulation, and relieve muscular pain. Massage can provide comfort and increased body awareness and can facilitate the release of emotional as well as bodily tension.
- *Movement therapy:* This modality involves guided series of movements and body work to open energy pathways and facilitate healing.

- *Neuromuscular therapy:* Neuromuscular therapy is a massage therapy in which moderate pressure over muscles and nerves, as well as on trigger points, is used to decrease pain and tension.
- *Physical therapy:* Physical therapy includes the treatment of physical conditions of body malfunction, damage, or injury using procedures designed to reduce swelling, relieve pain, strengthen muscles, restore range of motion, and return functioning to the patient.
- *Shiatsu:* Shiatsu is an energy-based system of bodywork using a firm sequence of rhythmic pressure held on specific pressure points on the body, designed to awaken acupressure meridians.
- *Trigger point therapy:* This is a method of compression of sensitive points in the muscle tissue, along with massage and passive stretches, for the relief of pain and tension. Treatment decreases swelling and stiffness and increases range of motion. Exercises may be assigned.

Mind–Body Medicine

- *Art therapy:* Art therapy incorporates the use of basic art materials to discover how to restore, maintain, or improve physical and mental health. Through observation and analysis, the art therapist is able to formulate treatment plans specific to the individual.
- *Color therapy:* Color therapy involves the use of electronic instrumentation and color receptivity, according to the work of Jacob Lieberman (1993), to integrate the nervous system and body–mind. It increases well-being, and can be helpful for many acute and chronic ailments.
- *Counseling/psychotherapy:* A broad category of therapies that treat individuals as a whole. Treatments and sessions are focused on integrated care on all levels, for individuals, families, or groups.
- *Eye movement desensitization and reprocessing (EMDR):* EMDR is an accelerated information-processing method using alternating stimuli—either eye movements or sounds—to desensitize and reprocess emotional wounds and install a healthier belief system. EMDR is effective with posttraumatic stress syndrome, childhood trauma, depression, addictions, compulsions, unhealthy patterns, and future-oriented solutions.
- *Guided imagery:* A holistic modality that assists clients in connecting with their inner knowledge at the thinking, feeling, and sensing levels, thus promoting their innate healing abilities. Together, guide and client co-create an effective way to work with pain, symptom, grief,

and stress management; conflict resolution; self-empowerment issues; and preparing for medical or surgical interventions.

- *Hypnotherapy:* A state of focused attention, achieved through guided relaxation, hypnotherapy is used to access the unconscious mind. Hypnosis is used for memory recall, medical treatment, and skill enhancement or personal growth.
- *Interactive imagery:* Fostering active participation, disease prevention, and health promotion, interactive imagery returns the focus of wellness to the individual.
- *Meditation:* A method of relaxing and quieting the mind to relieve muscle tension and facilitate inner peace. There are numerous forms of meditation, taught individually or in group settings, and it is thought that prayer for the self might have an effect similar to meditation. The nonsectarian form of prayer, which is akin to meditation and used for stress reduction, has long been recognized by clinicians to improve one's sense of well-being.
- *Music therapy:* An expressive art form designed to help the individual move into harmony and balance. Through the use of music, individuals explore emotional, spiritual, and behavioral issues. Musical skill is not necessary, as the process, rather than technique, is emphasized.
- *Neurolinguistic programming:* A systematic approach to changing behavior through changing patterns of thinking. Its originators, Dilts, Grinder, and Bandler (1980), propose *theoretical* connections between neurological processes (*neuro*), language (*linguistic*), and behavioral patterns that have been learned through experience (*programming*) that can be organized to achieve specific goals in life.
- *Stress management:* Any therapy or educational practice with the objective of decreasing stress and enhancing one's response to the elements of life that cannot be changed. This broad category may include bodywork, energy work, visualization, and counseling.
- *Tai chi (chuan):* A movement practice and Chinese martial art that enhances coordination, balance and breathing, and promotes physical, emotional, and spiritual well-being. Tai chi is taught in classes or as private lessons, and requires home practice to be effective.
- *Yoga therapy:* The use of yoga postures, controlled breathing, relaxation, meditation, and nutrition facilitates the release of muscular and emotional tension, improves concentration, increases oxygen levels in the blood, and assists the body in healing itself.

Biologically Based Practices

- *Biofeedback:* A relaxation technique involving careful monitoring of vital functions (such as breathing, heart rate, and blood pressure) in order to improve health. By conscious thought, visualization, movement, or relaxation, one can learn which actions result in desirable changes in these vital functions. Biofeedback is used for medical problems related to stress and for management of many health problems, including pain syndrome, migraine, and irritable bowel syndrome.
- *Herbal therapy:* The use of herbs and their chemical properties to alleviate specific conditions or to support the function of various body systems. Herbal formulas have three basic functions: elimination and detoxification, health management and maintenance, and health building. The scope of herbal medicine is sometimes extended to include fungal and bee products, as well as minerals, shells, and certain animal parts (Acharya & Shrivastava, 2008).
- *Hydrotherapy:* The use of water, ice, steam, and hot and cold temperatures to relieve pain, fever, inflammation, and maintain and restore health. Treatments include full-body immersion, steam baths, saunas, and the application of hot or cold compresses or both.
- *Nutritional counseling:* Nutritional counseling is performed by a practitioner who uses diet and supplementation therapeutically as the primary or adjunctive treatment for illness, as well as for maintaining good health. Nutritionists employ a variety of approaches, including food combining, macrobiotics, and orthomolecular theory.

Energy Medicine

- *Chi kung healing touch:* An Eastern method of healing involving breath and gentle movements that follows the Chinese five-element theory and works with the meridian system.
- *Energy work:* A broad category of healing influencing the seven major energy centers (chakras) and the flow of energy around and through this field.
- *Healing touch:* A therapeutic approach in which touch is used to influence energy systems. Healing touch is employed to affect physical, emotional, mental, and spiritual health and healing.
- *Magnetic therapy:* A modality using magnets to generate controlled magnetic fields. Magnetic therapy is used to improve the functioning of bodily systems and facilitate healing.

- *Reiki:* Using the hands and visualization, the Reiki practitioner directs energy to affected areas of the client's body to facilitate healing and relaxation.
- *Therapeutic touch:* A technique for balancing energy flow in the body through human energy transfer.

The DNP as Integrative Practitioner: Unique Aspects of DNP Preparation

The question will be asked, What advantage is there to having DNP preparation for an advanced practice nurse specializing in integrative health? Any registered professional nurse who takes a course in holistic nursing at the post-RN level should be able to function competently and therapeutically as an integrative practitioner. What, then, does the DNP bring to integrative health? And what is the advantage to seeking DNP preparation for this role?

The AACN addresses the competencies of the doctorally prepared APN (AACN, 2006). The DNP, a practice-focused terminal degree, prepares the APN to serve as an expert in nursing practice. Compared with the PhD and DNS degrees, which are research-focused degrees, the DNP is unique in providing education in those components of advanced nursing practice essential to practice at the highest clinical level. The skills gained in the DNP course of study will not only prepare the nurse for clinical competence but also prepare him or her for establishing a successful practice or business. As DNP programs proliferate in colleges and universities across the nation, and the world, certain states (e.g., Alabama and New York) are mandating that the curricula include a significant percentage of clinical content; indeed, some DNP programs (e.g., Columbia University, University of Wisconsin, University of Washington) include a clinical residency in the curriculum. Including clinical components in the DNP curriculum strengthens the DNP-prepared APN as a clinician. The University of Minnesota's Doctor of Nursing Practice Integrative Health and Healing area of concentration "prepares graduates with skills necessary for working with individuals, families, communities and health systems in developing holistic approaches to health promotion, disease prevention and chronic disease management, with a special emphasis on managing lifestyle changes and incorporating the use of complementary therapies" (University of Minnesota, n.d.). This program fully integrates the specialty courses relevant to integrative practice with those courses designed to meet the requirements of the AACN's *Essentials* competencies. These courses uniquely position the DNP graduate to succeed on many different fronts of integrative health.

DNP curricula are unique in other areas, in that they include coursework in the areas of business finance, health policy, human resource management, change, and leadership (Rush University, n.d.). The advanced practice nurse engaging in integrative health practice benefits from understanding past, current, and future trends in health policy. Healthcare legislation and regulation undergo frequent change, affecting the right to practice, scope of practice, definition of specialty, and related rights, privileges, and responsibilities. Legislation and regulation are influenced by many factors, including political, socioeconomic, and cultural. Advanced coursework in public policy provides the DNP with a firm foundation to clearly view the nuanced political landscape.

The number of APNs owning or directing solo practices remains small, due in part to the expensive and adventurous nature of being an entrepreneur. Because of the lack of research on APNs in private practice, it is not possible to quantify with any specificity the number of APNs who own their own businesses. However, one survey on nurse practitioners indicated that 3% are engaged in private practice (Rollet & Lebo, 2007). Given the nature and challenges of integrative health care (e.g., that health insurers do not consistently pay for holistic health services, that clients may be more inclined to pay for these services with disposable income, and that educated healthcare consumers are becoming increasingly interested in modalities that are more wellness oriented), it is reasonable to speculate that the numbers of APNs starting integrative health practices will increase. DNP programs provide the APN with education in health economics, financial management, budget creation and management, human resources, practice management, and business models.

In the case of the DNP as integrative or holistic practitioner, earning the DNP provides advantages in the areas of direct delivery of health care, practice development and management, and interpreting and synthesizing research. Although some will posit that enough is learned at the baccalaureate or master's levels, the competencies needed to provide health care to increasingly complex populations while managing a practice autonomously, using research for evidence-based care, and advocating for patient access to all relevant forms of interventions that promote wellness are all presented comprehensively in a DNP curriculum and provide the APN with the most optimal level of preparation for practice.

References

Abrams, S. E. (2008). The best of public health nursing, circa 1941. *Public Health Nursing, 25*(3), 285–291.

Acharya, D., & Shrivastava, A. (2008): *Indigenous herbal medicines: Tribal formulations and traditional herbal practices.* Jaipur, India: Aavishkar Publishers.

Acorn, S., Lamarche, K., & Edwards, M. (2009). Practice doctorates in nursing: Developing nursing leaders. *Nursing Leadership, 22*(2), 85–91.

Alabama Commission on Higher Education, Division of Instruction, Planning, and Special Services. (2006). *The doctor of nursing practice: A background paper for Alabama.* Retrieved from http://www.ache.state.al.us/Reports/Nursing%20Study%2015%20June %202007%20 Revision.pdf

American Academy of Home Care Physicians. (2009). *The Independent at Home Act (S. 1131, H.R. 2560).* Retrieved from www.aahcp.org/iahsummary.pdf

American Association of Colleges of Nursing. (2005). *Frequently asked questions concerning the AACN position statement on the practice doctorate in nursing.* Retrieved from http://www .aacn.nche.edu/DNP/AboutDNP.htm

American Association of Colleges of Nursing. (2006). *The essentials of doctoral education for advanced nursing practice.* Retrieved from http://www.aacn.nche.edu/DNP/pdf/Essentials.pdf

American Association of Colleges of Nursing. (2008). *Doctor of nursing talking points.* Retrieved from http://www.aacn.nche.edu/DNP/talkingpoints.htm

American Holistic Nurses Association. (n.d.). *Who we are.* Retrieved from http://www .ahna.org/Aboutus/tabid/1158/Default.aspx

American Nurses Association. (2007). *Public health nursing: Scope and standards of practice.* Silver Spring, MD: Author.

Americans continue to use complementary, alternative medicine. (2009, February 20). *NIH Record, 61*(4). Retrieved from http://nihrecord.od.nih.gov/newsletters/2009/02_20_2009/story8.htm

Association of Community Health Nursing Educators. (n.d.). *The Quad Council of Public Health Nursing Organizations.* Retrieved from http://www.achne.org/i4a/pages/index.cfm ?pageid=3292

Bishop, M. (2006, February 25). The rise of the social entrepreneur. *The Economist, 76*(8466), 12.

Boyer, E. L. (1990). *Scholarship reconsidered: Priorities of the professoriate.* Princeton, NJ: Carnegie Foundation for the Advancement of Teaching.

Boyer, E. L. (1996). The scholarship of engagement. *Journal of Public Service and Outreach, 1*(1), 11–20.

Brown, M. A., Draye, M. A., Zimmer, P. A., Magyary, D., Woods, S. L., Whitney, J., et al. (2006). Developing a practice doctorate in nursing: University of Washington perspectives and experience. *Nursing Outlook, 54*(3), 130–138.

Brown-Benedict, D. (2008). The Doctor of Nursing Practice degree: Lessons from the history of the professional doctorate in other health disciplines. *Journal of Nursing Education, 47*(10), 448–457.

Bullock, P. (2009). Practice snapshot: New genesis center. *Advance for Nurse Practitioners*. Retrieved from http://nurse-practitioners.advanceweb.com/Article/Practice-Snapshot-New-Genesis-Center.aspx

Caffrey, R. A. (2005). The rural community care gerontological nurse entrepreneur: Role development strategies. *Journal of Gerontological Nursing, 31*, 11–16.

Case Western Reserve University, Frances Payne Bolton School of Nursing. (2009). *Post-master's DNP* [Brochure]. Cleveland, OH: Author.

Castledine, G. (2006). The business habits of highly effective nurses. *British Journal of Nursing, 15*(20), 1143.

Center for Spirituality and Healing. (2008). *About us*. Retrieved from http://www.csh.umn.edu /about/home.html

Cohen, E., & Cesta, T. (2001). *Nursing case management* (3rd ed.). St. Louis, MO: Elsevier/Mosby.

Deming, W. (1986). *Out of the crisis*. Cambridge, MA: Massachusetts Institute of Technology, Center for Advanced Engineering Study.

Department of the Army. (1968). *FM 22-100*. Washington, DC: U.S. Government Printing Office.

Department of the Army. (2004). *The U.S. Army Leadership Field Manual*. Washington, DC: U.S. Government Printing Office.

Dilts, R., Grinder, J., Delozier , J., & Bandler, R. (1980). *Neuro-linguistic programming. Volume I: The study of the structure of subjective experience*. Cupertino, CA: Meta Publications.

Disease Management Association of America. (2009). *DMAA definition of disease management*. Retrieved from http://www.dmaa.org/dm_definition.asp

Dossey, B. (1997). *Core curriculum for holistic nursing*. New York: Aspen.

Dossey, B., & Keegan, L. (2008). *Holistic nursing: A handbook for practice* (5th ed.). Sudbury, MA: Jones and Bartlett.

Dossey, B., Selanders, L., Beck, D. M., & Attewell, A. (2005). *Florence Nightingale today: Healing, leadership, global action*. Washington, DC: Nursesbooks.org.

Douglas, W. (2005). Nursing considers clinical practice doctorate degree. *Texas Nurse, 79*(8), 6–14.

Draye, M. A., Acker, M., Zimmer, P. A. (2006). The practice doctorate in nursing: Approaches to transform nurse practitioner education and practice. *Nursing Outlook, 54*(3), 123–129.

Drucker, P. (1954). *The practice of management*. New York: Harper & Row.

Drucker, P. F. (1985). *Innovation and entrepreneurship: Practice and principles*. New York: Harper & Row.

Elango, B., Hunter, G. L., & Winchell, M. (2007). Barriers to nurse entrepreneurship: A study of the process model of entrepreneurship. *Journal of the American Academy of Nurse Practitioners, 19*, 198–204.

Ellis, L. (2007). Academics' perceptions of the professional or clinical doctorate: Findings of a national survey. *Journal of Clinical Nursing, 16*, 2272–2279.

Fain, J. A., Asselin, M., & McCurry, M. (2008). The DNP. . . why now? *Nursing Management, 39*(7), 34–37.

Falk, G. (2006). *Biography of Lillian Wald*. Retrieved from http://jbuff.com/c042706.htm

Faugier, J. (2005). Developing a new generation of nurse entrepreneurs. *Nursing Standard, 19*(30), 49–53.

Fitzpatrick, J. J. (2003). The case for the clinical doctorate in nursing. *Reflections on Nursing Leadership, 29*(1), 8–9, 37.

Fitzpatrick, J., & Wallace, M. (2009). *The doctor of nursing practice and clinical nurse leader: Essentials of program development and implementation for clinical practice.* New York: Springer.

Ford, J. (2009). DNP coming into focus. *Advance for Nurse Practitioners.* Retrieved from http://nurse-practitioners.advanceweb.com/Editorial/Content/Editorial.aspx?CC=191346

Green, A., Starck, P., & Long, K. (2006). *Doctorate of nursing practice (DNP): Talking points prepared for/responses to frequently asked questions.* Texas DNP Roadmap Taskforce. Retrieved from http://tobgne.org/download/DNP_Texas_Talking_Points.pdf

Hardy, E. (2008). Practice snapshot: Holistic Family Healthcare. *Advance for Nurse Practitioners, 16*(6), 16.

Hardy, E., DeBasio, N., Warmbrodt, L., Gartland, M., Bassett, W., & Tansey, M. (2004). Collaborative graduate education: Executive nurse practice and health care leadership. *Nursing Leadership Forum, 8*(4), 123–127.

Heller, B. R., Oros, M. T., & Durney-Crowley, J. (n.d.). *The future of nursing education: Ten trends to watch.* Retrieved from http://www.nln.org/nlnjournal/infotrends.htm

Helmstadter, C. (2002). Early nursing reform in nineteenth-century London: A doctor-driven phenomenon. *Medical History, 46*(3), 325–350.

Hirschman, D., & Morby, L. (2006). A study of the safety of continued anticoagulation for cataract surgery patients. *Nursing Forum, 41*(1), 30–37.

Hoffmann, R. L. (2005). The evolution of hospice in America: Nursing's role in the movement. *Journal of Gerontological Nursing, 31*(7), 26–34, 53–54.

Holland, B. (2005). *Community engagement and community-engaged scholarship: Clarifying our meanings when using these terms.* Teleconference call to the Community-Engaged Scholarship for Health Collaborative.

Houser, B. P., & Player, K. N. (2004). Loretta Ford. In *Pivotal moments in nursing: Leaders who changed the path of a profession.* Indianapolis, IN: Sigma Theta Tau International.

Howkins, E., & Thornton, C. (2003). Liberating the talents: Whose talents, and for what purpose? *Journal of Nursing Management, 11*(4), 219.

Institute of Medicine. (2003). *Crossing the quality chasm: A new health system for the 21st century.* Washington, DC: National Academies Press.

Jolley, J. (2007). Choose your doctorate. *Clinical Nursing, 16*(2), 225–233.

Kacel, B. (2008). NP practice snapshot: New Image Body and Wellness Clinic. *Advance for Nurse Practitioners.* Retrieved from http://nurse- practitioners.advanceweb.com/Editorial/Content/Editorial.aspx?CC=115800

Keyes, L. (2009). Business opportunities for nurses. *Nurse Entrepreneur Network.* Retrieved from: http://www.nurse-entrepreneur-network.com/public/281.cfm?sd=49

Kowal, N. (1988). Specialty practice entrepreneur: The advanced practice nurse. *Nursing Economics, 16*(5), 277–278.

Lieberman, J. (1993). *Light: Medicine of the future—how we can use it to heal ourselves now.* Santa Fe, NM: Inner Traditions/Bear & Company.

Long, K. A. (2006). *Background information: The DNP in Florida.* Retrieved from http://www.flbog.org/documents_meetings/0043_0135_1157_16%20- %20Strat% 20Plan%20Background%20Info—%20DNP%20bullet%20list-03-23- 06.doc

Mann, J. D. (2009). Practicing presence through Breema. *Spirituality and Health,* January–February, 1–2.

Marion, L., Viens, D., O'Sullivan, A., Crabtree, K., Fontana, & Price, M. (2003). The practice doctorate in nursing: Future or fringe? *Topics in Advanced Practice Nursing eJournal, 3*(2).

Marra, J., Jr. (2008). NP practice snapshot: Urgent Care Center. *Advance for Nurse Practitioners.* Retrieved from http://nurse-practitioners.advanceweb.com/Editorial/Content/Editorial .aspx?CC=122664

Merriam-Webster Online Dictionary. (2009). Retrieved from http://www.merriam-webster.com

Miller, J. (2008). The doctor of nursing practice: Recognizing a need or graying the line between doctor and nurse? *Medscape Journal of Medicine, 10*(11), 253.

Moen, G. (2009). Practice snapshot: Eagan Child and Family Care. *Advance for Nurse Practitioners.* Retrieved from http://nurse-practitioners.advanceweb.com/Editorial/Content /Editorial.aspx?CC=194750

National Center for Complementary and Alternative Medicine. (2007). *What is CAM?* Retrieved from http://nccam.nih.gov/health/whatiscam/overview.htm

National Center for Complementary and Alternative Medicine. (2009). *Homeopathy: An introduction.* Retrieved from http://nccam.nih.gov/health/homeopathy

National League for Nursing. (2007). *Reflection and dialogue: Doctor of nursing practice.* Retrieved from http://www.nln.org/aboutnln/reflection_dialogue/refl_dial_1.htm

National Organization of Nurse Practitioner Faculties. (2005). *The practice doctorate resource center: Recommendations.* Retrieved from http://www.nonpf.com/NONPF2005/Practice-DoctorateResourceCenter/PDrecommendations.htm

New York State Office of the Professions, State Education Department. (n.d.) *License requirements for nurse practitioner.* Retrieved from http://www.op.nysed.gov/np.htm

Osborne, K., & Dawley, K. (2005). Mary Breckenridge and the birth of the ACNM. *Journal of Midwifery and Women's Health, 50*(3), 257.

Otto, H. A., & Knight, J. W. (1979). *Dimensions in wholistic healing: New frontiers in the treatment of the whole person.* Chicago: Burnham.

Parry, M. S. (2006). Voices from the past: Dorothea Dix (1802–1887). *American Journal of Public Health, 96*(4), 622–624.

Partin, B. (2008). Update on the DNP degree. *Nurse Practice, 33*(3), 7.

Pennsylvania State Board of Nursing. (2005). Draft language for CRNP educational programs regulation. *Regulations of the State Board of Nursing,* 49 PA Code 21.1–21.607.

Pronsati, M. (2008). Some kinda miracle stuff. *Advance for Nurse Practitioners, 16*(12), 10.

Rector, C. (2010). The journey begins: Introduction to community health nursing. In J. Allender, C. Rector, & K. Warner (Eds.), *Community health nursing: Promoting and protecting the public's health* (7th ed., pp. 1–4). Philadelphia: Wolters Kluwer Health/Lippincott Williams & Wilkins.

Riley, E. (2009, March). New degree of doctor. *AZ Nurse Update*. Retrieved from: http://view .digipage.net/?userpath=00000001/00005932/00037812/&page=12

Rollet, J. (2008). Restoring dignity through dryness. *Advance for Nurse Practitioners*. Retrieved from http://nurse- practitioners.advanceweb.com/Editorial/Content/Editorial.aspx?CC=190253

Rollet, J., & Lebo, S. (2007). 2007 salary survey results: A decade of growth. Results of the 2007 national salary and workplace survey of nurse practitioners. *Advance for Nurse Practitioners*. Retrieved from http://nurse-practitioners.advanceweb.com/Article/2007-Salary-Survey-Results-A-Decade-of-Growth-3.aspx

Rollet, J., & Lebo, S. (2008). A decade of growth: Salaries increase as profession matures. *Advance for Nurse Practitioners*. Retrieved from http://nurse-practitioners.advanceweb.com/Article /A-Decade-of-Growth.aspx

Rush University. (n.d.). *Doctor of Nursing Practice degree program of study (beginning Winter 2009 for new matriculants)*. Retrieved from http://www.rushu.rush.edu/servlet/Satellite?Meta AttrName=meta_university&ParentId=1221491470501&ParentType=RushUnivLevel3 Page&c=content_block&cid=1211209856164&level1-p=3&level1-pp= 1221491470093&level1-ppp=1221491470093&pagename=Rush%2Fcontent_block %2FContentBlockDetail

Schiff, L. (2009). Practice snapshot: Advanced Practice Solutions. *Advance for Nurse Practitioners*. Retrieved from http://nurse-practitioners.advanceweb.com/Editorial/Content /Editorial.aspx?CC=196584

Scott, E. S., & Craig, J. B. (2008). Analysis of ANA's draft scope and standards of practice for nurse administrators. *Journal of Nursing Administration, 38*(9), 361–365.

Sgro, K. (2007). Reducing acute care hospitalization and emergent care use through home health disease management: One agency's success story. *Home Healthcare Nurse, 25*(10), 622–627.

Shirey, M. R. (2008). Endurance and inspiration for the entrepreneur. *Clinical Nurse Specialist, 22*(1), 9–11.

Smith, E. (2009). NP practice snapshot: Senior Moment Consulting. *Advance for Nurse Practitioners*. Retrieved from http://nurse-practitioners.advanceweb.com/Editorial/Content /Editorial.aspx?CC=193894

Sperhac, A., & Clinton, P. (2004). Facts and fallacies: The practice doctorate. *Journal of Pediatric Health, 18*(6), 292–296.

Stanhope, M., & Lancaster, J. (2006). *Foundations of nursing in the community: Community-oriented practice* (2nd ed.). St. Louis, MO: Mosby.

Stein, J. V. (2008). Becoming a doctor of nursing practice: My story. *Nursing Forum, 43*(1), 38–42.

Trivieri, L., & Anderson, J. W. (2002). *Alternative medicine: The definitive guide*. Berkeley, CA: Celestial Arts.

University of California, San Francisco, School of Nursing. (2009). *Leadership, nursing, and health systems (administration)*. Retrieved from: http://nurseweb.ucsf.edu/www/spec-adm.htm

University of Colorado at Denver, Health Sciences Center. (2008). School of Nursing [Brochure].

University of Kentucky, School of Nursing. (2009). *Post M.S.N.–Doctor of nursing practice (D.N.P. Degree)*. Retrieved from http://www.mc.uky.edu/Nursing/academic/dnp/default.html

University of Minnesota, Doctor of Nursing Practice Program. (n.d.). *Integrative health and healing.* Retrieved from http://www.nursing.unm.edu/DNP/ProspectiveStudent /Specialties/Integrative_Health_and_Healing/home.html

University of Tennessee. (2006). *Doctor of nursing practice.* Retrieved from http://www .utmem.edu/nursing/academic%20programs/DNP/index.php

U.S. Census Bureau. (1990). State population projections (based on 1990 Census released 1996). *U.S. Population Projections.* Retrieved from http://www.census.gov/population/www /projections/stproj1996.html

U.S. Department of Health and Human Services, Health Resources and Services Adminis- tration. (2004). *The registered nurse population: Findings from the March 2004 national sample survey of registered nurses.* Retrieved from ftp://ftp.hrsa.gov/bhpr/workforce/0306rnss.pdf

U.S. Department of Health and Human Services. (2008). *Phase I report: Recommendations for the framework and format of Healthy People 2020.* Retrieved from http://www.healthypeople.gov /hp2020/advisory/PhaseI/summary.htm

Veilleux, C. (2009). NP practice snapshot: Espanola Advanced Center for Healing. *Advance for Nurse Practitioners.* Retrieved from http://nurse-practitioners.advanceweb.com /Editorial/Content/Editorial.aspx?CC=193638.

Waddock, S. A., & Post, J. E. (1991). Social entrepreneurs and catalytic change. *Public Admin- istration Review, 51*(5), 393–401.

Wall, B. M., Novak, J. C., & Wilkerson, S. A. (2005). Doctor of Nursing Practice program devel- opment: Reengineering health care. *Journal of Nursing Education, 44*(9), 396–403.

Walton, M. (1986). *The Deming Management Method.* New York: Perigee.

Walton, M. (1991). *Deming Management at Work.* New York: Perigee.

West, W. D. (2008, March). Do you have to be a true entrepreneur to succeed? *Optometric Man- agement.* Retrieved from http://www.optometric.com/article.aspx?article=101462

Williams, S. (2006, September 11). *Game of strategy.* Retrieved from: http://news.nurse.com/apps /pbcs.dll/article?AID=2006609110343

Wilson, C. K. (1998). Mentoring the entrepreneur. *Nursing Administration Quarterly, 22*(2), 1–12.

Wilson, A., Averis, A., & Walsh, K. (2003). The influences on and experiences of becoming nurse entrepreneurs: A Delphi study. *International Journal of Nursing Practice, 9,* 236–245.

Yale Nursing. (2009). *DNP FAQs: Doctor of nursing practice degree.* Retrieved from http:// nursing.yale.edu/Academics/DNP_FAQs.html

PART III

THE DOCTOR OF NURSING PRACTICE SCHOLARLY PROJECT

CHAPTER 11

A Template for the DNP Scholarly Project

Kathryn Waud White and Mary E. Zaccagnini

Knowing is not enough; we must apply. Willing is not enough; we must do.
—Goethe

In 1995, Ernest Boyer delivered a landmark address to the American Association of Colleges of Nursing (AACN). In this widely cited address, he outlined a new paradigm for understanding scholarship in which he detailed the findings of a Carnegie Foundation report, *Scholarship Reconsidered: The Priorities of the Professorate* (Boyer, 1990). He outlined the evolution of American academic traditions from colonial times to 21st century America. Boyer argues that today the scholarship of discovery is disproportionately valued by academic institutions and that the scholarship of teaching and service is disregarded in many ways (Boyer, 1996). That plays out in the evaluation of professors for academic advancement and creates the curious situation in which it is far better for one's academic career to present a paper at a professional conference than it is to teach a class to undergraduate students and do it well. In his address to the AACN, Boyer proposed a reimagination of scholarship as a concept that has four interdependent aspects: the scholarship of discovery, the scholarship of integration, the scholarship of teaching, and the scholarship of application. He further proposed that each domain should be valued equally (Boyer, 1996).

Expanding on these thoughts and ideas, many nursing scholars and leaders began to believe that the scholarship of integration and application in the field of nursing could be best acknowledged through the development of a practice doctorate for advanced practice nurses. These practitioners would be prepared at the highest level of clinical practice and scholarship, integrating concepts of leadership and advocacy into the richness of nursing science and theory. The Doctor of Nursing Practice (DNP) course of study for advanced practice nurses was proposed as the terminal degree for clinical nurses by the AACN in 2004 after a long period of discussion and consensus building (AACN, 2004). At this writing, the AACN proposes that all advanced practice nursing programs be in the DNP framework by the year 2015.

The DNP course of study as proposed by the AACN culminates in a scholarly project, as should any doctoral education (AACN, 2006). The nature of the project should be commensurate with the domain of scholarship of the student. For PhD students, the domain of discovery of new knowledge dictates an original research project conducted and evaluated using traditional research methodologies, statistical analysis, and evaluation schemes. The Doctor of Nursing Practice degree focuses on the clinical scholarship of integration and application as elucidated by Boyer in 1996. Therefore, a project intended to discover new knowledge is an inappropriate vehicle for demonstration of the student's scholarship; scholarship for the DNP student is demonstrated through a project that reflects the breadth of the student's education and is a synthesis of the knowledge gained in the course of study (AACN, 2006). It should address a complex practice, process, or systems problem within the student's field of expertise, propose an evidence-based intervention to address that problem for a significant population, use doctoral-level leadership skills to implement and evaluate the efficacy of the intervention, and evaluate the outcomes of the intervention (National Organization of Nurse Practitioner Faculties [NONPF], 2007). The project may take on many forms, but the common element throughout the variety of DNP projects is the use of evidence to improve practice, processes, or outcomes (AACN, 2006). The structure and format of the final product will vary with the requirements of the degree-granting institution (AACN, 2006; NONPF, 2007).

Nature of the Project

Because the concept of the practice doctorate is relatively new to nursing, questions have arisen about the nature of the project. This is reflected in the many appellations given to this project: leadership project, scholarly project, capstone project, or, from the AACN, simply the DNP final project. What is this project? How can one discern what is and is not a DNP project?

We can gain insight from other disciplines that have used a project as evidence of scholarship. For example, projects are used in the fields of business and engineering as demonstration of mastery of the subject matter. The use of a capstone project as evidence of scholarship in the engineering field is particularly interesting because there are similarities between nursing and engineering. Both of these fields of study center on the application of evidence-based knowledge to practice problems, and they both integrate knowledge from other fields of scientific study as well as the base field to create interventions. In Ernest Boyer's definition of the scholarship of application, he states that this type of scholarship moves "from theory to practice and from practice back to theory" (Boyer, 1996). Both engineering and nursing take theories and new knowledge and test them in the gritty world of real life, real people, and real institutions.

Original research, even when illuminating and well executed, may languish for lack of application in the real world. In *Crossing the Quality Chasm* (2001), the Institute of Medicine (IOM) notes that the lag time from discovery of effective treatments to the integration and application of those treatments in clinical settings is 15 to 20 years. The IOM calls for development of an effective infrastructure to support the more rapid application of evidence to patient care. The Doctor of Nursing Practice is well positioned and educated to do just that: bring evidence to patient care. This is where the scholarship of integration and application brings life to theory and reality to research in the context of the real world.

In engineering and business, capstone projects are done most frequently at the baccalaureate and master's level. What distinguishes the doctoral project from the baccalaureate or master's project is the depth of inquiry, the depth of the literature reviewed, the scope of the project, the population served by the project, and the student's use of solid scientific evidence and theory as underpinnings of the project (AACN, 2006). Table 11-1 outlines Boyer's criteria by which we can evaluate scholarly work in any domain.

To date, no other fields of health care that require a practice doctorate for entry into practice require a capstone project similar to the DNP project. In a recent review of accreditation requirements for practice doctorates in 14 healthcare professions, the reviewers found that none of these programs required original research, as would be required in a PhD curriculum. Some accreditation requirements alluded to "opportunities" for research or access to faculty who are conducting research. The only other field of health sciences

■ Table 11-1   Boyer's Criteria for Evaluation of Scholarship

Are the goals of the project clearly stated?

Are the procedures well defined and appropriate for the project?

Are resources adequate for the stated goals of the project and utilized effectively?

Did the student communicate and collaborate effectively with others?

Are the results of the project significant?

Is there evidence of self-reflection and learning?

Source: Boyer, E. L. (1996). Clinical practice as scholarship. *Holistic Nursing Practice, 10*(3), 1–6. Adapted with permission.

that requires a clinical project for a practice doctorate is occupational therapy, but this practice doctorate is not required for entry into practice or certification as an occupational therapist. Practice doctorates in health care require a varying amount of exposure to research methodologies and evidence-based practice (Phelps & Gerbasi, 2009).

The DNP curriculum as outlined by the AACN in 2006 focuses on nursing practice, leadership, collaboration, and integration of science from many fields of study. This curriculum prepares advanced practice nurses to evaluate evidence for the implementation of best practices and the improvement of patient care. The PhD course of study focuses on vigorous research, generation of new knowledge, and the scholarship of discovery. Therefore, the DNP project should be the demonstration of the scholarship of integration and application as first discussed by Boyer in 1995. Although the DNP project is quite different from a PhD thesis (Table 11-2), it is a rigorously executed project that is described and the results documented in a paper or product of doctoral quality (AACN, 2006).

When evaluating the differences between the PhD thesis and the DNP project, it is useful to consider the desired outcomes. The PhD-prepared nurse will likely conduct his or her career in the academic or research setting. The DNP-prepared nurse will almost certainly conduct his or her career in clinical practice. To that end, the emphasis of the PhD thesis is on the rigorous application of standard methodologies and the meticulous evaluation of results using generally accepted scientific analysis techniques that can be reliably reproduced and are generalizable. The DNP project focuses on a practice problem and the evidence-based solutions for that problem. It

■ Table 11-2 Comparison of DNP Scholarly Project and PhD Research Project

PhD Dissertation	DNP Project
Systematic search for an answer to a research question	Systematic investigation of a practice issue
Outcome is an answer to the research question that is generalizable beyond current study; reproducible	Outcome is a solution to a practice problem that usually involves systems change; may be reproducible in other systems
Not specific to a time or place	Limited to a place and a time
Based in theory and literature	Based in theory and literature
Uses rigorous methodology that is unbiased and can be reproduced	Uses rigorous methods that are appropriate to the scope of the problem

Source: Edwardson, S. (2009, January 14). MN/DNP colloquium. Colloquium conducted at the University of Minnesota School of Nursing, Minneapolis, MN. Reprinted with permission.

is specific to a place or a system and may be applied to other settings, but this is not the goal of the project. Rather, the project focuses on the application of evidence to the problem that was identified. Results may be analyzed using standard statistical methods, but this is not strictly necessary (Edwardson, 2009).

Some important similarities between the PhD thesis and DNP capstone project emerge as well. Both approaches to problems need to be systematic and rigorous. The literature review should be in depth and rigorous. The PhD dissertation topic is necessarily narrow; the investigation is tightly controlled to eliminate extraneous influences. The DNP project is a real-world project and cannot control those influences. The DNP project seeks to adapt the research to real situations. Both the PhD thesis and the DNP project are based in theoretical concepts and literature. The PhD will be focused; the DNP will be broader and have many different points at which a discussion of theory is appropriate. The final product should meet all of the academic institution's requirements for scholarly work (AACN, 2006).

Because this scholarly project is a synthesis of the student's work in the DNP program, it should be related to the student's advanced practice specialty (NONPF, 2007). The problem to be addressed usually arises from clinical practice issues observed by the student. The process or practice improvement project is often conducted at the student's clinical practice site. It can also be done in partnership with an agency of the community (e.g., school, health agency, church, nonprofit organization). The leadership of the project is typically handled by the student alone, but the project may be conducted in collaboration with another student if the institution permits it. The project should engage a team of professionals to accomplish the change, demonstrating the student's leadership and collaboration skills (AACN, 2006; NONPF, 2007). The demonstration of doctoral-level leadership and collaboration are important aspects of the DNP student's scholarship.

Structure of the Project

A needs assessment and literature review should be conducted to support the need for improvement. The improvement should benefit a significant population instead of a single patient or practitioner (NONPF, 2007). The review of literature for the DNP project is not done to identify gaps in the body of knowledge as one would do for the PhD research project. Rather, the DNP project proposes to fix a gap in a system given the available research. One dimension of this review of literature is to support the need for the practice or process improvement. Another important dimension is in support of the structure of the particular intervention used in the DNP project and support of the rationale for selection of that specific intervention. The literature review should support the validity and reliability of assessment tools, specifically surveys and data collection methodologies. Scholarly support for the project includes the use of nursing theories and theories from other fields of study to describe the conceptual framework of the project. The student may find the need to integrate several theories from different fields of study in order to adequately describe this framework.

The implementation of the DNP project should meet all of the ethical standards for conducting any research or quality improvement project. Review by an institutional review board (IRB) is dictated by the nature of the project and the policies of the academic institution. As the lines between quality improvement activities and research blur, the tendency for these projects to undergo review by IRBs is stronger than in the past. The expected outcomes of the project should be defined when constructing the project. They should be measurable in the time frame of the project. The elements for the successful implementation of the project should also be described to an extent such that the project could be implemented at other clinical sites (NONPF, 2007).

Data collection during the project should be rigorous and structured. The tools and methods for data collection should meet accepted standards of practice (NONPF, 2007). They should be defined early in the project for best-practice and best-outcomes evaluation. It is helpful to consult with a statistician early in the project if statistical analysis is anticipated. Data collected can be qualitative or quantitative. Statistical analysis is useful as a measure of change but is not the only measure. The time frame of these projects often does not permit the collection of enough data points to achieve statistical significance. Other measures of change may include graphs, trends, attitudes, cost analysis, narrative data, and patterns of practice.

The development, implementation, and outcomes of the project should be reviewed by an academic panel or committee per the academic policies of the degree-granting institution, and disseminated in a public forum (NONPF, 2007). Modalities for dissemination are diverse and vary from project to project.

Advising the DNP project is somewhat different from the PhD dissertation and is a highly debated topic in nursing academia at this writing. If the DNP is to be the required degree for all advanced practice nurses by 2015 (AACN, 2004), there may be a faculty workload issue (Cartwright & Reed, 2005). Advising is often quite intense because of the condensed time frame of the project. Instead of one or two PhD advisees, faculty in schools of nursing that house advanced practice programs may have 10, 15, or 20 DNP advisees. Various strategies have been suggested to account for faculty workload, but in this economic climate it is unlikely that workload accounting practices will be altered to allow for more advising time. Some suggest that the DNP degree will only make the faculty shortage all the more acute in the short run (Fulton & Lyon, 2005).

As nursing progresses toward the goal of educating all advanced practice nurses in a DNP framework, projects are evolving. It is reminiscent of the Indian fable of the six blind men examining an elephant to ascertain what an elephant is. Each one felt a different part and came to different conclusions about what the elephant was because they could not see the whole. In the remainder of this chapter, the authors lay out a schema for the DNP project. The authors' graphic representation of the process is shown in Figure 11-1. This model is one framework for the development, implementation,

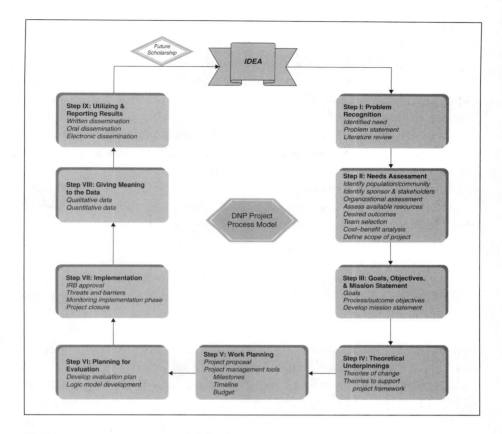

■ Figure 11-1   Process Model for the DNP Project

and evaluation of DNP projects. This section is primarily written to assist the DNP student but can be used by any practitioner who is developing a new project or program.

The Project

Step I: Problem Recognition

Project ideas typically emanate from a clinical issue or opportunity identified by the nurse who has critical thinking skills, that is, the skills to step back from clinical practice and analyze "what is" and ask "what could be." The critical thinker identifies a need or change required in a practice environment. The problem could be brought forth by an individual, a group, the

■ Table 11-3   Internal and External Drivers for Projects

Internal Drivers	External Drivers
Administration	Public policy
Healthcare professionals	Standards of practice
Budgetary issues	Evidence-based guidelines
Customer needs	Accreditation organizations
Quality improvement programs	Third-party payers
Safety issues	Government regulations
Staffing issues	Mandatory education
Educational requirements	

administration of the facility, regulatory bodies, accreditation organizations, or governmental agencies. Drivers for the project can be internal or external (Table 11-3).

The problem must be articulated clearly to the academic advisor working with the student's project. The academic advisor and student must focus the project enough so that it can be accomplished within the period of time defined by the academic institution. The project should be in the student's area of practice scholarship (NONPF, 2007). It also must fit into the mission of the organization in which the project will be developed and implemented, as well as the constraints of that organization. The next step is to develop a problem statement.

DEVELOPING THE PROBLEM STATEMENT

A problem statement identifies a situation that requires change and puts it into an organized form. It answers the questions "Why this project?" and "Why now?" Clarity is the key. The following is a framework for developing a problem statement.

1. Identify the deficits in the current circumstances.
2. Describe the milieu of the problem.
3. Define the magnitude of the problem in measurable terms.
4. Characterize the impact of the problem on the population or organization.
5. Outline evidence-based solutions. (Waddick, 2009; Polit & Beck, 2008)

At this juncture, a literature review must be done to support the problem statement and should be able to answer the questions posed earlier: "Why this project?" and "Why now?"

Step II: Needs Assessment

POPULATION IDENTIFICATION

A needs assessment is done to gather the information required to develop a plan for the project. That information begins with an assessment of the population affected by the problem. Tools for this assessment may include demographic data from public sources, consultations, surveys, interviews, chart reviews, focus groups, internal organizational data, and external data from government websites.

IDENTIFICATION OF PROJECT SPONSOR AND KEY STAKEHOLDERS

The next phase of the needs assessment is identification of individuals who have a vested interest in the outcome of the project. Those vital individuals include a project sponsor who can partner with the academic institution to address institutional barriers and help the student navigate the matrix of the project setting. This person could be an administrator in the institution where the project is being conducted or a similar individual with the authority to facilitate accomplishment of the project goals.

Stakeholders are key individuals who will be affected one way or another by the project. To identify the stakeholders, consider the individuals who are not only affected by the work but who may have an interest in its outcomes. Table 11-4 lists examples of potential stakeholders (Mind Tools, 2009).

ORGANIZATIONAL ASSESSMENT

The organizational setting and culture should be assessed. This assessment should answer these questions: What are the values of the organization in which the project will be conducted? Are the values of the organization consistent with the values of the project and the project leader? To what extent is the mission of the project consistent with that of the organization in which the project will take place (W. K. Kellogg Foundation, 1998)? The evaluation of the setting may identify challenges and stumbling blocks for the program. When such stumbling blocks are identified, plans can be made to address them or implement the project in a different setting. If the values of

■ Table 11-4   Identifying Key Stakeholders

Internal	External
Site administrator	Insurers
Chief financial officer	Regulatory agencies
Medical director	People in the community
Chief nursing officer	Suppliers
Department or program director	Interest groups
Project team members	Families in the community
Nurses	Health advocacy organizations
Ancillary staff	Community health organizations
Patients or residents	Support groups

Source: Mind Tools. (2009). The Mind Tools e-book (6th ed.). London: Mind Tools. Adapted with permission.

the project or the project leader are not consistent with the organization, the project is likely to fail.

ASSESSMENT OF AVAILABLE RESOURCES

A thorough assessment of available resources should be conducted early in the project development and planning. These resources could include but are not limited to the following: financial support, personnel, materials for the project, marketing, statistical analysis support, office space and materials, communication costs, consulting costs, grant writing support, travel expenses, survey costs, and copyright costs. The cost of the resources must be thoroughly investigated, understood, and documented before moving on to develop a cost–benefit analysis for the project proposal.

IDENTIFICATION OF DESIRED OUTCOMES

Early in the project, the project leader (DNP student) must develop a reasonable estimate of the desired outcomes. These can be defined through the literature review done for the problem statement; alternatively, this may be a point at which the literature review needs expansion to search for predictable outcomes based on other similar projects. In either case some outcome statements should be developed. The project is developmental, and these outcomes statements at this phase of project development are brief and will need refinement before the implementation phase. Nevertheless, the remainder of the project plan cannot proceed without clear outcomes in mind (Mind Tools, 2009).

TEAM SELECTION AND FORMATION

At this point the DNP student should assemble a team of individuals with the correct skills to conduct the project. There is no defined number or recommended composition for the team. The team membership is dictated by each individual project. These team members may or may not come from the list of stakeholders; however, the project leader is always the team leader.

Team formation is a process well defined in the literature that proceeds through four phases: forming, storming, norming, and performing. In the *forming* stage, the people on the team are getting to know each other and may be hesitant to offer opinions. This is a good time to evaluate individual skills and personalities. The team leader should be directive during this phase. In the *storming* phase, team members may jockey for position and authority. At this point, some team members may feel overwhelmed by the scope of the project and the tasks necessary to complete the project. Some may be resistant to the project and express doubts about it. At all times the DNP student should remember that she or he is the project and team leader, is ultimately responsible for the project, and that the end product will reflect upon her or his scholarship. The project leader should support those team members who feel less secure, work to build positive relationships among team members, and remain positive but firm when the goals of the project or his or her leadership is challenged. *Norming* brings the team's strong commitment to the project goals, and as the team socializes more, the members are more agreeable to take on the tasks of the project and work together as a unit. The leader of the team should facilitate the development of collaboration between team members. The last stage of team development is *performing*. In this stage, the team makes rapid progress toward the goals of the project. The team leader may be able to delegate much of the work but remains ultimately responsible for the outcome. The team leader must remain cognizant of the constraints of the team members. In many cases, the members are staff members with other responsibilities. If the project is not dictated by the needs of the institution or community in which it is being conducted, there may be constraints on the time that team members can commit to the project. Be respectful of the delegation of tasks to team members (Mind Tools, 2009).

Closure is an important part of the project because there is a beginning and an end to each project. This allows the project leader to revisit the project goals with the team members and closes the partnerships with the team and the sponsoring institution or organization (Mind Tools, 2009).

COST–BENEFIT ANALYSIS

A cost–benefit analysis is a powerful tool to promote the project to sponsors and others with vested interests. The development of this analysis simply adds up the real costs of the project and subtracts them from the benefits gleaned from the project. The point of the analysis is to demonstrate that the benefit of solving the problem is worth the costs experienced (Mind Tools, 2009). For most projects, it is important that both costs and benefits be quantifiable. It is often easy to quantify costs and relatively difficult to measure benefits that are intangible and are realized over a period of time. Table 11-5 provides an example of benefits that are difficult to quantify but useful to name.

In some instances projects are dictated by regulatory requirements, governing bodies, or organizational administration. In this case, it is still feasible to do a cost–benefit analysis. If the cost–benefit analysis demonstrates more cost than benefit, the analysis will demonstrate how the costs will affect the budget. This does not imply that the project will not be done; often the institution has no choice. For example, regulatory issues may dictate the implementation of the project regardless of the cost. At times the project will proceed simply because it is the right thing to do. Examples of this might be a project that is done to benefit the community served by the organization to improve community relationships or provide service to the community.

DEFINING THE SCOPE OF THE PROJECT

Now the scope of the project statement can be written. A well-crafted project scope statement is essential for the project to stay on track. The scope statement will clearly state what the project will and will not do (Luecke, 2004). The project manager uses the scope statement to make well-informed decisions throughout the life of the project. The scope will help to identify potential barriers to the project. The scope statement will bind the agreement between the project leader, the project sponsor, and the organization (Microsoft Office Online, 2009a).

Table 11-5 Example of a Cost–Benefit Analysis for a DNP Project

Reducing Social Isolation and Loneliness Through the Development of a Computer Resource and Communication Center

Benefit Analysis	Costs of Intervention	Percent of Residents Needing Service (national average)	Number of Nursing Home Residents	Private Room Cost Per Day	Semiprivate Room Cost Per Day	Annual Private Room Cost	Annual Semiprivate Room Cost	Goals/Assumptions	Calculated hours of care per day/person	Hours of care per day/sample	Total cost of nursing care*/day/person	Total cost of nursing care*/day/sample	Goal: Hours of care per day/person with intervention	Hours of care will decrease by 5%	Cost of care	PRO-JECTED annual savings for the sample
Nursing Home Care MPLS Area*			119	$228	$191	$83,220	$69,715									
Indirect Expenses Room and board (space, lights, heating, Internet, housekeeping)		100%														
Direct Expenses Medication management		100%	Possible random sample of personal care													
Personal care**		44%	22						3.07	68	$51.19	$3,457.37	Maintain—Improve—Decrease hours of care 3.07	2.92	$3,288	$61,658

■ Table 11-5 Example of a Cost–Benefit Analysis for a DNP Project (CONTINUED)

Reducing Social Isolation and Loneliness Through the Development of a Computer Resource and Communication Center

Benefit Analysis	Costs of Intervention	Percent of Residents Needing Service (national average)	Number of Nursing Home Residents	Private Room Cost Per Day	Semiprivate Room Cost Per Day	Annual Private Room Cost	Annual Semiprivate Room Cost	Goals/Assumptions
Personal care with one or more ADL**		51% (+ 7% of pc)	25					Maintain—Improve—Decrease
Social and recreational activities**		40%	24					Increase use
Cost of Intervention								
Cognitive Assessment/ Rescreening/ Analysis— Investigator grant funded	$6,750	at 45/hr (3 hours/ client— if hired outside agency						**Improved mental cognition**
Mini-Mental Exam								Improved mental cognition
MDS								Improved mental cognition
Depression Scale								Improved mental cognition

(continues)

■ Table 11-5 Example of a Cost–Benefit Analysis for a DNP Project (CONTINUED)

Reducing Social Isolation and Loneliness Through the Development of a Computer Resource and Communication Center

Benefit Analysis	Costs of Intervention	Percent of Residents Needing Service (national average)	Number of Nursing Home Residents	Private Room Cost Per Day	Semiprivate Room Cost Per Day	Annual Private Room Cost	Annual Semiprivate Room Cost	Goals/ Assumptions
Facility Costs for Intervention								
Space/rental	0	In kind						
Equipment for the Intervention	$8,540							
Computer (includes software)								
Headphones								
Microphone								
Printer/fax								
Equipment already purchased	$(2,696)							
Remaining Equipment Costs	$5,844							
Supplies								
Paper	$1,000							
Toner	$1,500							
Ink cartridges	$1,020							
Total Annual Supply Costs	$3,520							

■ Table 11-5 Example of a Cost–Benefit Analysis for a DNP Project (CONTINUED)

Reducing Social Isolation and Loneliness Through the Development of a Computer Resource and Communication Center

Benefit Analysis	Costs of Inter-vention	Percent of Residents Needing Service (national average)	Number of Nursing Home Residents	Private Room Cost Per Day	Semiprivate Room Cost Per Day	Annual Private Room Cost	Annual Semiprivate Room Cost	Goals/ Assumptions
Teaching computer skills to the elderly	$4,320.00			($15/hr 6 hrs/week/ 48 weeks)				
Staff salary savings attributable to student volunteers	**$(11,520.00)**			($15/hr 8 hrs/week/ 48 weeks/ 2 students) —not included in calculations				
Total Cost of Intervention	**$13,684**							
PROJECTED Annual Savings (Benefit)	$61,658							
Possible annual cost savings of the intervention	**$47,974.35**							

* The MetLife Market Survey of Nursing Home & Home Care Costs Nursing Sep-06.

Source: Zaccagnini, M. (2007). *The development of a computer resourced communication center in a long-term care facility* (Unpublished DNP project paper). University of Minnesota, Minneapolis, MN.

The scope statement summarizes the work done thus far, includes the problem statement and the expected outcomes, defines the boundaries of the project, the sponsor, and selected team members, and provides the bottom line of the cost–benefit analysis. It should be written in the style of an executive summary that does not exceed one page (Microsoft Office Online, 2009a).

Step III: Goals, Objectives, and Mission Statement Development

GOALS

The entire topic of goals and objectives is complicated by confusing and overlapping terminology. For the purposes of this chapter, we define *goals* as broad statements that identify future outcomes, provide overarching direction to the project, and point to the expected outcomes of the project. Goals should be written first. Typically a project has several goals, and each goal will need different objectives to support its achievement. Institutional demands may dictate that the goals of the project be prioritized according to financial savings, safety, or the institutional mission. Simply stated, goals are where you want to be; objectives are how you get there.

OBJECTIVES

Objectives are clear, realistic, specific, measurable, and time-limited statements of the actions which, when completed, will move the project toward its goals. In the business literature, the commonly used template for crafting objectives is SMART, which stands for specific, measurable, attainable, realistic, and timely (Lewis, 2007). In the case of the DNP project, *specific* means being precise. It is not enough to state that you want to improve a process or practice, you must name the who (target population), what (what will the project accomplish), where (project setting), and when (creation of a specific timeline) (Issel, 2004). *Measurable* implies that there are collectible data adequate for measuring change. *Attainable* and *realistic* mean that the scope of the project has been focused so that the project is feasible and meaningful with the resources at hand. Will the project really make a difference or is it simply an exercise to attain a degree? *Timely* refers to the ability to realistically get the project accomplished in the time allotted by the academic institution. This can be an opportunity to recheck whether the scope of the project is attainable. The objectives should be rigorous but not impossible to achieve (Lewis, 2007).

In this conceptualization of the DNP project, there will be two types of objectives, although there are many other types found in the literature:

outcomes objectives and process objectives. *Outcomes objectives* simply address the outcomes of the project as they were defined earlier but state a specific time frame for accomplishment of the desired outcome. The *process objectives* define the steps needed to accomplish the outcomes objectives. The process objectives are the actions or activities of the team required to implement the project in the time frame stated. Process objectives should be succinct and clear. They function as a real-time check on the progress of the project so that course corrections can be made in a timely manner (Burroughs & Wood, 2000).

MISSION STATEMENT

The mission statement is a succinct paragraph that accurately describes why the project is being conducted. The academic institution determines whether a mission statement will be included in the DNP project. The benefit of a mission statement is that it helps clarify the purpose of the project and the methods of getting the project accomplished. Writing a mission statement is an opportunity for the project leader to take all of the information gathered thus far and focus on the problem to be solved and the methods of solving it in two or three sentences (Allison & Kaye, 2005). A mission statement can be used to solicit support for the project. It can be used as an explanatory statement for "elevator conversations," well-rehearsed 30-second conversations that the project leader can turn into an opportunity to inform a person or group of people about the project. A well-crafted mission statement can help keep the project focused throughout the entirety of the project.

To draft a succinct mission statement, the project manager or project team needs to answer three questions: What is the purpose of the project? (The answer should use an infinitive verb and a statement of the problem to be addressed.) What is the population to be addressed in solving the problem? What are the methods to be utilized in addressing the problem? It is often helpful to engage the project team in developing the mission statement to help clarify the mission to the team itself and cultivate buy-in from the team members and other stakeholders (Allison & Kaye, 2005).

The mission statement for this book is as follows:

This book is intended to serve as a core textbook for DNP students and faculty to use to achieve mastery of the American Association of Colleges of Nursing essentials as well as a shelf reference for practicing DNPs. The DNP essentials are all covered herein; each essential is covered in adequate detail to frame the foundation of the DNP educational program. This book provides the infrastructure for students, faculty, and practicing DNPs to achieve and sustain the highest level of practice.

Step IV: Theoretical Underpinnings of the Project

THEORETICAL UNDERPINNINGS OF CHANGE

The DNP project leader now has completed the work necessary to begin implementing the project plan. Each project will by definition involve change in a system or practice (NONPF, 2007). Change is notoriously difficult to achieve. The change will be made easier by using a theory to support the change process and build a model of the planned change. Planning expedites change and improves the likelihood of long-term success. Theories of change come from many different fields of study: sociology, psychology, organizational psychology, business management, and health care. A literature review will assist the project leader to identify theoretical supports for the project. The DNP project leader will utilize the scholarship of integration to select a theory of change that best describes the change that will occur as a result of the project.

Kurt Lewin is noted as the first change theorist. His work had a profound impact on the field of psychology and organizational psychology. His force field analysis is still used to create force field diagrams. He theorized that issues are held in balance by those forces that maintain the current state and those forces that advance change, which he called restraining forces and driving forces, respectively. Until the driving forces exceed the restraining forces, change will not occur. Lewin also created tools to map the driving forces and restraining forces. The resulting force field diagram (also called a force field analysis) is a powerful tool to understand the environment in which the project will take place.

Kurt Lewin was also the first person to develop a model of the change process, and it is regarded as one of his strengths. His model of the change process has three stages: unfreezing, movement, and refreezing. Most other theories of change are based in part on Lewin's theory. The first step entails an "unfreezing" of the current status or state. This can be achieved by convincing people to let go of the status quo or old way of doing something. The second step involves movement toward a new state. In this phase people are persuaded to take a fresh look at problems from a different perspective and move toward a new paradigm. Movement of the group is supported by respected leaders who understand the need for change. In the final or third step, the change becomes the new norm for the population affected by the change. One mechanism for accomplishing this is to reinforce the new behaviors and institutionalize ("refreeze") them through formal and informal mechanisms. This reinforcement is done to ensure that the change will endure past the project implementation and become incorporated into the organizational culture.

There are many other change theorists in addition to Lewin, such as Lippitt, Watson, and Westley; Wheatley; Haverlock; Rogers; Kotter; and Prochaska and DiClemente. For additional information and resources on change theories in the business and education literature, please refer to Appendix 11-1.

THEORY TO SUPPORT PROJECT FRAMEWORK

Essential I (scientific underpinnings) of the *Essentials of Doctoral Education for Advanced Nursing Practice* supports the notion of utilizing theory to create a framework for the project. It states that "[t]he DNP program prepares the graduate to . . . [u]se science-based theories and concepts . . . [and] [d]evelop and evaluate new practice approaches based on nursing theories and theories from other disciplines" (AACN, 2006). The theoretical framework helps the project leader to conceptualize the project and supports it throughout the course of the project.

Theoretical frameworks can be constructed using concepts from fields of study other than nursing. Often theories from different fields will need to be integrated into a theoretical framework that describes the unique project. For example, a framework developed by Dr. Kathleen Casey incorporated a change theory and a nursing theory to support her DNP project. Casey (2007) used Kotter's theory of change and the American Association of Critical Care Nurse's synergy theory to create a theoretical framework for her project, "Development of an Innovative Staffing Model: Nurse Practitioner (NP) Hospitalist/Intensivist."

Step V: Work Planning

PROJECT PROPOSAL

Typically, a formal project proposal will be required by the academic institution or the organization where the project will take place. Minimally, the expectation would be to develop an executive summary. The amount of detail required varies from institution to institution. Most proposals will include a synopsis of the problem recognition and the problem statement, a summary of the significant findings from the scope of the project and its mission state-ment, the desired outcomes, the goals and objectives, and, most important, the cost–benefit analysis. It is incumbent upon the project leader to check with the organization for the details required for the project proposal.

Templates for project proposals can be found online. One such website is www.klariti.com/templates/Proposal-Template.shtml. Another source for templates is Microsoft Office Online. We do not support any one software package or website; many good sources exist. If you decide to use additional software, you must find a package that meets your needs. Many of these software packages include project management tools that will be helpful in the next phase of work planning.

PROJECT MANAGEMENT TOOLS

Project management is a body of specialized knowledge and skills that equips project managers with skills often developed in parallel with large govern-ment projects, beginning with the transcontinental railroad and continuing through the projects of the National Aeronautics and Space Administration (NASA) that eventually landed people on the moon. The common theme is that these projects employed thousands or hundreds of thousands of people who needed to complete highly accurate work on time and within budget. To manage these requirements, the field of project management was born. Around the turn of the 20th century, Frederick Taylor studied work effi-ciency in detail and demonstrated that output can be improved by studying the work and breaking it down into small tasks that can be made more effi-cient (Microsoft Office Online, 2009b). One of Taylor's peers, Henry Gantt, studied the order of tasks, primarily in shipyards during World War I (Microsoft Office Online, 2009b). Any project developed today is likely to include a Gantt chart, which details the timeline for the project as well as which tasks can be done in parallel and which are sequential. An example of a Gantt chart is shown later in this chapter. Today the field of project man-agement is a distinct field of scholarship and certifications. Using the schol-arship of integration (Boyer, 1990), the DNP project leader can borrow knowledge, skills, and tools from the field of project management that will serve the field of healthcare projects as well as NASA space projects.

Baker, Baker, and Campbell (2003) define a project as "a sequence of tasks with a beginning and an end that is bounded by time and resources and that produces a unique product or service" (p. 404). From this definition, the DNP student can discern where these tools might help the DNP project and where the DNP student will need to select different tools. For example, in the project management literature, the project is typically deemed to be assigned to someone who is designated as the team leader. For the DNP project, considerable time and effort are expended on the needs assessment, which is then used to persuade the leadership of the organization that the project is necessary for improvement of patient or process outcomes.

Defining the scope of the project; identifying key stakeholders; assessing resources, goals, and objectives; and writing a mission statement are project management tools that have already been discussed in this chapter. Additional tools that can be helpful to the DNP project leader include work breakdown, timeline tools, and project milestones. These three tools will help the project manager determine the flow of the project, predict when resources are needed, and estimate time to completion, which will in turn help the project leader to estimate whether the project can be done in the allotted time. These tools will identify which project tasks need to be done sequentially and when tasks can be done in parallel.

Work Breakdown and Milestones

Accurate planning of work requires that the work be broken down into small packages that can be easily monitored. Each task of the project is broken down into levels and sublevels or subprojects. Each subproject is then examined for milestones. Milestones identify when an important or large part of the project is completed (Baker, Baker, & Campbell, 2003). The subproject is further broken down into major activities and then into work packages (Figure 11-2). The purpose of this activity is to systematically identify all of the work that needs to be done to execute the project. Table 11-6 identifies the benefits of a work breakdown structure (WBS).

The WBS can be diagrammed as a simple tree diagram (Baker, Baker, & Campbell, 2003). Templates are available online, some at no charge to the user. The work breakdown does not have to be perfect. The amount of detail will vary from project to project and from institution to institution. The project leader will know that the work is broken into small enough tasks when a task can be done by one individual in a defined amount of time and that task will produce a distinct product (Baker, Baker, & Campbell, 2003).

Once the WBS is completed in sufficient detail, the project leader can begin to estimate the time required to complete the subprojects and tasks. At this time it is essential to begin to identify whether tasks can be done in parallel or whether they are sequential to other tasks. This can be done by

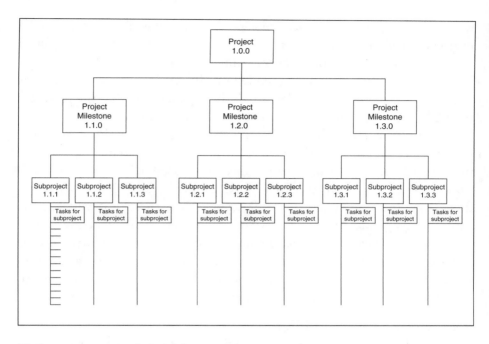

■ Figure 11-2   Work Breakdown Structure Template

■ Table 11-6   Benefits of Work Breakdown Structure

Identifies all of the work needed for the project to be completed

Organizes the work in a logical sequence

Predicts when work may be completed

Identifies team members who have the best skills for the tasks

Identifies which resources are needed and when

Helps to prepare budget

Provides a communication tool for all team members

Keeps team members attuned to the work of all team members

Organizes work tasks with milestones

placing the activities into a simple table such as the one in Table 11-7 (Mind Tools, 2009). The information in the table can then be placed into a Gantt chart (Figure 11-3).

Other types of charts can be used to diagram the timeline. Some of the more common types of charts are the PERT chart and the critical path dia-

■ Table 11-7   Task Length Table

Task	Estimated Start	Estimated Length to Completion	Sequential or Parallel	Dependent on
A	Week 1	Four weeks	Parallel	None
B	Week 1	One week	Parallel	None
C	Week 2	Two weeks	Sequential	Task B
D	Week 5	One day	Sequential	Task A
E	Week 6	One week	Sequential	Task D

gram (Lewis, 2007). Examples of these can be found in many project management books and websites. The point of the activity is to gain benefit from careful work planning and scheduling.

Budget Development

Developing a budget is an important step in project management. Administrators, funding agencies, and project stakeholders will need to know the costs associated with the project in order to decide whether to proceed with the project. Making a detailed and accurate budget and staying within the project budget will gain the project manager credibility within the organization. Here are a few pitfalls to avoid when developing a budget:

■ *Underestimating labor costs.* Even though some of the team members may be salaried by the sponsoring institution, the project manager must include these costs in the project budget. Employee benefits, often estimated as a percentage of employee salary, must also be included in the calculations. They are not free.

Task	Wk 1	Wk 2	Wk 3	Wk 4	Wk 5	Wk 6
Task A				*		
Task B						
Task C				*		
Task D						
Task E						

*Milestone event

■ Figure 11-3   Gantt Chart Developed from Table 11-7

- *Neglecting to add in the costs of equipment in use at the institution.* Use of computers, copiers, and other business equipment should be accounted for in the budget.
- *Neglecting to add in the cost of business space.* Estimates for business space can be found from many different sources online for each city or town in the United States.
- *Underestimating the costs of external consultants and supplies.* Most professionals will provide an hourly estimate for services.
- *Forgetting about travel costs.* Mileage rates for various purposes can be found at IRS.gov if the institution does not have a set rate for mileage.
- *Forgetting to include all of the costs for materials.* The team will need supplies such as paper and pencils, pens, and folders. (Baker, Baker, & Campbell, 2003; Luecke, 2004)

Calculating Direct and Indirect Costs The budget must account for both direct and indirect costs. Direct costs are those that are specifically attributable to the project. This would include items such as labor, materials, supplies, equipment for the project, travel, consultant fees, project training, and marketing. Indirect costs would include items that are shared by many different entities in the institution, such as business space, Internet access, information technology services, internal communications such as telephones and pagers, and support staff (Baker, Baker, & Campbell, 2003; Luecke, 2004). Indirect costs are often expressed as a percentage of the direct costs. A more experienced colleague or manager at the institution may be able to assist with the development of the budget.

Templates for Budgeting Most institutions have a template they prefer to use for developing a budget. If the institution does not have a template that it prefers, templates can be found online. Microsoft Excel and Word also provide templates within the programs. Once the budget is developed and final project approval is obtained, the plan for evaluation can now be created.

Step VI: Planning for Evaluation

In today's healthcare environment, funds for projects are limited and competition for funding is fiercely competitive. To get the best funding for your project, you must have a strong evaluation plan with clearly identified outcomes from the start. It is also an ethical imperative to demonstrate the efficacy of programs and practice changes (W. K. Kellogg Foundation, 1998). It is no longer acceptable to present materials, give a post-test, and count participants. Evaluation is a far broader range of data collection involving both quantitative and qualitative data. The focus of evaluation is not simply the DNP project: these methods should become ingrained into the framework of the professional practice of the DNP.

Unlike research that has a prescribed protocol, evidence-based practice or process improvement programs are applied broadly and thus do not have a defined research question. We are not collecting data to make the project reproducible, we are collecting data to measure change in a population or practice. Although some statistical methods may be useful for evaluation of the DNP project, many of the methods for evaluation will be different from those of the research project. The purpose of data collection is different as well. Evaluation provides accountability to the stakeholders, demonstrates quality improvement, demonstrates effectiveness in the population involved in the study, and provides clarity of purpose to the program (W. K. Kellogg Foundation, 1998).

This section presents tools, methods, and resources that can be used for evaluation of the program or project. It is the responsibility of the project leader to select the correct tools and methods for evaluation of the project in a coherent plan for evaluation. This section also presents logic models that will assist in the development of the plan. Like any other skill, development of an evaluation plan requires both tools and practice. As the DNP utilizes these tools and methods, confidence and competence in project planning, implementation, and evaluation will develop. These are skills that will be necessary past the educational program into DNP practice. They define clinical scholarship.

DEVELOPMENT OF EVALUATION METHODS

Evaluation should be thoughtfully designed so that it measures the degree to which the outcomes were or were not met. The evaluation design should fit the unique project. The project leader must determine the appropriate methods and types of data to be collected that best demonstrate the outcomes. The evaluation plan could consist of qualitative methods, quantitative methods, or a mix of both. When choosing the methods, there are some indications of whether quantitative or qualitative methods are most appropriate for measurement of your outcomes. If the outcome is to identify how much, how many, how often, or an average response, then the best method is quantitative. If the outcome is to identify what worked, what the numbers mean, how the project was useful, what it meant to the participants, or what factors influenced success or failure, then one should select qualitative methods (Olney & Barnes, 2006a, 2006b). Qualitative data can provide contextual meaning to the quantitative data in a project that uses both. For example, it is useful to know the number of diabetic patients in a population that develop diabetic retinopathy; it is another thing to understand the impact of blindness in a person's life. Qualitative data provide meaning to the people affected by the project, the stakeholders, the organization, and possibly outside audiences (W. K. Kellogg Foundation, 1998). Regardless of which approach is used for evaluation, the methods should be chosen before implementation of the project.

Tools for qualitative evaluation may include observations, ethnographic interviews, structured interviews, written questions, and document review. Issues of cultural sensitivity should be kept in mind when developing survey or interview questions. Tools for quantitative data collection include surveys, health factors, laboratory test results, and chart reviews. No matter which methods the project leader selects for evaluation data collection, they should be reliable and valid (Olney & Barnes, 2006a, 2006b).

LOGIC MODEL DEVELOPMENT

Basically, a logic model is a systematic and visual way to present and share your understanding of the relationships among the resources you have to operate your program, the activities you plan, and the changes or results you hope to achieve.
—W. K. KELLOGG FOUNDATION (2004)

The first logic models were developed in the 1970s. *Evaluation: Promise and Performance* by Joseph S. Wholey was the first text to use the term *logic model* (Taylor-Powell & Henert, 2008). Logic models have evolved since the introduction of the Government Results and Performance Act of 1993. This act was intended to improve the effectiveness of federal programs through requirements for strategic planning and program evaluation. It shifted the focus of evaluation onto results and not simply activities. The models identified in this chapter were developed in part in response to this act (Streeter, 1998).

A logic model (Figure 11-4) is a picture of how the project developer believes the program will work. It uses a series of diagrams to indicate how parts of the program are linked together or sequenced. There is no one correct way to diagram the logic model. It depends in large part on the purpose of the model. If the diagram is used to describe the entire project plan, it should be detailed. If it is used for communication among team members, it should be less complex. The project developer may need several models for various parts of the pro-

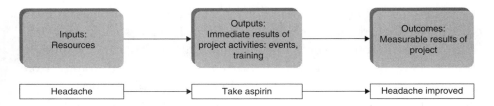

■ **Figure 11-4   Simple Logic Model**

Source: Taylor-Powell, E., & Henert, E. (2008). *Developing a logic model: Teaching and training guide*. Retrieved from the University of Wisconsin–Extension website: http://www.uwex.edu/ces/pdande. Adapted with permission.

ject (Taylor-Powell & Henert, 2008). Logic models all have similar components: inputs, outputs, and outcomes (Taylor-Powell & Henert, 2008).

Only the simplest of programs will be adequately described by this model. For example, if you had a headache, it would describe the input as "headache," the output as "take an aspirin," and the outcome as "headache is better." This simple model does not identify how projects get from inputs to outputs. No activities are defined in the model. Most programs will require more detail to adequately describe the project.

The logic model template presented in this chapter is an assimilation of several models: the Kellogg Foundation logic model, the United Way program outcome model, and the University of Wisconsin Extension Service logic model. Resources, templates, designs, and worksheets for development of these models are available online at no charge to the individual. Figure 11-5 is a template created by the authors.

Inputs	Constraints	Activities	Outputs	Outcomes		
				Short Term	Long Term	Impact
Personnel	Budget	Events	Number of participants	Knowledge improvement	Behavior improvement	Long-term results of the change
Financial	Physical space	Training	Amount of education delivered	Skill improvement	Motivation improvement	
Time	Law, regulations, local policy	Education	Number of hours of service	Improved level of functioning		
Materials	Timeframe	Media/Technology				
Equipment	Existing culture	Meetings				
Facilities		Development of processes				

■ **Figure 11-5   Template for Logic Model of Project**

Source: White & Zaccagnini, 2009.

In the template, *inputs* are the resources required to implement and evaluate the project. Those resources may include personnel, facilities, equipment, time, and finances. Resources could be constrained by laws, regulations, funding, time, existing culture, and local policy. *Constraints* can prevent the project from advancing or limit the project in some manner. For example, financial resource allocations may be less than what was originally proposed to support the project. The project leader may either redefine the budget or reexamine the project activities that affect the budget. *Activities* are what the project does with the resources to achieve the intended outcomes: events, training and education, meetings, development of media and technology, and development of the processes necessary to implement the project. *Outputs* are the immediate results of the project. They could include the number of participants, the number of hours of instruction, the number of meetings, participation rates, and the number of hours of each service provided. *Outcomes* can be considered at three levels: short-term, long-term, and impact outcomes. In short-term outcomes, the project leader measures the effect of the activities on the knowledge base and skills or level of functioning. The long-term outcomes reflect a change in behavior or motivation. Impact outcomes describe the results of the change on the population served by the project.

Figure 11-6 demonstrates an application of the logic model to a more complex project completed in 2007 as part of the requirements of the DNP curriculum at the University of Minnesota School of Nursing. This model describes a DNP project completed by Mary Zaccagnini, "Development of a Computer Assisted Communication Center in a Long Term Care Facility." This project addressed the problem of social isolation within a long-term care facility and the resultant problems caused by the isolation. The project leader developed a computer center and trained the staff and volunteers to assist the residents. It demonstrated that the residents who used the computer center experienced an increase in socialization and communication via email and a decrease in loneliness.

> Thinking about a program in logic model terms prompts the clarity and specificity required for success, and often demanded by funders and your community. Using a simple logic model produces (1) an inventory of what you have and what you need to operate your program; (2) a strong case for how and why your program will produce your desired results; and (3) a method for program management and assessment. (Kellogg Foundation, 2004)

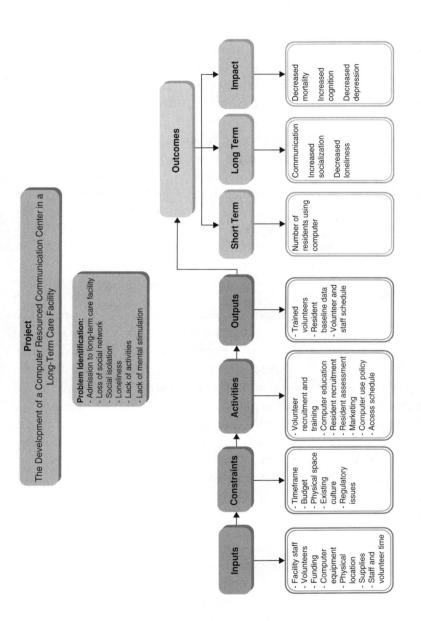

■ Figure 11-6 Logic Model for Actual DNP Project

Source: Zaccagnini, 2007.

Step VII: Implementation

INSTITUTIONAL REVIEW BOARD PROCESS

If steps I through VI went well, the DNP project is ready to be implemented. Most institutions will require a review from the institutional review board or human subjects committee. These reviews are a mechanism to ensure that human subjects are protected and have given fully informed consent when required. It also ensures that patient privacy issues are addressed and that the data collected are secure and used correctly. Some projects may require just one review through the academic institution; other projects and settings may require an academic review and a review by the IRB of the institution where the project will be conducted. The timeline and manner in which this review is conducted will be dictated by the institutions that complete the review. Because these reviews can take some time to process, the DNP project leader must be certain to account for this time in the project timeline. Projects cannot be implemented until the IRB review is completed.

GETTING THE PROJECT STARTED

The IRB review is a good opportunity to review all of the project steps taken thus far. The DNP project leader should review the goals, objectives, and work plans to be certain that they are appropriate to the problem identified in the needs assessment. The project leader should reflect on her or his own leadership style and the team she or he will be leading. In addition this is a good time to review the evaluation plan to be certain that it will measure the correct data points to determine whether the project addressed the problem. It is a good idea to plan a formal kickoff event to reenergize the team at this time because enthusiasm can wane over the time it takes to plan the project. The team should select a firm start date for the project and avoid wavering on this date. All of this involves clear and frequent communication. This is a time when every team member should be fully informed and knowledgeable about the project plan.

THREATS AND BARRIERS TO PROJECT SUCCESS

The project leader should think very carefully about threats and barriers to the project. Threats can be divided into those that can be predicted and those that cannot. Foreseeable threats to the project are those threats that the project leader and team members can identify as potential barriers at the beginning of the planning. The threats to the project might include lack of or decreased funding, employee turnover, disinterest over time, time frame barriers, and technology challenges. Unforeseen threats are events that just happen and over which the project leader has no control. Events such as a change in institutional leadership, new regulations or policies that affect the project, changes in the economy, business failures, and "acts of God" such as Hurricane Katrina are examples of unforeseen threats (Baker, Baker, & Campbell, 2003).

Although it is impossible to predict unforeseen events, the foreseeable threats and barriers should be addressed with alternative plans for implementation. The project leader should consult with the team to develop different strategies, taking the available resources into consideration. For example, if funding is less than anticipated, the project leader will need to work with the team on a scaled-back plan. Ultimately, if the project is successful, the project can be expanded when additional funding is available (Baker, Baker, & Campbell, 2003).

MONITORING THE IMPLEMENTATION PHASE

Project implementation is the exercise of leadership and control of the project. This is the time when the DNP has to be the explicit project leader to monitor every step of implementation and measure progress against the goals and objectives, mission statement, evaluation plan, and timeline. This is the time when the project leader must have a clear vision of the project. The leader cannot vacillate on the goals and objectives or the direction of the project. The project leader cannot relinquish the leadership role to another team member or show diminished enthusiasm. Implementation is the time to showcase all of the previous work and to turn ideas into reality.

PROJECT CLOSURE

Every project has a beginning and an end. A good project leader plans for project closure. Closure should include a meeting with stakeholders and an acknowledgment that the project is completed, summarizing the results, plans for sustaining the changes due to the project, and plans for transfer of leadership to the institution. The project leader should meet with team members and celebrate the accomplishments of the project team. The well-done project will sustain itself after implementation.

Step VIII: Giving Meaning to the Data

QUANTITATIVE DATA

Quantitative data collected in the DNP project serve a different purpose from those collected for the PhD thesis. They serve to demonstrate the efficacy of the project, and are not intended to meet rigorous statistical tests for significance. Nevertheless, funders and other stakeholders will be interested in the project's results, and the correct data must be collected in sufficient amounts to demonstrate the outcomes of the project. Data that describe the outcomes of the project must be collected, organized, and presented to peers, the academic community, and other parties of interest. These data will also help other clinicians with similar issues select an intervention that is likely to address the problems they are experiencing in a similar setting.

Descriptive statistical analysis is the traditional method for bringing meaning to data. This type of statistical analysis describes the population in which data were collected and what was observed in the population. The authors recommend engaging a statistician early in project planning if the plan for evaluation includes statistical analysis. Mahn-DiNicola (2009) advises likewise: "The APN may wish to enlist the support and guidance of a statistician or doctorally prepared nurse researcher to insure the end product is methodologically sound and contains the information necessary to convince others" (p. 764). In addition to statisticians, statistical analysis software programs are available. Microsoft Excel has some tools for statistical analysis built into the program.

Even if the project design and sample size do not permit the application of inferential statistical analysis, there are other ways in which the project leader can bring meaning to the data. The project leader can present the findings with other visual tools and techniques, such as charts, graphs, and diagrams. Many of these tools are used for quality assurance. Examples of these could be run charts that display a change in response over time, pie charts that show relative proportions in relationship to the whole, or flowcharts that diagram processes (Mahn-DiNicola, 2009).

QUALITATIVE DATA

The analysis of qualitative data can be daunting because of the sheer volume of records, narratives, and interviews. An organized and logical approach is needed to gain meaning from this kind of data. The process for analysis of qualitative data includes revisiting the data, placing the data into focus areas, coding the data looking for themes and patterns, identifying common themes and patterns across data sets, and interpreting the results.

Step 1 is to review all documents, tapes, videos, surveys, and field notes to get an overall sense of the data. This step will also help the project leader eliminate unnecessary or extraneous information. As this review is under way, the themes or focus areas can be identified. Step 2 is sorting the information into the categories and themes identified in step 1. Step 3 is to code the information, naming the themes identified in a systematic manner. Step 4 is to look for common threads of meaning or patterns within and across the coded data sets. Step 5 is to interpret the data by returning to the outcomes for the project and evaluating whether the qualitative data collected and organized reflects the desired outcomes.

Programs exist to help project leaders assess and interpret qualitative data, such as ATLAS.TI. Microsoft Word also has some qualitative analysis tools built into the program (Taylor-Powell & Renner, 2003). Resources for beginners include "Analyzing Qualitative Research" at the University of Wisconsin–Extension website (http://learningstore.uwex.edu/pdf/G3658-12.pdf) and the National Library of Medicine's *Planning for Evaluating Health Information Outreach Projects Booklet 3: Collecting and Analyzing Evaluation Data* (http://nnlm.gov/evaluation/booklets/booklet3/booklet3_whole.pdf).

Step IX: Dissemination and Utilization of Results
WHY DISSEMINATE YOUR SCHOLARLY OUTCOMES?
There are two purposes for dissemination of the project results: reporting the results of the project to stakeholders and the academic community, and dissemination to other professionals in similar settings. The information and results of the successful DNP project will have application beyond the immediate practice environment. It is very likely that the problem you identified at the beginning of the project is experienced by others as well. Therefore it is important to share the findings of the project whether the project produced the results you expected or different results. There are many venues for dissemination of the project results.

WRITTEN DISSEMINATION
Written dissemination is a time-honored method of sharing information. Considerations for selection of the best place to disseminate the information include the targeted audience, the environment in which the project is most likely to be helpful, and the forum in which the project should be published. If the project leader simply wants to communicate the outcomes of the project, an executive summary is a good mechanism for this purpose.

Executive Summary
An executive summary is a one-page document that summarizes the results of the project. It typically has a problem statement, a short description of the background, a summary of results when applicable, and recommendations.

The executive summary is used quite differently from an abstract. The executive summary provides the project leader with a chance to present important information to a group that may be able to fully fund a project or continue it past the immediate project. This one-page document provides an opportunity to sell the project. Viewed in that light, the executive summary must be very well done, succinct, and smooth and polished. When creating an executive summary, reread the project paper. Identify and extract the main themes. Create a rough draft from the ideas you have identified as the major points in each category or heading. Reread the summary until you are certain that every word in it is important and clearly communicates the outcomes of the project.

Abstracts

An abstract is a very short description of the project and significant results. The purpose of an abstract is for readers to get a glimpse of the main published work to decide whether it contains information they would find interesting or informative. Most journals are very prescriptive about the number of words and characters that may be included in an abstract. Look in the "Information for Authors" section of the journal. Some journals require as few as 200 words, making it difficult to discern which main concepts should go into this type of abstract. The author should keep in mind the purpose of the abstract: What would colleagues find interesting or informative about the project? Focusing on that will help create a succinct and engaging abstract.

Peer-Reviewed Journals

If the audience for dissemination of the results of the project is a group of professionals in a similar practice setting, a peer-reviewed journal is an appropriate medium. There are thousands of journals on the market. The project leader must select the most appropriate. If it is a more general project, select a journal that targets a broad base of professionals, such as the *American Journal of Nursing* or *Advanced Practice Nursing*. A more focused project should be submitted to the appropriate specialty journals. Look at several recent issues of the journal you believe may be the best for publication. Find articles that have similar subject matter to the topic you are presenting and read them to discern the style, format, and themes. Authors can also contact the editor-in-chief with the topic idea to see whether she or he believes it will be appropriate for the audience targeted by the journal.

The authors of this chapter suggest the following methodology for writing for publication. Readers may find some of these tips to be helpful.

- Set a goal for publication that includes the desired journal, the target publication date, and how the author will manage her or his time for writing.
- Good writing takes time. Set aside regular time when you can write quietly.
- The most difficult task will be to convey the most important findings in a four- to five-page article. Go through the major sections of your project and select the key highlights of each section to create an outline.
- Keep a folder of articles that you have cited. Make the citations in the text as you write. This is far easier than trying to go back and remember which articles support what sentences.
- Keep the material engaging. This is the author's chance to share important material with other professionals so that they can learn about a project that improved a practice or some outcomes.
- Manuscript preparation is crucial to getting the article published. Most journals have information for authors that details how the manuscript must be prepared for that journal's editors to review. Carefully follow those guidelines when preparing the manuscript. If questions arise, contact the journal's editorial assistant.
- Journals also have specific requirements for the abstract and keywords. Carefully follow the journal's requirements.
- Be meticulous about grammar and style. The editors will not accept an article with multiple grammar or style errors, and such errors diminish the scholarly quality of the work.
- After submission, expect feedback from expert reviewers. The feedback to the author is not intended to make the author feel good: it is intended to make the article stronger and more meaningful to the audience. In general, editors know their business well, and if you incorporate reviewer suggestions into the manuscript it will be a better article.
- Be patient. This is a process that will take some time.
- Enjoy the results.

Other Professional Publications

There are many other types of publications that are not peer reviewed but may have a far larger audience. These include nonsubscription journals that come in the mail to practitioners, local publications, public media, and newspapers. All of these will be appropriate vehicles for dissemination of your outcomes if the audience is identified correctly. In general, the suggestions for peer-reviewed journals also apply to these types of publications. Reflect the scholarly nature of the project in all forms of communication.

ORAL DISSEMINATION

Nurses disseminate much information orally, and clear communication is imperative. Leaving a voice mail for a patient requires careful thought and consideration of the content and anticipated outcome of the communication. Oral dissemination to professional audiences can be effective as well, and oral communications give the author the chance to express passion for the topic through voice tones and gestures. Oral dissemination opportunities include poster sessions, presentations or lectures for professional meetings at the local, state, or national level, and presentations to population-based groups.

Preparing for oral presentations is a bit different from preparing written materials. Nevertheless, the successful presenter must identify the audience before beginning preparation, just as if the materials were being submitted to a peer-reviewed journal. Here are some tips from the authors on preparing oral presentations.

- Understand the setting for your presentation. If you are not familiar with the organization that requested the presentation, find out about the organization by visiting its website or reading the materials published by that organization.
- Contact an organizational officer or member of the board of directors for questions. Know why you were asked to present, what issues may underlie the presentation, the knowledge level of the audience on the topic, the organizational context, the topics of other speakers before or after the presentation, the timing of the presentation, and what is happening before or after the presentation (for example, if there a business meeting preceding or following the presentation, the audience may be anxious about the impending meeting) (Guffey, 2003).
- Review your project for main points and create an outline. Remember that the criteria for citations in oral presentations are the same as for written work. All of the points in the presentation will need the same kind of strong support from the relevant literature. Do not use figures or tables unless you get permission from the authors. Cartoons also need permission from the author of the cartoon.

- Recognize that listening is different from reading and that it is difficult for most people to sit and listen for long periods of time. Thus, it is useful to change the style of presentation by interspersing scientific content with stories or case reports that break up the presentation but still present useful information in a different manner.
- Fill in the outline with the most important findings and results of the project. Be succinct.
- The rule of thumb is that every presentation should have three parts (Guffey, 2003):
  □ Tell the audience what you are going to say in the introduction.
  □ Tell the audience the information most relevant to the project in the body of the presentation.
  □ Recap what you presented in the conclusion.

Presentation Software Packages

There are many presentation software packages on the market. They will assist you in creating slides for your presentation, but the point of the slides is to enhance the oral presentation with a visual component, not to replace the oral materials. The slides should be simple and easy to read so as to not distract the listeners from the oral materials. The slides should cover one major point per slide and have no more than seven lines with seven words on a line (Guffey, 2003). Remember that many figures and tables are difficult to read when projected, so keep the tables simple and readable or consider the use of bar graphs or pie charts instead of tables. Avoid the use of all caps—IT LOOKS AGGRESSIVE. The font size should be 24 points or higher for best readability (Guffey, 2003). The slides should be free of grammatical errors just as if the presentation were being published (often the presentation slides will be published for the attendees). Plan on no more than one slide per minute of presentation (Guffey, 2003).

Tips for presenting to professional audiences include the following (adapted from Guffey, 2003):

- Time your presentation carefully and rehearse it meticulously.
- Preparation is the key to a successful presentation. You cannot possibly rehearse too much.
- Learn to speak to the audience, not the slides.
- Check that all of the embedded links work with the equipment at the site before the presentation begins.
- Bring a backup disc with the presentation materials on it.

- Get instruction on how to use the audiovisual equipment prior to the presentation.
- Establish a routine of self-care for the evening before the presentation to get a good night's rest and appear enthusiastic about the materials.
- Avoid drinking caffeinated beverages immediately before the presentation.
- Dress professionally but comfortably.

ELECTRONIC VENUES FOR DISSEMINATION

Electronic venues for dissemination are exciting recent phenomena. Our society has quickly incorporated these forms of communication into our culture and language. One astounding example is social networking sites. SixDegrees.com was the first identifiable social network, established in 1997 (Boyd & Ellinson, 2007). Since that time the use of social networks has exploded and taken off into many different directions from the original intent of connecting friends electronically. At this writing there are literally hundreds of social networking sites with different purposes. Many professional organizations maintain a Facebook site, and there are thousands of informal social networking groups of professionals. This is just one example of an electronic dissemination venue. Many more are available to the DNP student or practitioner who wants to disseminate project results to a specific audience. Table 11-8 lists some of the available venues.

Use caution when publishing to social networks and other electronic media. There is little quality control over content, and most of these types of electronic tools are not peer reviewed. Once an article is published to many of these sites, the author has no control over where it goes or how it is used. Until some of these issues are resolved, be cautious in publishing articles to a website or other electronic medium.

Conclusion

The DNP project is not simply a requirement for a degree. At its finest it should reflect a synthesis of all of the knowledge and skills gained by the DNP student in the course of studies (AACN, 2006). It should also establish the basis for the student's future scholarly work—the scholarship of integration and application. The state of American health care will benefit enormously from a cadre of expert clinicians who can utilize evidence-based projects and tools to improve the outcomes of care delivered by advanced practice nurses.

■ Table 11-8   Electronic Dissemination Venues

Formal
Peer-reviewed electronic journals
Adobe Presenter or other voice over network (VON) programs
Teleconferencing
Podcasts
Videoconferencing
Organizational/professional websites
Patient education websites
Websites with evidence-based guidelines (e.g., NIH, AHQR)

Informal
Blogs
Twitter
Social networks
Wikis

References

Allison, M., & Kaye, J. (2005). *Strategic planning for nonprofit organizations*. Hoboken, NJ: Wiley.

American Association of Colleges of Nursing. (2004). *AACN position statement on the practice doctorate in nursing*. Washington, DC: Author.

American Association of Colleges of Nursing. (2005). *AACN comparison of DNP and PhD/DNSc/DNS programs*. Washington, DC: Author.

American Association of Colleges of Nursing. (2006). *The essentials of doctoral education for advanced practice nursing*. Washington, DC: Author.

Baker, S., Baker, K., & Campbell, G. (2003). *The complete idiot's guide to project management*. Indianapolis, IN: Alpha.

Bandura, A. (1977a). *Social learning theory*. Englewood Cliffs, NJ: Prentice-Hall.

Bandura, A. (1977b). Self-efficacy: Toward a unifying theory of behavioral change. *Psychological Review, 84,* 191–215.

Boyd, D. M., & Ellison, N. B. (2007). Social network sites: Definition, history, and scholarship. *Journal of Computer-Mediated Communication, 13*(1), article 11. Retrieved from http://jcmc .indiana.edu/vol13/issue1/boyd.ellison.html

Boyer, E. (1990). *Scholarship reconsidered: Priorities of the professorate*. San Francisco: Jossey-Bass.

Boyer, E. L. (1996). Clinical practice as scholarship. *Holistic Nursing Practice, 10*(3), 1–6.

Burroughs, C., & Wood, F. (2000). *Measuring the difference: Guide to planning and evaluation of health information outreach*. Seattle, WA: National Network of Libraries of Medicine.

Cartwright, C., & Reed, C. (2005). Planning and policy perspectives for the doctorate in nursing practice: An educational perspective. *Online Journal of Nursing, 10*(3). Retrieved from http://nursingworld.org/MainMenuCategories/ANAMarketplace/ANAPeriodicals/OJIN/TableofContents/Volume102005/No3Sept05/tpc28_616030.aspx

Casey, K. (2007). *Development of innovative staffing model: Nurse practitioner (NP) hospitalist/intensivist* (Unpublished DNP project paper). University of Minnesota School of Nursing, Minneapolis, MN.

Edwardson, S. (2009, January 14). MN/DNP colloquium. Colloquium conducted at the University of Minnesota School of Nursing, Minneapolis, MN.

Fulton, J., & Lyon, B. (2005). The need for some sense making: The doctor of nursing practice. *Online Journal of Nursing, 10*(3). Retrieved from http://nursingworld.org/Main MenuCategories/ANAMarketplace/ANAPeriodicals/OJIN/TableofContents/Volume102 005/No3Sept05/tpc28_316027.aspx

Guffey, M. (2003). *Business communication: Process and product* (4th ed.). Mason, OH: South-Western.

Institute of Medicine. (2001). *Crossing the quality chasm: A new health system for the 21st century*. Washington, DC: National Academies Press.

Issel, L. (2004). *Health program planning and evaluation: A practical, systematic approach for community health*. Sudbury, MA: Jones and Bartlett.

Kotter, J. (1996). *Leading change*. Boston: Harvard Business School Press.

Kritsonas, A. (2004). Comparison of change theories. *International Journal of Scholarly Academic Diversity, 8*(1), 1–7.

Lane, A. (1992). Using Havelock's model to plan unit-based change. *Nursing Management, 23*(9), 58–60.

Lewis, J. (2007). *Fundamentals of project management* (3rd ed.). New York: American Management Association.

Luecke, R. (2004). *Managing projects large and small*. Boston: Harvard Business School Press.

Mahn-DiNicola, V. A. (2009). Outcomes evaluation and performance improvement: Using data and information technology to improve practice. In A. Hamric, J. Spross, & C. Hanson (Eds.), *Advanced practice nursing: An integrative approach* (4th ed., pp. 733–768). St. Louis, MO: Elsevier Saunders.

Microsoft Office Online. (2009a). *Write a scope statement*. Retrieved from http://office.microsoft.com/en-us/project/HA01142721033.aspx

Microsoft Office Online. (2009b). *A quick history of project management*. Retrieved from http://office.microsoft.com/en-us/project/HA011353421033.aspx

Mind Tools. (2009). *The Mind Tools e-book* (6th ed.). London: Mind Tools.

National Organization of Nurse Practitioner Faculties. (2007). *NONPF recommended criteria for NP scholarly projects in the practice doctorate program*. Retrieved from http://www.nonpf.org/associations/10789/files/ScholarlyProjectCriteria.pdf

Olney, C., & Barnes, S. (2006a). *Collecting and analyzing evaluation data*. Seattle, WA: National Network of Libraries of Medicine.

Olney, C., & Barnes, S. (2006b). *Including evaluation in outreach project planning*. Seattle, WA: National Network of Libraries of Medicine.

Outcomes Measurement Resource Network. (n.d.). *Measuring program outcomes: A practical approach*. Retrieved from http://www/lineunited.org/outcomes/resources/mpo/model.cfm

Peterson, S., & Bredow, T. (2004). *Middle range theories: Application to nursing research.* Philadelphia: Lippincott Williams & Wilkins.

Phelps, M. R., & Gerbasi, F. (2009). Accreditation requirements for practice doctorates in 14 health care professions. *AANA Journal, 77*(1), 19–26.

Polit, D., & Beck, C. (2008). *Nursing research: Generating and assessing evidence for nursing practice.* Philadelphia: Wolters Kluwer/Lippincott Williams and Wilkins.

Prochaska, J., & Velicer, W. (1997). The transtheoretical model of health behavior change. *American Journal of Health Promotion, 12*(1), 38–48.

Rogers, E. (1995). *Diffusion of innovations* (4th ed.). New York: Free Press.

Schein, E. (n.d.). *Kurt Lewin's change theory in the field and in the classroom: Notes towards a model of managed learning.* Retrieved from http://www.a2zpshchology.com/articles/kurt_lewin%27s_change_theory.htm

Streeter, S. (1998). *Government Performance and Results Act and the appropriations process.* CRS Report for Congress. Retrieved from http://www.rules.house.gov/archives/98-726.htm

Taylor-Powell, E., & Henert, E. (2008). *Developing a logic model: Teaching and training guide.* Retrieved from the University of Wisconsin–Extension website: http://www.uwex.edu/ces/pdande/evaluation/pdf/lmguidecomplete.pdf

Taylor-Powell, E., & Renner, M. (2003). *Analyzing qualitative data.* Madison, WI: Cooperative Extension Publishing.

Value Based Management. (2009). *Force field analysis and diagram—Kurt Lewin.* Retrieved from http://www.valuebasedmanagement.net/methods_lewin_force_field_analysis.html

W. K. Kellogg Foundation. (1998). *Evaluation handbook.* Battle Creek, MI: Author.

W. K. Kellogg Foundation. (2004). *Logic model development guide.* Battle Creek, MI: Author.

Waddick, P. (2009). *Six sigma DMAIC quick reference: Define phase.* Retrieved from http://www.isixsigma.com/library/content/six_sigma_dmaic_quickref_define.asp

Wheatley, M. (2007). Fearlessness: The last organizational change strategy. *Business Executive, the Journal of the Association of Business Executives* (England). Retrieved from http://www.abeuk.com

Wheatley, M., & Frieze, D. (2008). *Using emergence to take innovation to scale.* Retrieved from Berkana Institute website: http://www.berkana.org/articles/lifecycle.htm

White, K. (2005). *A model for evaluating the cost-effectiveness of various staffing patterns at a Veteran's Affairs anesthesia department* (Unpublished DNP project paper). Rush University, Chicago, IL.

Zaccagnini, M. (2007). *The development of a computer resourced communication center in a long term care facility* (Unpublished DNP project paper). University of Minnesota, Minneapolis, MN.

Change Theorists

	Lewin	Lippitt	Rogers	Havelock
Dates of contributions	1890–1947	1950–2004	1960s	Mid-1970s
Name of model	Change	Phases of change	Diffusion of innovations	CREATER model
Focus	Change	Role of change agent	Innovation adoption in populations	Relationship with client
Main features of model	Three-phase model: unfreezing, movement, and freezing	Phases: 1) Diagnose the problem in need of changing 2) Assess change motivation 3) Assess resources 4) Develop action plans and strategies 5) Select role of change agent; clarify expectations 6) Change maintenance 7) Termination of helping relationship as change incorporates into organizational culture	Adopters of any change can be divided into *innovators, early adopters, early majority, late majority,* and *laggards.* Also proposes that these are best described by a bell curve.	Six-part model to create change: 1) Establish a relationship 2) Diagnose the needs 3) Assess and procure resources 4) Select a change strategy 5) Gain acceptance for the solution 6) Establish self-renewal
Other important work	Force field analysis: drivers and inhibitors of change	Authored many books on organizational psychology and consulting	Three types of innovation decisions within diffusion of innovation: optional innovation decision, collective innovation decision, and authority innovation decision	Steps: care, relate, examine, acquire, try, extend, renew (CREATER)
Source	Schein (n.d.)	Kritsonas (2004)	Rogers (1995)	Lane (1992)

(continues)

	Proschaska & DiClemente	Bandura	Wheatley	Kotter
Dates of contributions	1977–present	1962–present	1970–present	Present
Name of model	Stages of change; transtheoretical model (TTM)	Social cognitive theory	Life's change process	Kotter's eight-step change model
Focus	Movement of the individual to change behavior	Self-efficacy	People in organizational change	Planning for change
Main features of model	Stages of change: 1) Precontemplation 2) Contemplation 3) Preparation 4) Action 5) Maintenance	Behavior change is driven by environmental influences, personal characteristics, and the behavior itself. Individuals' outcome expectations are based largely on their perceived self-efficacy.	Life's change process takes place in the context of interwoven relationships. Life change happens through emergence.	Eight steps: 1) Create a sense of urgency 2) Form a powerful coalition 3) Create a vision 4) Communicate the vision 5) Remove obstacles 6) Create short-term wins 7) Build on change 8) Anchor change in corporate culture
Other important work	Important constructs within TTM: decisional balance, self-efficacy, temptation	Important influence on Pender's health promotion model	Important constructs: emergence, networking for social change, fearlessness	Companion book: *Our Iceberg Is Melting*, an allegory of change theory
Source	Prochaska & Velicer (1997)	Kritsonas (2004), Bandura (1977a, 1977b), Peterson & Bredow (2004)	Wheatley (2007), Wheatley & Frieze (2008)	Kotter (1996)

Process Model for the DNP Project

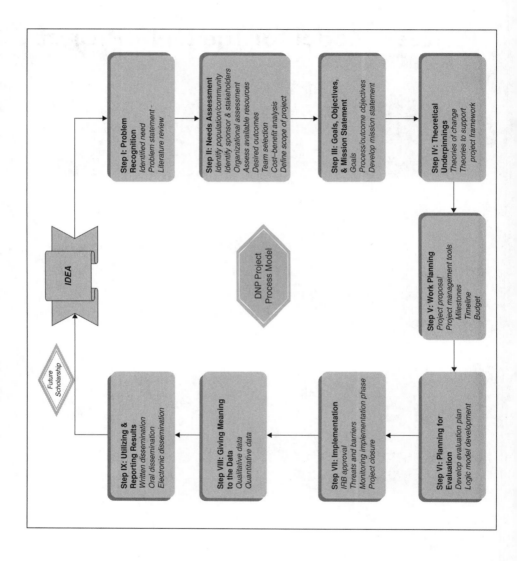

INDEX

Italicized page locators indicate a figure; tables are noted with a *t*.